NURSING CARE OF THE TRANSPLANT RECIPIENT

KATHERINE M. SIGARDSON-POOR, RN, MS

LINDA M. HAGGERTY, MS, RN, CCTC

1990

W.B. SAUNDERS COMPANY

Harcourt Brace Jovanovich, Inc.

Philadelphia / London / Toronto / Montreal / Sydney / Tokyo

W. B. SAUNDERS COMPANY
Harcourt Brace Jovanovich, Inc.

The Curtis Center
Independence Square West
Philadelphia, PA 19106

Library of Congress Cataloging-in-Publication Data

Nursing care of the transplant recipient.

1. Transplantation of organs, tissues, etc.—Nursing.
   I. Sigardson-Poor, Katherine M.   II. Haggerty, Linda M.
   [DNLM: 1. Nursing Care. 2. Transplantation. WY 161 N9742]

RD129.8.N87   1990   610.73′677   89–10641

ISBN 0–7216–2882–6

Editor: Thomas Eoyang
Manuscript Editor: Barbara Hodgson
Production Manager: Frank Polizzano
Indexer: Ellen Murray

Nursing Care of the Transplant Recipient   ISBN   0–7216–2882–6

Copyright © 1990 by W. B. Saunders Company.

All rights reserved.   No part of this publication may be reproduced or transmitted in any form or by any means, electronic or mechanical, including photocopy, recording, or any information storage and retrieval system, without permission in writing from the publisher.

Printed in the United States of America.

Last digit is the print number: 9   8   7   6   5   4   3   2   1

Contributors

LOIS BARTELL, R.N., B.S.N.
Organ Transplant Clinical Nurse Specialist, The University of Minnesota Hospitals and Clinics, Minneapolis, Minnesota
Patient Education: Theory and Strategies

JOANNE E. BARTOSH, R.N., B.S.N., C.N.N.
Clinical Educator for Hemodialysis, The Methodist Hospital, Houston, Texas
Transcultural Nursing and Transplantation

MARILYN ROSSMAN BARTUCCI, R.N., M.S.N., C.S., C.C.T.C.
Clinical Instructor, Medical-Surgical Nursing, Frances Payne Bolton School of Nursing, Case Western Reserve University; Head Nurse Manager, Transplant Center, University Hospitals of Cleveland, Cleveland, Ohio
The Immunology of Transplant Rejection

ELIZABETH J. BUCHAN, R.N., M.S.N.
Formerly Head Nurse, Neurology-Neurosurgery Unit, Vanderbilt University Medical Center, Nashville, Tennessee
Autotransplantation of the Adrenal Medulla

VIRGINIA H. CARR, R.N., M.S.
Psychiatric Liaison Nurse, Rush-Presbyterian-St. Luke's Medical Center; Practitioner/Teacher, Rush University, Chicago, Illinois
Managing the Psychosocial Responses of the Transplant Patient

PATRICIA CHALUPSKY, R.N., B.S.N.
Manager, International Patient Services Department, Methodist Hospital, Houston, Texas
Transcultural Nursing and Transplantation

JANICE A. COPELAND, R.N., B.S.N.
Transplant Coordinator, University of Arizona, Tucson, Arizona
Heart-Lung and Unilateral Lung Transplantation

BETTY C. CRANDALL, M.S., R.N., C.N.N.
Formerly Clinical Nurse Specialist, Transplantation, Johns Hopkins Hospital, Baltimore, Maryland; Faculty Associate, State University of New York at Plattsburgh; Clinical Director, Medical/Surgical Nursing, CVPH Medical Center, Plattsburgh, New York
Immunosuppression

MARY BETH DANNEFFEL, R.N., B.S.N., C.P.T.C.
Senior Vice President, Michigan Eye-Bank and Transplantation Center, Ann Arbor, Michigan
Corneal Transplantation

NANCY S. DAVIS, R.N., C.P.T.C.
Certified Procurement Transplant Coordinator, Tennessee Donor Services, Nashville, Tennessee
Legal and Ethical Issues

EILEEN M. DeMAYO, R.N., B.S.N., C.C.T.C.
Renal Transplant Service, Division of Nephrology, UCLA Medical Center, Los Angeles, California
Pancreas Transplantation

BARBARA A. ELICK, R.N., C.C.T.C., C.P.T.C.
Chief, Transplant Coordinator, Department of Surgery, University of Minnesota Hospitals and Clinics, Minneapolis, Minnesota
Pancreas Transplantation

ELIZABETH ERB, R.N., M.S.N., C.A.N.P.
Formerly Program Coordinator, Parkinson's Disease Center, Department of Neurology and Neurosurgery, Vanderbilt University Medical Center; now Program Coordinator, National Parkinson's Disease Brain Bank, Nashville, Tennessee
Autotransplantation of the Adrenal Medulla

PATRICIA GAMBERG, R.N., C.C.T.C.
Nurse Educator, Stanford University, Stanford, California
Heart Transplant

LINDA M. HAGGERTY, M.S., R.N., C.C.T.C.
Transplant Clinical Specialist, Rush-Presbyterian-St. Luke's Medical Center; Practitioner/Teacher, Rush University, Chicago, Illinois
Kidney Transplantation; Extended Role of the Nurse

BECKY A. HARRIS, R.N., B.S.N., C.C.T.C.
Transplantation Coordinator, William Beaumont Hospital, Royal Oak, Michigan
Extended Role of the Nurse

MARY C. HOFFMAN, R.N., B.S.N., M.M.

Formerly Regional Director, Musculoskeletal Transplant Foundation, Chicago; now Manager, Extramural Grant Program, Renal Division, Baxter Healthcare Corporation, Round Lake, Illinois

Organ Procurement and Preservation

PATRICIA F. JASSAK, M.S., R.N.C.S.

Clinical Assistant Professor, Marcella Niehoff School of Nursing, Loyola University; Oncology Clinical Nurse Specialist, Foster G. McGaw Hospital, Loyola University Medical Center, Chicago, Illinois

Bone Marrow Transplantation

MINDY MALECKI, R.N.

Formerly Regional Director, Musculoskeletal Transplant Foundation; now Risk Manager, Rush-Presbyterian-St. Luke's Medical Center, Chicago, Illinois

Organ Procurement and Preservation

SUSAN J. NEELY, R.N., B.S.N.

Formerly Administrative Director, Transplantation Services, Baylor University Medical Center, Dallas, Texas. Currently residing in Tunis, Tunisia.

Legal and Ethical Issues

MARY ANN PALUMBI, R.N., C.C.T.C.

Director, Transplantation Services, Allegheny General Hospital, Pittsburgh, Pennsylvania

Historical Perspective

PATRICIA PIASECKI, R.N., M.S.

Clinical Coordinator, Orthopedic Oncology, Rush-Presbyterian-St. Luke's Medical Center, Chicago, Illinois

Bone Transplantation

NANCY L. PORTER, R.N., M.S., O.C.N.

Head Nurse, Bone Marrow Transplant Unit, Foster G. McGaw Hospital, Loyola University Medical Center, Chicago, Illinois

Bone Marrow Transplantation

MARY A. ROVELLI, R.N., B.S.N.

Senior Transplant Coordinator, Hartford Hospital, Hartford, Connecticut

Infectious Disease and Transplantation

BARBARA A. SCHANBACHER, R.N., B.S.N., C.C.T.C., C.P.T.C.
Transplant Coordinator, Department of Surgery, University of Iowa Hospitals and Clinics, Iowa City, Iowa
Pancreas Transplantation

MARY CUSELLA SELLER, R.N., M.S.N., C.S.
Clinical Instructor, Medical-Surgical Nursing, Frances Payne Bolton School of Nursing, Case Western Reserve University; Clinical Nurse Specialist, Renal/Pancreas Transplant, University Hospitals of Cleveland, Cleveland, Ohio
The Immunology of Transplant Rejection

KATHERINE M. SIGARDSON-POOR, R.N., M.S.
Formerly Renal Transplant Clinical Specialist, Foster G. McGaw Hospital, Loyola University Medical Center, Maywood, and Edward Hines, Jr. Veterans Administration Hospital, Hines, Illinois; now Consultant and Lecturer, Bettendorf, Iowa
Kidney Transplantation; Patient Education: Theory and Strategies

SANDRA M. STASCHAK, R.N., C.C.T.C.
Senior Transplant Coordinator, Department of Surgery, University of Pittsburgh, Pittsburgh, Pennsylvania
Liver Transplantation: Nursing Diagnosis and Management

KIMBERLY DIANE WALTON, R.N., B.S.N., M.P.H.
Clinical Transplant Consultant, Nurse Epidemiologist, Jefferson Park Hospital and Children's Rehabilitation Hospital, Philadelphia, Pennsylvania
Heart Transplant

MARYA L. WEIL, R.N., C.C.T.C.
Renal Transplant Coordinator, St. Joseph Hospital BioEthics Committee, St. Joseph Hospital, Orange, California
Infectious Disease and Transplantation

VIRGINIA WILLIAMS, R.N., M.S.N.
Formerly Clinical Nurse Specialist, Vanderbilt University Medical Center, Nashville, Tennessee
Autotransplantation of the Adrenal Medulla

KAREN ZAMBERLAN, R.N., Ph.D.
Clinical Research Associate, Department of Transplant Surgery, University of Pittsburgh; Clinical Nurse Specialist, Children's Hospital of Pittsburgh, Pittsburgh, Pennsylvania
Liver Transplantation: Nursing Diagnosis and Management

Acknowledgments

This endeavor would not have been possible without the support of many people in many different ways. Your caring concern helped us through the process of preparing this text. We are fortunate and grateful.

To Curt, without whose support for this project from the beginning I could not have finished. Your loving prodding enabled me to find the energy to finish (KSP).

To Rachel Poor: your mother and godmother gave up many hours we would much rather have spent with you. However, we had a goal—to share our knowledge to help others as we hope we have helped our patients over our years in transplant.

To Kevin, thanks for your patience, love, and laughter (LMH).

To Steve Jensik, M.D., under whose teaching I've grown in experience, expertise, and appreciation for the field of transplantation and holistic patient care (LMH).

To NATCO: your initial financial contributions helped us put together this text and enabled us to get many of our contributors working early in this project. Many NATCO members encouraged us to finish this project by asking to buy the book.

To Thomas Eoyang, our editor at W. B. Saunders: your faith and encouragement saw us through many difficult periods in the publication process. Somehow you always knew when to call.

We greatly appreciate the many contributions of Radiology Group, P.C., S.C. of Davenport, Iowa. You gave us the space on your computer for preparation of this manuscript, and initially our typist. We especially thank Maxine Schroeder for her generous cooperation and for locating our second typist when the first had other commitments. Maureen Lemek, our second typist, did an outstanding job, not only in typing our manuscript, but also in correcting our grammar, punctuation, and word usage. You were truly an asset to this project. Dr. Robert Hartung of Radiology Group deserves special thanks for helping the typists make the computer produce in ways it usually does not!

Our contributors deserve many kudos for their efforts; some have been particularly memorable. During our manuscript preparation we shared the births of four babies, one marriage, several relocations—one international—and other life events.

KSP & LMH

Foreword

Transplantation has brought medical technology to heights previously unknown. Organ and tissue transplantation is one of the most rapidly growing specialties in modern medicine, and from this rapid growth has emerged a new health care professional, the transplant coordinator.

The role of the transplant coordinator evolved out of a need to provide expertise in the procurement, preservation, and distribution of transplantable organs and tissue and to ensure continuity of patient care throughout the transplant process. Transplant coordinators also provide public and professional education regarding organ and tissue donation and transplantation.

Transplant coordination has become a profession. Transplant coordinators are highly skilled health care professionals involved in every aspect of organ and tissue donation and, as such, are a vital element in the transplant process.

In 1979, the North American Transplant Coordinators Organization (NATCO) became the professional society for transplant coordinators. NATCO's mission is ". . . to influence and increase procurement in the utilization of transplantation tissue . . . and . . . support and enrich the high quality patient care delivered by its members. . . ."

NATCO as an organization is committed to excellence. NATCO created the first national extrarenal organ sharing system in the United States and Canada. NATCO participated in the deliberations of the National Task Force on Organ Transplantation, established as a result of passage of the 1984 National Organ Transplant Act. In addition, NATCO holds a seat on the board of directors of the United Network for Organ Sharing (UNOS), the federally mandated nationwide organ procurement and transplantation network.

NATCO also holds a prominent position in the field of transplant education. NATCO conducts university-affiliated education training programs in transplant coordination and is developing residency programs for the future education of professional transplant coordinators. Further, through the establishment of a national accreditation program for transplant coordinators, NATCO has provided a mechanism to ensure competency, safeguard the quality of performance, and promote standards of practice within the field of transplant coordination.

In keeping with this tradition of high-quality accomplishment, NATCO takes special pride in sponsoring this textbook on clinical transplantation. This book reflects the advanced body of knowledge and level of practice of the transplant coordinator. It stands as a state-of-the-art resource in transplantation and the care of the transplant recipient.

It is a privilege to acknowledge the contributors as distinguished members of our profession, and I am pleased to recognize the co-editors, Kay Sigardson-Poor and Linda Haggerty, for their outstanding achievement. During my tenure as president, it has been a distinct honor to witness their dedication and concern for excellence, without which so notable an accomplishment would not have been possible.

This book is a tribute to the professional transplant coordinator.

ANITA L. PRINCIPE, R.N., B.S.N., M.P.A.
President
North American Transplant
Coordinators Organization

Preface

Both of us had been interested for quite some time in producing a text about transplantation, primarily for nurses, because no reference was available. We discussed possible topics based on our experience and the questions that we commonly encountered in our individual practices. Later, we narrowed the list of topics and divided them into general areas common to all transplant recipients and their organ specific content. We later began contacting those in the field of transplantation who are preeminent experts in these specific areas. Many are associated with transplant surgeons who are, and continue to be, pioneers in their specialty.

The goal of this project was always to produce a book for nurses, by nurses. Invariably, we discovered that much of the information can be utilized by other health care professionals who come in contact with transplant patients. We also have known a few patients who would find this a valuable resource.

Of course, not all aspects of transplantation can be covered in a single text. One area we attempted to incorporate was financial concerns. We found that each state was so different and insurance trends changing so rapidly that it was not possible. However, as nurses, we do deal daily with patients who are faced with tremendous financial burdens. These occur not just in transplantation but certainly are more intense and magnified because of the life or death option decided by whether a procedure can be performed or a medication purchased. Society as a whole will have to come to grips with this problem and the percentage of gross national product consumed by health care dollars.

Staff nurses, transplant coordinators, and clinical specialists interact in many areas of patient concerns. These may include family and psychosocial responses to illness and the transplant process and physical needs in the various phases of transplantation. All interact and become a focus for nursing care at all levels. This book will provide much of the information important to holistic care of the organ/tissue transplant recipient.

Contents

xiii

1

Historical Perspective

Mary Ann Palumbi

Transplantation of solid organs and tissues has become a viable form of therapy for many life-altering and life-threatening disease entities. The acceptance of this form of therapy by both the medical community and the lay population has only become evident in the 1980s. To many, the "overnight success" of transplantation belies the eighty or more years of research that preceded this highly visible and, in some cases, controversial form of therapy (see Table 1–1).

No form of medical treatment has ever received the extensive media coverage that transplantation has. Early milestones received little public attention, with the exception of the first heart transplant, heralded as the "miracle in South Africa." To this day, the name of Dr. Christiaan Barnard, the doctor who performed that transplant in 1967, is recognizable to a major portion of the public. For one not to have been exposed to news of transplantation in this decade is virtually impossible.

The media has been obsessed with this procedure. From national television networks to local radio stations, from nationally circulated weekly newsmagazines to small-town papers—all have at one time covered some aspect of transplantation. The stories range from local coverage of the tragic death of a young man whose family donated his organs to the national plea of distraught parents for an organ donor for their dying child.

There are a number of reasons for the media's obsession. The major reason appears to be the lack of available donors and, therefore, the inability to control the outcome. In addition, because organs are considered a scarce commodity, the drama and potential for corruption of the system increase the public's interest. This close scrutiny has resulted in programs being held accountable for the patient selection process and the distribution of organs; it also has been partly responsible for the increased interest by the federal government, resulting in investigations, hearings, and, eventually, the passage of the National Organ Transplant

1

Act of 1984. The media attention has also made the public and the medical community more aware of transplantation and organ donation. This awareness has resulted in an increase in organ donation, although the demand still far exceeds the supply. Whether it is a help or a hindrance, media attention will probably continue.

RESEARCH AND PRESERVATION

Research in transplantation, unlike that in any other form of surgical therapy, has required not only the refinement of the technical aspects, but also the study of the immune system and various means of controlling the immune response. In addition, methods of preserving the organs have created areas of concern and complications.

The primary goal of organ preservation is to maintain the cellular integrity and function of the organ for a specific amount of time, to allow selection and preparation of the recipient (Belzer, 1988). The sensitivity of the vascular organs, as well as that of all tissue, to the lack of perfusion is a well-recognized problem for the transplant team.

There are two objectives of organ preservation: (1) to avoid ischemic damage before the recovery of the organs by donor maintainance (Marshall, 1984) and (2) to diminish ischemia after recovery by reducing the metabolic demands of the tissue and supplying the vital substances and nutrients necessary to prevent cellular swelling and acidosis (Belzer, 1988).

Donor management has evolved from no involvement, followed by rapid recovery of organs after cessation of cardiac function, to a sophisticated method of brain death determination with maintainance of good perfusion. The basic concept of donor management is to maintain fluid

TABLE 1–1. LANDMARKS IN ORGAN TRANSPLANTATION

1909	First kidney transplant (xenograft) (Berlin)
1933	First human kidney transplant (USSR)
1948	Development of first renal transplant program (Boston)
1953	First living-related donor (Paris)
1958	First description of HLA antigen
1961	Development of azathioprine
1962	First use of tissue typing between donor and recipient
1963	First human liver transplant (Denver)
1966	First clinical trials in pancreas transplantation (Minnesota)
1967	First human heart transplant (South Africa)
1973	First description of transfusion effect on graft survival
1973	Passage of Uniform Anatomical Gift Act
1976	Creation of North American Transplant Coordinators Organization
1978	First clinical use of cyclosporine (England)
1978	Identification of DR antigen
1984	Passage of Organ Procurement and Transplantation Act

and electrolyte balance, prevent hypotension, and maintain cardiac output (Wicomb, 1984).

Preservation of organs after recovery relies primarily on cooling to diminish metabolic activity, including oxygen consumption. However, cooling alone is not sufficient to prevent ischemia with long-term preservation (Belzer, 1988); nutrients need to be supplied in conjunction with the cooling (Marshall, 1984). Preservation begins with flushing the organ free of all blood with a cold solution. Initially, the organ was flushed after removal, or ex vivo. Recent studies have shown, however, that immediate flushing after cessation of blood flow to the organ, or in situ, decreases ischemic damage (Lee, 1984). Since the 1970s the composition of the flushing solution has undergone changes in attempts to improve cellular metabolism and control cellular volume. Solutions have ranged from Ringer's lactate (Calne, 1983) to more iso-osmolar or hyperosmolar types, such as Collins, Eurocollins, and Sacks solutions (Marshall, 1984). The use of hyperosmolar solutions has proved to be successful in lengthening preservation times in liver, kidney, and pancreas studies (Marshall, 1984). Cardiac preservation requires hypothermia, but also the ability to induce cardiac arrest, which further decreases metabolic activity (Wicomb, 1984).

Long-term storage of organs has included (1) pulsatile perfusion methods, which literally pump the cold solution through the vasculature of the organ, and (2) simple storage of the organ in a portable cooler, surrounded by a cold solution, usually the same solution as that used in the flushing process. Early attempts at renal perfusion were made by Carrell in 1938 (Marshall, 1984). Machine preservation was not considered reliable until Belzer succeeded in preserving kidneys for three days (Marshall, 1984). Belzer's concepts are still used in many programs today. Lindbergh, in 1938, also tried pulsatile perfusion of the heart, as well as of the kidneys (Wicomb, 1984). Since that time modifications and adjustments to the system have been attempted. Cardiac pulsatile perfusion, however, remains under laboratory investigation owing to technical problems that result in coronary vascular resistance and myocardial damage (Wicomb, 1984). Both Starzl and Belzer attempted perfusion of the liver, with limited success (Belzer, 1984). The method of choice for liver preservation continues to be cold storage (Calne, 1983). All vascular organs are currently preserved in cold storage, with the exception of several programs that maintain kidney perfusion. Researchers at the University of Wisconsin have recently reported success in prolonged cold storage with the use of UW (Viaspan) solution (Belzer, 1984). This solution has allowed prolonged cold storage with initial graft function seen in clinical trials of the liver, kidney, and pancreas. This prolonged time allows for optimal recipient selection and preparation, improved tissue-typing techniques, and operative procedures performed under less stressful conditions. Research in preservation, as well as in the immune response and technical aspects, continues today in the attempt to further the efficacy and safety of transplantation.

KIDNEY TRANSPLANTATION

Animal experiments in kidney transplantation were documented in 1902 by Ulmann in Vienna and in 1905 by Carrel in the United States. This early work primarily dealt with the technical aspects of the procedure (Hamilton, 1984). Early success in vascular surgery led to the interest in transplant surgery and the ability to determine the immediate outcome of the procedure. Initial surgery consisted of the anastomosis of the animal's renal vessels to its carotid vessels. Many of these early procedures actually resulted in the production of urine by the graft (Hamilton, 1984). At this time, technical achievements overshadowed the rejection process. Unger, however, first made note of the rejection process in 1909. He had performed more than 100 renal transplants in animals, and in 1909 he transplanted a kidney from an ape into a young girl who was dying of renal failure. The graft never functioned, and Unger concluded that there was a "chemical barrier" to transplantation (Hamilton, 1984).

The next several decades saw little activity in transplantation, except for that being generated by Voronoy of the Soviet Union (Hamilton, 1984). Voronoy's initial work with blood transfusions was carried over into transplantation. He performed six cadaver transplants in humans, but without success.

Interest did not peak again in the United States until shortly after World War II. In 1946 a group of surgeons headed by David Hume in Boston transplanted a cadaver kidney into a young woman with acute renal failure. The graft functioned for only a short time, but this was sufficient to support the patient through the oliguric phase of acute tubular necrosis. Hume and associates performed a number of cadaver transplants, some of which functioned well. These early successes were attributed to the use of corticosteroids in the postoperative phase (Hamilton, 1984). Hume's group also was responsible for one of the most dramatic events: the transplant of a kidney between identical twins in 1954 (Hamilton, 1984). Of note is that the surgical technique used by Hume has essentially remained unchanged. Placement of the kidney extraperitoneally into the iliac fossa, with the anastomosis to the iliac vessels, is still the most common approach (Lee, 1984).

Living-related transplantation was considered an optimal form of therapy as early as 1953, despite limited knowledge of the immune system (Hamilton, 1984). Living-related transplants continued to be the optimal choice throughout the 1960s and 1970s. The use of cyclosporine and the increased success rates with cadaver transplants have prompted many programs to limit living-related transplantation. However, recent long-term studies again support the greater success rates achieved in well-matched living-related transplants (Takiff, Mickey, Cicciarelli, & Terasaki, 1987). Controversy regarding the potential risks to the donor versus the improved graft survival still exists.

Intense study of the immune system and of methods of controlling rejection was undertaken between 1955 and 1962. The use of total-body irradiation and 6-mercaptopurine resulted in poor graft survival and high patient mortality. The introduction of azathioprine, however, and its pairing with prednisone, dramatically increased graft survival and began the era of transplantation as it is known today (d'Apice, 1984).

Increased patient and graft survival have resulted in tremendous growth in kidney transplantation, from four centers in 1961 to more than 120 centers in 1985 (Grzelka, 1986) (see Figure 1–1). Renal transplantation is the most common of the solid organ transplants, with more than 7000 performed in 1986 (Grzelka, 1986).

LIVER TRANSPLANTATION

Research into liver transplantation began in 1955, much later than the initial studies in renal transplantation. Results of heterotopic transplants were first reported by Welch in 1955 (Calne, 1983). This method was found to be useful in treating those patients with debilitating enzyme

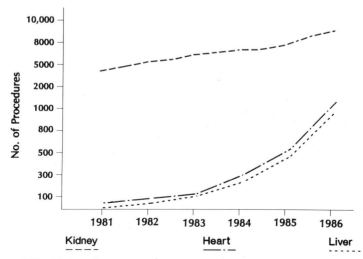

FIGURE 1–1. Growth in transplant procedures in the United States.

deficiencies; however, the dismal results have led to little research in this branch of the field since the late 1970s. The major problems are technical, primarily the inability to place such a large organ into the abdominal cavity. In addition, vascular and ductal anastomoses were found to be extremely difficult in heterotopic transplantation.

Orthotopic liver transplantation was developed independently in 1959 by both Moore in Boston and Starzl in Chicago. The major problems were, again, of a technical nature. Early difficulties included vascular problems, such as poor flow in the splenic artery and inferior vena cava, and inadequate biliary drainage (Calne, 1983).

The first human liver transplant was performed in 1963 by Starzl, in Denver. Immunosuppressive therapy consisted, as in renal transplantation, of azathioprine and high-dose steroids. The first five patients died, and success rates remained poor, at approximately 35 per cent (Starzl, 1969). Mortality and morbidity were caused by infection, rejection, and technical complications. Starzl and Calne continued their clinical work throughout the 1970s with emphasis on improvement of the technical aspects. The introduction of cyclosporine, combined with technical improvements, has nearly doubled the success rates, with one-year graft survival of approximately 75 per cent (Calne, 1983).

From 1963 to 1983 approximately 200 transplants were performed in the United States and 125 in England (Calne, 1983). However, from 1983 to 1985 close to 1100 liver transplants were performed in the United States at 40 centers (Grzelka, 1986) (see Fig. 1–1). Liver transplantation is now considered a viable form of therapy for end-stage liver failure.

HEART TRANSPLANTATION

Carrell and Guthrie reported the first experimental work in heart transplantation in 1905 (Cooper, 1984). In 1933 Mann developed a technical method, anastomosis of the donor heart to the recipient's carotid vessels, that maintained the coronary circulation and a normal electrocardiogram. Most research from 1933 to the early 1950s dealt with auxiliary transplantation (Cooper, 1984). Demikhov performed the first laboratory orthotopic transplant in 1951. Extensive animal research continued through the mid-1960s. In 1964 Hardy performed the first human transplant, in a 68-year-old man. The patient had deteriorated suddenly, secondary to severe coronary artery disease, but no human donor was available. The heart of a large chimpanzee was transplanted orthotopically. Unfortunately, the heart was not able to support circulation, and the patient died (Cooper, 1984).

No form of transplantation carried such impact as that of the first human heart transplant in Cape Town, South Africa, in December 1967.

The attention of both the lay and the medical communities was focused on the recipient as well as on the surgeon, Dr. Christiaan Barnard. At that time Dr. Barnard was chief of surgery, and had done extensive research in cardiac surgery as well as in transplantation.

In the next 12 to 18 months more than 100 heart transplants were performed worldwide. As with previous organ transplants, initial success rates were poor, prompting most programs to abandon this form of transplantation. The major problems were immunologic, with graft loss primarily caused by rejection, and recipient death from infection (Cooper, 1984).

In the United States most of the heart transplants were performed by Dr. Norman Shumway at Stanford University from 1967 to 1975. Shumway was the first to report the use of steroids in combination with azathioprine or mercaptopurine, which improved success rates (Cooper, 1984). The Stanford group also was the first to note the correlation between diet and early death owing to advanced coronary artery disease (Jamieson, Oyer, Bieber, Hunt, Billingham, et al., 1983). In addition, the group pioneered the development and use of the endomyocardial biopsy for early diagnosis of rejection (Caves, Stinson, Graham, Billingham, Grehl, & Shumway, 1973).

Renewed interest in the late 1970s, as well as improved success rates, have resulted in a proliferation of heart transplant programs. In 1981 there were 15 active heart transplant programs in the United States. This number increased in 1986 to 120 programs with a corresponding increase in the number of procedures (Solis & Kaye, 1986) (see Fig. 1–1).

By 1986, 94 per cent of all heart transplants were orthotopic; the remaining 6 per cent were heterotopic (Solis & Kaye, 1986). This latter method, developed in 1974, was thought to be advantageous in preventing death from acute rejection. The major complication with this procedure is the formation of thrombus in the recipient's poorly contracting left ventricle, which can break away and become systemic. The use of cyclosporine has resulted in limited use of heterotopic transplantation owing to the improved success rate of orthotopic transplantation (Becerra, Cooper, Novitsky, & Reichert, 1987).

Although prosthetic devices have not been used successfully in other forms of vital organ transplantation, the artificial heart has been a viable concept outside the laboratory. As early as 1969 an artificial heart was implanted at the Texas Heart Institute (Cooley, 1982). In the 1980s DeVries replaced the heart of a dentist with a device developed by Jarvik at the University of Utah. The patient, Barney Clark, lived for 112 days before succumbing to progressive renal failure and refractory hypotension (DeVries, Anderson, Joyce, Anderson, Hammond et al., 1984). Subsequent recipients have suffered multiple complications, including stroke and infection. Despite research in this area, the use of a total artificial heart as a permanent form of therapy is questioned by most practitioners today. It has been accepted as an adjunct to human transplantation, with its use limited as a "bridge" to maintain the recipient until a donor is located (Barnard, 1984).

As with the other organ transplants, increased graft survival has resulted from improvements in immunosuppression, as well as from the early detection and treatment of rejection. The most current national statistics show a one-year graft and patient survival of 75 per cent to 80 per cent (Grzelka, 1986). Heart transplantation, like that of the liver and kidney, is now an accepted form of therapy for end-stage heart disease.

PANCREAS TRANSPLANTATION

Diabetes mellitus, especially type I, continues to be a devastating disease that afflicts more than 12 million persons in the United States. The use of insulin and dietary control have been ineffective in preventing the debilitating and sometimes fatal sequelae of diabetes mellitus.

Initial clinical trials in pancreas transplantation were undertaken by Lillehei in 1966. As in the case of liver transplantation, technical problems resulted in poor success rates, a high incidence of complications, and delayed progress and research in the field (Lillehei, Simmons & Najarian, 1970).

Clinical work in this area was limited in the United States until 1980, with the majority of research being presented by Groth in Sweden and Dubernard in France. However, throughout the 1970s Lillehei and colleagues established an aggressive pancreas program in Minnesota that involved both cadaveric and living-related transplantation (Sutherland & Chinn, 1984).

The primary technical concern was the disposition of the gland's exocrine secretions. Early methods of control consisted of segmental transplantation with occlusion of the severed area by synthetic agents or simply ligation of the section (Dubernard, Traeger, & Bosi, 1984). Whole-pancreas transplants, with diversion into the enteric system, and most recently into the bladder, have resulted in an increase in the success rate and a decrease in complications.

The advent of cyclosporine helped to renew interest in pancreas transplantation throughout the United States, as well as the world, in the mid-1980s. This interest and research, as with other organ transplants, have increased the technical success of pancreas transplantation from 33 per cent to 35 per cent in 1977 to more than 60 per cent in 1986 (Nghiem, Shulak, & Corry, 1987).

Pancreas transplants have most often been performed either in conjunction with a renal transplant or after a successful renal transplant.

Improved graft and patient survival, as well as control or reversal of some of the diabetic complications, have prompted increased interest in those patients who have not yet reached end-stage renal disease. By 1987 approximately one-fifth of all patients listed in the Pancreas Transplant Registry had received only the pancreas graft and had not yet reached end-stage renal failure (Sutherland & Moudry, 1986). The success in these patients, as well as in the combined pancreas-renal transplant recipients, will now begin to move pancreas transplantation from the realm of an experimental procedure to an accepted form of therapy.

IMMUNOLOGY

Throughout all the early clinical trials in transplantation, primarily those of the kidney, the recognition of the immune response to foreign tissue was outweighed by the technical problems. Research into the correlation between the immune system and rejection of the graft coincided with the initial successes in kidney transplantation.

The primary goal of immunology in transplantation is simply to understand the immune response and be able to determine a method of controlling it, while causing the patient the least amount of harm.

In 1957 the initial work of Jean Dausset resulted in the identification of a human leukocyte antigen, which is known today as A2 (Hamburger, Crosnier, Bach, & Kress, 1981). This led to the identification of other antigens and, eventually, to clarification of the body's response to foreign antigens. The ability to control this response in a safe and efficacious manner continues to be one of the main focuses of transplant research.

Early attempts at controlling the immune system consisted of total-body irradiation (1959–62), as well as the use of potent anticancer drugs such as 6-mercaptopurine and methotrexate (1959). The development of azathioprine (in 1961) and its subsequent combination with steroids (in 1962–63) resulted in markedly improved graft survival. However, although graft survival and control of rejection improved, the incidence of morbidity and mortality from fulminent infections increased. Throughout the 1960s the primary cause of death in kidney transplant recipients was infection. Profound leukopenia frequently resulted in the rapid onset of pneumonia, wound infection, and, eventually, systemic infections that usually were not responsive to conventional therapy (Calne, 1967).

The first use of tissue typing, or antigen matching, between donor and recipient occurred in 1962 and has since become routine. In 1978 the identification and clinical application of the DR antigens were first seen, and again, these have become routine (Hamburger et al., 1981).

The most exciting development, and the one with the greatest clinical application, was the introduction of cyclosporine in 1978. Borel first reported the potent immunosuppressive qualities of this drug in 1976. Clinical trials in kidney transplantation were begun by Calne in 1978. Over the next five years extensive clinical trials, first in Europe and then in the United States, reported major improvements in graft survival, with less morbidity (Morris, 1984). The availability of cyclosporine initially with kidney transplantation, as well as the major increase in graft and patient survival, has resulted in the prolific growth of extrarenal transplantation in the 1980s.

The development of polyclonal and monoclonal antibodies has further increased the success of transplantation. The striking advances since the late 1970s have prompted continued and aggressive studies to develop the ultimate method of controlling the immune system.

TISSUE TRANSPLANTATION

The transplantation of skin, bone, and other tissue was first considered in ancient Greek and Chinese civilizations. Later history speaks of St. Thomas More's attempt to transplant a leg from one man to another. Serious research in this field was begun in the mid-nineteenth century.

Transplantation of the cornea to reverse blindness was first attempted by von Hippel in Berlin, in 1930. Sir Tudor-Thomas further developed the procedure in England in the 1930s. The first successful clinical cornea transplant was performed by Stocker in 1952. Stocker used topical steroids in an attempt to control edema. This may have been the reason for this early success (Borushoff & Thoft, 1987). Although acute rejection is rare in corneal transplants, owing to the lack of direct blood supply, a lymphocytic accumulation can be documented approximately three weeks post transplant (Borushoff & Thoft, 1987).

The transplantation of bone and tendons was first used in the early 1950s to prevent the crippling effects of polio (Edmonson & Crenshaw, 1980). Transplantation is now a commonly used treatment for congenital defects, as well as for the disfigurement and crippling caused by arthritis, trauma, and cancer (Edmonson & Crenshaw, 1980).

SUMMARY

The tremendous strides that have been made in transplantation since the 1960s have resulted in acceptable forms of treatment for end-stage organ failure; however, there are still a number of areas in which transplantation is restricted.

Exorbitant cost and limited financial coverage remain major barriers for many potential recipients. Kidney transplantation is covered under the federal End-Stage Renal Disease Program, which was enacted in 1973. This program covers 80 per cent of all costs incurred in the treatment of renal failure, including both dialysis and transplantation, under Medicare. It is available to all people, regardless of age, who qualify for the program. Because of the extensive success rate in renal transplantation, private insurors and state assistance are usually available for the remaining 20 per cent of medical coverage. Major financial problems still exist for liver, heart, and pancreas recipients. Medicare has recently agreed to fund heart transplants, but only at certain centers and only in patients who qualify for routine Medicare coverage. Many insurance companies, unfortunately, continue to consider transplantation of the liver in adults, and heart and pancreas transplantation, as experimental procedures and, therefore, do not offer coverage. In addition, a number of state-aid programs have begun to eliminate coverage of transplantation for eligible patients because of the high costs and the programs' limited budgets. Financial coverage remains a stumbling block to many seeking transplantation. Decreases in morbidity and in hospital costs may increase coverage by both state and private insurance programs in the future.

Other factors that limit transplantation are the need for complete and safe control of the immune system and the problem of rejection. Exhaustive research in this area continues at centers throughout the world in an attempt to further improve graft and patient survival, as well as the quality of life for the recipients. An aspect somewhat unique to transplantation is the cooperative sharing of research strategies from one center to another. This cooperation is evident in the multicenter studies that have been done both in the United States and in Canada, as well as throughout Europe. National and international meetings encourage this sharing of knowledge.

The care of transplant recipients and their families offers one of the most exciting challenges in the nursing profession. This book examines these challenges, as well as the rewards associated with transplant nursing.

References

Becerra, E., Cooper, D.K.C., Novitsky, D., & Reichert, B. (1987). Are there indications for heterotopic heart transplantation today? *Transplantation Proceedings, 19*(1), 2512–2513.

Belzer, F.O. (1988). Principles of organ preservation. *Transplantation Proceedings, 20*(1), 925–927.

Barnard, C.N. (1984). The future of heart replacement. In D.K.C. Cooper & R.P. Lanza (Eds.), *Heart Transplantation* (pp. 341–349). Boston: M.T.P. Press.

Borushoff, S.A. & Thoft, R.A. (1987). Therapeutic keratoplasty. In G. Smoolin & R.A. Thoft (Eds.), *The Cornea: Scientific Foundations and Clinical Practice* (pp. 543–545) Boston: Little, Brown.

Calne, R.Y. (Ed.). (1983). *Liver Transplantation.* New York: Grune & Stratton.

Caves, P.K., Stinson, E.B., Graham, A.F., Billingham, M.E., Grehl, T.M., & Shumway, N.E.

(1973). Percutaneous transvenous endomyocardial biopsy. *Journal of the American Medical Association, 22*(3), 288–291.

Cooley, D.A. (1982). Staged cardiac transplantation: Report of three cases. *Heart Transplantation, 1*, 145–148.

Cooper, D.K.C. (1984). Experimental development and early clinical experience. In D.K.C. Cooper & R.P. Lanza (Eds.), *Heart Transplantation* (pp. 1–21). Boston: M.T.P. Press.

d'Apice, A.J.F. (1984). Nonspecific immunosuppression: Azathioprine and steroids. In P.J. Morris (Ed.), *Kidney Transplantation: Principles and Practices* (2nd ed.) (pp. 239–241). Orlando, Grune and Stratton.

DeVries, W.C., Anderson, J.L., Joyce, L.D., Anderson F.L., Hammond, E.H., Jarvik, R.K., & Knolff, W.J. (1984). Clinical use of the total artificial heart. *New England Journal of Medicine, 310*, 273–278.

Dubernard, J.M., Traeger, J., & Bosi, E. (1984). The technique of neoprene injection for human pancreatic transplantation: Experience in 40 cases. *Transplantation Proceedings, 16*, 685–686.

Edmonson, A.S. & Crenshaw, A.H. (Eds.). (1980). *Campbell's Operative Orthopedics*. St. Louis: C.V. Mosby.

Grzelka, C. (1986). Organ donation laws create demand for education. *Healthlink, 2*(3), 11–13.

Hamburger, J., Crosnier, J., Bach, J.F., & Kress, H. (1981). *Renal Transplantation: Theory and Practice*. Baltimore: Williams & Wilkins.

Hamilton, D. (1984). Kidney transplantation: A history. In P.J. Morris (Ed.), *Kidney Transplantation: Principles and Practices* (2nd ed.) (pp. 4–8). Orlando: Grune & Stratton.

Jamieson, S.W., Oyer, P.E., Bieber, C.P., Hunt, S.A., Billingham, M., Miller, J., Gomberg, P., Stinson, E.B., & Shumway, N.E. (1983). Cardiac transplantation at Stanford. *Heart Transplantation, 2*, 243–244.

Lee, H.M. (1984). Surgical techniques of renal transplantation. In P.J. Morris (Ed.), *Kidney Transplantation: Principles and Practices*. (2nd ed.) (pp. 199–218). Orlando: Grune & Stratton.

Lillehei, R.C., Simmons, R.L., & Najarian, J.S. (1970). Pancreaticoduodenal allotransplantation: Experimental and clinical experience. *Annals of Surgery, 172*, 405–436.

Marshall, V.C. (1984). Renal preservation. In P.J. Morris (Ed.), *Kidney Transplantation: Principles and Practices* (2nd ed.) (pp. 129–148). Orlando: Grune & Stratton.

Morris, P.J. (1984). Cyclosporine. In P.J. Morris (Ed.), *Kidney Transplantation: Principles and Practices* (pp. 261–264). Orlando: Grune & Stratton.

Nghiem, D.D., Shulak, J.A., & Corry, R.J. (1987). Duodenopancreatectomy for transplantation. *Archives of Surgery, 122*, 1201–1206.

Solis, E., & Kaye, M.P. (1986). The registry of the International Society for Heart Transplant: third official report. In P. Terasaki (Ed.) *Clinical Transplants, 1986* (pp. 1–5). Los Angeles: UCLA Tissue Typing Laboratory.

Starzl, T.E. (1969). *Experience in Hepatic Transplantation*. Philadelphia: W.B. Saunders.

Sutherland, D.E.R. & Chinn, P.L. (1984). Minnesota experience with 85 pancreas transplants between 1978 and 1983. *World Journal of Surgery, 8*, 244–252.

Sutherland, D.E.R. & Moudry, K. (1986). Report of pancreas transplant registry. In P. Terasaki (Ed.), *Clinical Transplants, 1986* (pp. 7–15). Los Angeles: UCLA Tissue Typing Laboratory.

Takiff, H., Mickey, M.R., Cicciarelli, J., & Terasaki, P.J. (1987). Factors important in ten-year kidney graft survival. *Transplantation Proceedings, 19*(1), 666–668.

Wicomb, W.N. (1984). Donor heart storage. In D.K.C. Cooper & R.P. Lanza (Eds.), *Heart Transplantation*, (pp. 51–70). Boston: M.T.P. Press.

2

Organ Procurement and Preservation

Mary Hoffman and Mindy Malecki

Nurses are frequently involved with patients and families who want to donate organs and tissues after their own deaths or the deaths of loved ones. Advances in the transplantation of kidney, heart, liver, pancreas, lung, bone, skin, and cornea and the resultant publicity surrounding the successes have increased the demand for these organs and tissues. In addition, relatively more experimental transplants are on the horizon, such as bowel, brain, and limb, offering even greater hope for patients with end-stage organ and tissue disease.

Nurses are a vital part of the procurement process. They work with the donor family and assist in maintaining the cadaveric donor. Specific skills and background knowledge are required to expedite the donor process while showing the utmost respect for the donor and the donor's family. This chapter addresses pertinent issues involved in donation that are relative to nursing practice, including donor identification and maintenance, presenting the option of donation to a bereaved family, and professional education. Information about donation and transplantation as social issues is given to provide continuity and a more complete understanding of the total picture.

LEGISLATIVE BACKGROUND

The Uniform Anatomical Gift Act

First proposed in 1968, the Uniform Anatomical Gift Act (UAGA) has been adopted in all 50 states. It allows that at the time of death, an anatomical gift may be executed by the donor or the donor's next of kin as defined by the Act.

If the donor has signed a donor card (in many states some form of donor consent appears on the driver's license) and the signature is witnessed by two persons, the card is considered a legal document. However, out of respect for the donor's family, organs are not removed without signed consent from the legal next of kin. Consequently, the donor card functions primarily as a means of educating the public about organ and tissue donation and often prompts family discussion before death occurs.

The National Organ Transplant Act

Because organs for transplantation are considered a scarce national resource, in 1984, Congress enacted the National Organ Transplant Act (NOTA). The Act directed the Secretary of Health and Human Services to establish a Task Force on Organ Transplantation. This task force was charged with making a comprehensive examination of the medical, legal, ethical, economic, and social issues presented by human organ procurement and transplantation. NOTA also established a national organ procurement and transplantation network to maintain a national list of people who are in need of transplants and to assist organ procurement organizations (OPOs) in matching and equitably distributing donated organs. In 1986, the government contract for a national sharing system was awarded to United Network of Organ Sharing (UNOS) of Richmond, Virginia. Finally, NOTA made the buying and/or selling of organs for transplantation unlawful in the United States. See Chapter 18 for additional details.

Task Force Recommendations

The Task Force report stated that "physicians and nurses are in a position to facilitate organ donation, but frequently do not" (Organ Transplantation Issues and Recommendations, Department of Health and Human Services, 1986, p. 32). The majority of state legislatures, recognizing the need for donations, had already passed what were known as "Required Request" or "Routine Inquiry" laws. Oregon was the first to enact such laws, in 1985, closely followed by New York. The state laws require that when a person dies in a hospital, the administrator or the administrator's designee must ask the deceased's next of kin if he or she wants to make an anatomical gift. State laws vary but generally allow three exceptions to the law: (1) the deceased is known by the administrator or the administrator's designee to have objected to donation; (2)

the deceased was of a religion known to object to donation; and (3) the deceased does not meet the general medical criteria for donation.

THE ROLE OF THE ORGAN PROCUREMENT ORGANIZATION

Federal law in 1986 deemed that there will be one federally approved OPO per service region. A statute of NOTA provides that a qualified OPO must be a not-for-profit entity, have a defined geographical area that includes at least 50 potential donors each year, and have enough trained personnel to obtain donation within the service area.

The responsibilities of an OPO are to coordinate, procure, and distribute organs and tissues for and within its designated service area. Some states may have more than one OPO per service area for various reasons, such as geographical size of the area and the number of transplant centers located within the area. Nurses must be able to access their hospital's OPO quickly, since time is of the essence in the procurement process. Additional responsibilities of the OPO include education of hospital personnel regarding donor criteria and provision of guidance in discussing the option of donation with a grieving family. Some state regulations require that hospital personnel involved in the donor process receive training.

OPOs are governed by a board of advisers from various medical specialties and lay organizations. Each OPO has a medical advisory board made up of transplant surgeons who are the actual procurers of the recovered organs and tissues. Transplant surgeons determine the medical suitability of potential donors referred to the OPO by area hospitals.

The organ procurement coordinator is an essential member of the procurement team. Coordinators are specialized health care professionals who manage all aspects of donation, including public and professional education. Under the supervision of transplant surgeons, procurement coordinators screen potential donors for medical suitability. If a potential donor meets the necessary criteria, the coordinator will facilitate the donation process.

DONOR IDENTIFICATION

To identify a potential donor, the nurse must first distinguish between organ and tissue. All solid organs, such as the heart, liver, kidneys, pancreas, and bowel, must be donated by people who have suffered irreversible brain injury. These potential donors must meet the criteria for brain death. They are maintained on life support to allow the organs to remain viable. Tissues, such as bone, skin, and corneas, are removed once oxygenation has stopped; therefore, people who have suffered cardiorespiratory arrest can be evaluated for tissue donation.

Brain Death

As respiratory ventilators and total-system monitoring became more sophisticated, health care workers were able to maintain patients for longer periods. The medical definition of death became an issue. The first documented report on the diagnosis of brain death was published by an ad hoc committee of the Harvard Medical School. This report did not define brain death, but rather presented physicians with guidelines to determine the level of brain activity. The committee recommended that the diagnosis be made through the confirmation of four tests: (1) no response to painful stimuli, (2) absence of spontaneous respirations, (3) absence of all reflex activity, and (4) a flat electroencephalogram. These tests were to be repeated 24 hours apart before brain death was declared (Report of the Ad Hoc Committee of the Harvard Medical School, 1968).

These guidelines were used by physicians as the medical standard until 1981, when the President's Commission submitted a report stating that "if the brain stem completely lacks function, the brain as a whole cannot function" (Report of the Medical Consultants on the Diagnosis of Death to the President's Commission for the Study of Ethical Problems in Medicine and Biomedical and Behavioral Research, 1981). Determination of brain death could be made with a thorough clinical, bedside examination. Electroencephalograms were no longer considered necessary because of the technical difficulties in administration and the lack of accuracy in assessing the total absence of brain activity.

Although this report was published nationally, many physicians continued to use the electroencephalogram as a diagnostic tool. Many times a cerebral blood flow study is ordered, which can objectively determine whether there is any blood flow to the brain. A lack of blood flow signifies the absence of brain function.

Currently there is no nationally accepted definition of brain death. Brain death is, however, medically defined as the irreversible cessation of all brain activity, including that of the brain stem. This differs from a persistent vegetative coma in that patients in a coma do maintain some level of brain stem activity, for example, spontaneous respirations. In brain death there is no essential brain cell activity, and therefore no chance of recovery.

To clinically assess for brain death, all signs of brain stem activity are evaluated. This bedside examination includes the criteria listed in Table 2–1.

TABLE 2–1. BRAIN DEATH CRITERIA AND ASSESSMENT

SYMPTOM	TEST
Absence of all respirations	Apnea test: Place patient on 100% oxygen for 15 minutes. Turn off ventilator, while closely monitoring vital signs. Arterial blood gases should be drawn every minute. Because the stimulus to breathe is activated by an increase in CO_2, if the patient does not breathe on her own within 3 to 4 minutes, the respirator is turned back on. This test must be carefully monitored to prevent the patient from going into cardiac arrest.
No response to painful stimuli	Deeply pinch the patient's arm or leg.
Fixed and dilated pupils	Check for reactivity to light.
Absent gag or cough reflex	While suctioning, assess for reflex.
Absent corneal reflex	Gently raise eyebrow and brush sclera with cotton wisp.
Absent doll's eye reflex	Hold the patient's eyelids open and gently turn her head to each side. In brain death the patient's eyes don't move.
No ocular movement	Cold calorics test: Inject 20 ml of ice cold water onto the tympanic membrane. In brain death there is no ocular movement.

In caring for a patient with a severe neurologic injury, the nurse should document any change in neurologic response that is manifested by the patient. Clinical evaluative tests must be done in the absence of hypothermia and an elevated barbiturate level. These two conditions can clinically mimic brain death and must be corrected before an accurate diagnosis can be made.

The physiology of brain death can be simply explained by referring to Figure 2–1. When the brain is injured (e.g., trauma, cerebral aneurysm, or tumor), the cells react by swelling. As the swelling accelerates, the tissue being confined in the skull has no area in which to expand. This physiologically increases cerebral pressure. As the pressure increases, further tissue injury ensues. The cycle is repeated; unless the swelling is controlled, permanent damage results. In brain death, the extraneous medical measures used to control swelling are ineffective in preventing further cellular injury. The result is irreversible cessation of all brain activity.

Once brain death criteria are met, the diagnosis is made. The physician must document the death on the chart with a date and time. This is the legal time of death, and it will be placed on the death certificate. Once the death is declared, the option of organ and tissue donation should be offered to the family.

DONOR EVALUATION

Identification of a potential organ donor is generally confined to a previously healthy person, 70 years or younger, who has suffered irre-

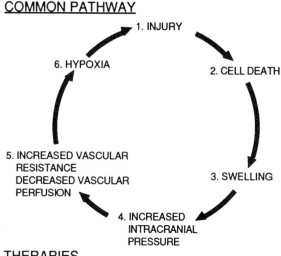

COMMON PATHWAY

1. INJURY

6. HYPOXIA

2. CELL DEATH

5. INCREASED VASCULAR
RESISTANCE
DECREASED VASCULAR
PERFUSION

3. SWELLING

4. INCREASED
INTRACRANIAL
PRESSURE

THERAPIES

STEROIDS
VASODILATORS
ACID-BASE MANIPULATION
BARBITURATES

FIGURE 2–1. Pathophysiology of brain death.

versible, catastrophic brain injury leading to brain death. The injury is confined to the head and neck, allowing the internal visceral organs to remain healthy. The patient is often brought to the hospital neurologically injured, but with some reflexes present. However, as discussed previously, the cellular damage expands, and the brain stem herniates and ceases to function.

Potential causes of injury leading to brain death are:

1. Acute head or neurologic trauma
2. Subarachnoid hemorrhage
3. Cerebrovascular accident
4. Primary brain tumor
5. Drug overdose
6. Smoke inhalation.

The cause of death must be known in evaluating for donation. If the cause of death cannot be determined, most transplant centers will decline the donation. This conservative approach is maintained in order to protect the recipients. Causes of death that are contraindications to donation are noted in Table 2–2.

If previous medical charts are available, they are reviewed. Fre-

TABLE 2–2. CONTRAINDICATIONS TO DONATION

Acute bacterial meningitis and cerebritis
Subdural emphysema
Brain abscess
Acute viral encephalitis
Aseptic meningitis
Slow virus infection of the central nervous system
Malignant neoplastic disease
Guillain-Barré syndrome
Amyotrophic lateral sclerosis
Reye's syndrome
Systemic viral diseases
Bacteremia
(*Note:* Some centers will consider donors with *Haemophilus* influenza or pneumococcal meningitis if they have been appropriately treated with antibiotics and have had subsequent negative cultures.)

quently the family will be the main source of information regarding the donor's medical history. The nurse performs a visual examination of the donor, assessing for signs of intravenous drug abuse, previous surgery, and preexisting illnesses. Systemic illnesses, such as hypertension and diabetes mellitus, do not automatically rule out donation. Cancer, with the exception of a primary brain tumor, is a contraindication to donation. Systemic illnesses are further evaluated in terms of duration, severity, treatment, and history of compliance.

The family is questioned regarding the donor's social history. Intravenous drug use, alcoholism, homosexuality, smoking, and current medications are assessed. Although this is a traumatic time for the family, obtaining an accurate social history is crucial in evaluating the donor. If this is done in a sensitive, caring way, the family will realize the importance of protecting the recipient.

The course of the current hospitalization must also be closely evaluated. The most critical assessment is that of the cardiopulmonary system. This includes detailing any cardiac arrests for duration and response to cardiopulmonary resuscitation, amount of blood loss and replacement, range of blood pressure readings, heart rate, use of vasopressors, arterial blood gas (ABG) values, and urine output. The nurse must also assess the donor for any signs of systemic infection. Laboratory values are monitored for increased total white blood cell count (WBC) and an increase in the absolute number of lymphocytes. It must be noted that when there is a severe neurologic injury, the elevated WBC count can be due to the injury, and not to infection. It is important not to isolate the WBC count reading, but to combine it with other clinical data when assessing for infection. Because of injury to the brain, body temperature is not always an accurate sign of infection.

If surgery or other invasive procedures were performed during the current hospitalization, the records are reviewed. This is particularly true in trauma cases in which abdominal injury is suspected but may not be confirmed. Abdominal drains, gastrostomies, and colostomies are generally contraindications to donation. This decision, however, is made by the individual procuring physician. Surgeries to the limbs to repair or immobilize fractures are to be noted but are not a contraindication to organ donation. Any type of cranial surgery, such as an evacuation of a hematoma, must also be evaluated but will not necessarily inhibit donation. All medications that the donor is receiving should be evaluated at the time the donation process begins. Most medications used to treat neurologic injuries are discontinued at this time.

Certain laboratory values are needed to determine the status of all organs. These are blood type (needed for recipient matching), chemistry profile, ABG measurement, complete blood count (CBC) with platelets, blood cultures, urine cultures, and urinalysis.

The culture results may not be available at the time of the procurement, but they will be evaluated when the 24-hour results are completed. If any cultures are positive, the sensitivity results will direct appropriate antibiotic therapy.

The following tests for infectious diseases are also performed: human immunodeficiency virus (HIV), hepatitis B surface antigen (HbsAg), and rapid plasma reagent (RPR). If any of these tests are positive, transplantation cannot occur.

Once the donor has been assessed for general medical status, specific criteria for each organ must be met. The following required laboratory and clinical tests will be ordered by the procurement center and evaluated by a transplant physician. These requirements may vary, depending on the transplant surgeon and the donor. Other tests specific to each organ or tissue are discussed below and summarized in Table 2–3.

Kidney Evaluation

The acceptable age range for a kidney donor is between 2 and 70 years of age. Urine output should average at least 50 cc/hr during the entire course of hospitalization. The serum blood urea nitrogen (BUN) and creatinine levels should be within normal range. On initial evaluation of the donor, the BUN level may be slightly elevated owing to the dehydrated status, but it should return to normal with adequate fluid replacement. The urinalysis is also a critical tool used in evaluating renal function. Any abnormalities must be further assessed.

Although the kidneys are more resistant to episodes of hypoxia and hypotension, it is still important to maintain a stable cardiorespiratory status. Dopamine doses greater than 30 μg/kg/min, however, can cause renal damage.

TABLE 2–3. ORGAN- AND TISSUE-SPECIFIC EVALUATIVE TESTS

ORGAN	AGE RANGE (in years)	SPECIFIC TESTS
Kidneys	2–70	Urine output greater than 50 ml/hr BUN Creatinine Urinalysis
Liver	Less than 50	Height and weight SGOT SGPT PT/PTT
Heart	Less than 40	Height and weight 12-lead EKG Echocardiogram Chest x-ray Cardiac enzymes Cardiac catheterization Cardiology consult
Lungs	Less than 40	All heart tests plus sputum Gram stain and culture
Pancreas	3–40	Amylase Lipase

TISSUE	AGE RANGE (in years)	SPECIFIC TESTS
Bone	15–65	X-rays of limbs if questionable closure of growth plate
Skin	12–70	None
Eyes	1–75	None

Liver Evaluation

The generally accepted age criterion for a liver donor is less than 45 years, although some centers accept livers from donors up to 50 years of age. The lower age cutoff depends on the age of the recipient population. In addition to blood type, the donor and recipient are matched for height and weight. The donor liver must be of compatible size in order to fit into the recipient's abdominal cavity. In pediatric cases, abdominal circumference is often used as a measurement in matching size. ABO blood group barriers may be crossed in emergencies. Chronic alcohol abuse usually rules out liver donation. A complete liver profile should be done to assess for specific liver damage.

The liver is an extremely vascular organ, and is sensitive to variations in blood pressure. A cardiac arrest or hypotensive episode (less than 30 minutes in duration) may not necessarily rule out donation but must be further evaluated. Adequate oxygenation is critical, with the PaO_2 minimally maintained at greater than 70 mm Hg. If the hemoglobin is less than 10 g/dl, a transfusion may be ordered.

Dopamine dosage greater than 10 μg/kg/min may compromise hepatic perfusion and contraindicate donation. Other vasopressors, such as norepinephrine injection (Levophed), metaraminol bitartrate (Aramine), and phenylephrine (Neo-Synephrine), have a vasoconstricting effect on hepatic circulation and are also considered a contraindication to donation.

Cardiac Evaluation

The generally accepted age criterion for a heart donor is less than 40 years of age for females and less than 35 years of age for males. The lower age range varies, depending on the recipient need. As with livers, the height and weight of the donor must match that of the recipient in order for the heart to fit into the chest cavity and fulfill the cardiovascular needs of the recipient. ABO compatibility between donor and recipient is a strict criterion. When the recipient has a high percentage of reactive antibodies (PRA >50%) the risk of immediate rejection is greater. A donor-recipient lymphocyte crossmatch is then performed before cardiac donation. In all cases a retrospective crossmatch is performed by the transplant center.

Stable donor hemodynamics are essential in assessing for heart donation. All periods of arrhythmias or hypotension must be assessed. In general, a cardiac arrest does rule out donation for whole-heart transplant. Accepted dopamine use varies; however, the upper limit usually ranges from 10 to 20 µg/kg/min. The duration of vasopressor administration often affects the amount accepted.

Alterations in heart rate are closely evaluated. Brief periods of tachycardia are generally not of concern. Prolonged tachycardia can result in cardiac exhaustion. If the tachycardia is considered to be neurologic in origin, propranolol (Inderal) or verapamil (Isoptin) may be ordered. Sinus bradycardia is usually well tolerated if maintained between 50 and 60 beats per minute (BPM). If heart rate declines to less than 50 BPM, a dobutamine drip may be ordered. Atropine is generally ineffective in donors because of the lack of vagal stimulation.

Maintenance of adequate oxygenation is critical in assuring the viability of the heart. Any hypoxic episodes are assessed for duration and severity. Chest tube acceptance varies, depending on the transplant surgeon. In general, chest tubes that have been inserted for a pneumothorax, induced from a central venous pressure line insertion, are acceptable. Chest tubes inserted for other reasons should be further evaluated. Blunt chest trauma implies potential cardiac damage, as does severe abdominal trauma, which may force the visceral organs into the chest cavity, ruling out donation.

Lung Evaluation

The generally accepted age criterion for a lung donor is the same as for a heart donor. Again, donor size is critical in matching the lung to the recipient so that the lung will fit into the recipient's chest cavity and will meet her ventilatory needs. Usually only a single lung is transplanted. A current chest x-ray is needed to evaluate for pulmonary injury or infection. The diameter of the main stem bronchus is often measured on x-ray and compared with recipient size. A Gram stain is also required, owing to the high risk of infection from prolonged intubation. ABG values are closely monitored for signs of pulmonary dysfunction. The donor should be placed on 100% oxygen for 15 to 30 minutes, followed by an ABG measurement. A PaO_2 of greater than 300 mm Hg is generally preferred. Chest tubes are a contraindication to lung donation.

If the heart and both lungs are removed from the donor and transplanted into the same recipient, the criteria for both organs are used in donor evaluation.

Pancreas Evaluation

For a pancreas donor the generally accepted age range is between 3 and 40 years. Donor size is not a criterion in matching the pancreas with a recipient. The donor should have no history of diabetes, chronic pancreatitis, or chronic alcoholism. A family history of diabetes must also be ruled out. Laboratory values should include normal amylase and lipase levels.

An accurate abdominal physical assessment is required in order to evaluate for pancreatic injury. Such injury could include trauma, or adhesion secondary to previous surgeries.

Other Organ Evaluations

At this time experimental transplantation of small bowel, stomach, large intestine, brain, and limb is being performed. No standard criteria are yet established for donation of these organs. They are currently removed infrequently and only when there is a specific need.

Tissue Evaluation

The general criteria used in evaluating a potential tissue donor are (1) absence of all cancer (except for corneas), (2) absence of systemic infection, (3) no active viral disease, and (4) no history of intravenous drug abuse. The generally accepted age range for a tissue donor varies, depending on the tissue. For eyes it is between 1 and 65 years; for bone, between 15 and 60 years; and for skin, between 12 and 70 years. The age criterion is established by the tissue-procuring center and may differ from these ranges.

The extensive laboratory tests needed to evaluate for organ donation are not mandatory; however, the HIV, HBsAg, and RPR must be done. Blood type is generally required for retrospective data evaluation. The family should be asked for a brief social history, to include possible homosexuality and drug abuse, and a medical history to ascertain any chronic illnesses.

The tissue donor is normally a healthy person who has suffered a sudden cardiac or respiratory arrest owing to trauma or natural causes. The cause of death must be known before a donation is accepted. If the donor was also an organ donor, the tests done for that purpose are not repeated. For bone donations that are done in the operating room, blood cultures may be ordered.

In evaluating for an eye donation the nurse should note any signs of trauma to the ocular area. A history should be obtained from the family specific to any eye injuries or illnesses the donor may have had. Visual acuity has no impact on donation. While waiting for the technician to arrive, the eyelids should be kept closed and wet, with moist gauze pads placed over them. This prevents any abrasions caused by dryness.

In evaluating for skin, the amount and quality of the area should be examined. Skin must be procured from large surface areas so that the skin pieces are large enough to transplant. The skin should be assessed for any abnormalities or unusual growths that could indicate infection.

For bone and skin donations there are no special interventions for the care of the donor. The body should be placed in the morgue as quickly as possible until the procurement team arrives.

OFFERING THE OPTION OF DONATION

Asking a family if they want to donate the organs and tissues of a loved one who has suddenly died is not easy. Often the deceased is a young, previously healthy person who died suddenly in a tragic accident. This task is even more difficult for a nurse who has no background information about the donor process. Educational preparation allows the nurse to communicate with a potential donor family in an informed, confident manner.

A 1987 study of 124 nurses showed that those who personally felt uncomfortable about requesting donation received a significantly higher

TABLE 2–4. CONSOLATION VS. IMPOSITION: THE NURSING DILEMMA

Breakdown of nurses surveyed*

ICU	56% (70)
ER	11% (14)
OR	2% (3)
Medical	23% (29)
Other†	6% (8)
Total	124

*Percentages rounded to nearest whole number.
†Nursing education and house supervisors.

Level of discomfort
Question: How did you feel when approaching the families?

	Sad/ Comfortable but Confident	Very Uncomfortable
Tissues		
ICU (30/35)	19	11
ER (3/3)	3	0
OR (1/1)	1	0
Medical (2/6)	2	0
Other (4/4)	3	1
Total (40/49)	28/40 (78%)	12/40 (30%)
Organs		
ICU (27/31)	24	3
ER (2/2)	2	0
OR (1/1)	1	0
Medical (1/2)	1	0
Other 5/5)	4	1
Total (36/41)	32/38 (89%)	4/36 (11%)

Responses to requests for donation
Question: How many of the families said yes?

	Yes	No
Tissues		
Sad/comfortable but confident (28)	24 (86%)	4 (14%)
Very uncomfortable (12)	5 (42%)	7 (58%)
Organs		
Sad/comfortable but confident (32)	27 (84%)	5 (16%)
Very uncomfortable (4)	0	4 (100%)

From Malecki, M. & Hoffman, M. (1987). Getting to yes: How nurses' attitudes affect their success in obtaining consent for organ and tissue donations. *Dialysis and Transplantation, 16*(5) 276–278.

number of negative responses from potential donor families than did nurses who were sad, but comfortable and confident (Hoffman & Malecki, 1987) (Table 2–4). After specific training aimed largely at, but not limited to, working with potential donor families, nurses were more willing to broach the subject of donation. Aside from clinical information, training about the donor process should include where to approach a family, nonverbal communication techniques, language choices, common family concerns, and legal implications. Trained nurses attribute their rise in confidence to increased knowledge about the actual procurement process, combined with communicating skills that involve interactions with donor families.

The argument for organ donation lies essentially in the good it does those who receive an organ transplant. Their benefit is unequivocable. Many, however, believe that families of donors also benefit. To test this assumption, in a 1987 study (Table 2–5) donor families were asked if they thought that donation had made coping with their loss any easier. The data indicated that donation had been helpful for most people (Batten & Prottas, 1987). Therefore, the option of organ and tissue donation is most often a consolation, not an imposition, for a grieving family.

There is no "comfortable" time to ask a family for a donation. Because of the sadness of each situation, it is never easy to ask the question, and doing so can engender tension and anxiety. The nurse's feelings should be recognized as part of a genuine concern for the grieving family and should not become an excuse to avoid the request. In the spirit of continuing care, it is necessary to remember that although the donor has expired, the nurse can still offer consolation to the surviving family. Donation allows the family to take something positive from an otherwise tragic situation. In addition, it is the family's right to be offered a choice.

Table 2–5. DONOR FAMILY REFLECTIONS

Very important reasons for donating relative's organs

	Coping Somewhat Easier (n = 159)	Coping Not Any Easier (n = 105)
Organ donation can help someone else live	91%	77%
Functioning organs should not be wasted	84	58
Organ donation makes something positive come out of death	96	70
Relative could live on in someone else through donation		48

Differences between the two groups statistically significant, p = 0.01.

Percentage of groups that believe organ donation helps families in their grieving process

Group	Percentage	Total Sample
Hospital administrators	82	227
Intensive care unit nurses	79	919
Neurosurgeons	66	246
General public	81	750
Donor family members	79	264

From Batten & Prottas (1987). Reprinted by permission of *Health Affairs*, Project HOPE, Millwood, VA 22646.

Suggested Methods of Approach

Below are some guidelines on how one might offer the option of organ and tissue donation to a bereaved family:

- Take the family to a quiet, private area without distraction. Asking for donation at the bedside of the deceased is poor nonverbal communication. It shows disrespect for the donor as a person, emphasizing instead the organs and tissues in question.

- Once in a private location, the nurse should be conscious of appearing physically comfortable. Openness and empathy can be conveyed with relaxed body language, such as uncrossed legs and open hands placed in the lap. A nurse's personal discomfort with the issue may convey disapproval. The information then loses its necessary objectivity. An obviously uncomfortable nurse puts herself in an unnecessarily stressful role of "persuader" or "nonpersuader." The role of the nurse is to present information, not to persuade. A nurse who is opposed to donation should not be put in the position of requesting it.

- Begin the discussion by offering sympathy to the family member(s) about the death in one's own words. For example, "I'm sorry that your husband has died," or "I'm sorry that John has been pronounced dead."

- Focus on the deceased's wishes. Had the deceased ever signed a donor card? Had he or she ever discussed organ donation? This can lessen the stress on the survivor if a decision had already been made.

- Answer questions simply and honestly. In order to do this, nurses do not need to be experts on procurement. A nurse who needs assistance should contact the OPO. Donor families have common concerns about donation. Nurses should be generally familiar with these areas of concern.

- Consent for any type of donation must be obtained from the next of kin or guardian. Consent forms can be obtained from the OPO, and signature must be witnessed by two persons. When the next of kin is not present, a consent may be obtained over the telephone with two witnesses to the conversation. If the next of kin cannot be located, the OPO and the hospital will make a decision in conjunction with the medical examiner or coroner.

- The medical examiner or coroner must give final consent in cases of death under their jurisdiction (e.g., homicides, suicides, or any questionable death). It may be prudent to first obtain the medical examiner's or coroner's consent before approaching the family in case the postmortem investigation precludes donation. In "John Doe" cases, in which the identity of the potential donor is unknown, donation will usually not occur because of the lack of available medical history.

- To avoid nonverbal pressure on the family, keep the consent form out of sight until the decision to donate has been made.

COMMON CONCERNS

Many donor families have the following concerns about donation.

- Many families require repeat explanations of brain death. The nurse should be prepared to discuss the definition of brain death in simple terms. For example: "Brain death means total, irreversible loss of brain function. Your loved one appears to be breathing but is being mechanically maintained. If we were to turn off the ventilator, he would not even be able to take a breath. We have performed a number of tests to come to this conclusion. Do you have any questions or concerns about brain death that I can help clarify?"

- Donor families fear that their loved ones will be disfigured by the surgical recovery of the organs and tissues. All organs and tissues are removed under sterile conditions in an operating room, just as they would be on a living person, with the utmost respect for the donor's body. Funeral arrangements, including an open casket, are not affected by donation. Because some families may not broach this issue, it is helpful to say, "In case you were wondering, there will be no disfigurement. You will be able to have an open-casket viewing if you so choose."

- All of the major religions support donation and transplantation. Enlist the counseling support of hospital clergy when necessary.

- Cultural differences play a part in the decision-making process of donor families, particularly among minority groups. It is important to keep their orientation in mind, including their views of the American health system. Enlist support of a social worker and interpreter when necessary.

- Once a donor is accepted by the OPO and the family consents, all costs incurred related to the donation are the responsibility of the OPO. The family incurs no costs involved in donation. They are, however, still responsible for funeral costs.

- Families may ask if the donation will delay their funeral plans. The best person to answer such a question is the procurement coordinator. The answer will depend on which teams are retrieving organs and tissues and what their travel time will be to the donor hospital. It is best to be as honest as possible with the family about this issue, reassuring them that the OPO will do everything possible to be efficient.

- The OPO will send a follow-up letter to the next of kin shortly after the organs and tissues are transplanted. This letter contains general but anonymous information about the recipients, such as sex, age, and medical condition. Families should be informed of this after giving consent so that they can expect future closure on the issue.

- It is often difficult for family members to decide when to "say good-bye" to their loved one. It may be helpful for the nurse to determine when the family can do no more (possibly after consent has been obtained) and to gently suggest that the family go home. Under no circumstance should family members be forced to leave before they are ready. Every consideration should be given to their comfort.

- The family may ask to view the body after the organs have been removed. The procurement coordinator should be advised of this request to ensure that the body is properly prepared for viewing.

DONOR MANAGEMENT

Management of the donor is crucial in preserving the viability of organs for transplant. Evaluation and coordination of the various surgical teams can take from 8 to 12 hours, depending partly on the travel time of the participating teams. The role of the critical care nurse is to maintain the donor until surgery occurs. Nursing activities required for donor management are summarized in Table 2–6. The orders for all donor care are given by the procurement surgeon through the procurement coordinator.

SURGICAL RETRIEVAL

Once the evaluation process is complete and the surgical teams have arrived, the donor surgery begins. In most cases the surgery occurs at the donor hospital, although in rare instances the donor is flown to the recipient center. The surgical teams come prepared with their own specialized solutions and equipment. They will require the assistance of a scrub nurse, a circulating nurse, and anesthesia personnel. No anesthetic agent is required, but a paralyzing agent may be administered initially to inhibit spinal reflexes during the incision. Typically, a multiple-organ procurement procedure will last approximately three to five hours, depending on which organs are being removed.

The operating room nurse prepares the room as for any large abdominal and thoracic case. Additionally, there is need for a back table with a sterile basin for each organ being removed (Fig. 2–2).

Surgery for multiple organ donation routinely includes the removal of the heart, liver and/or pancreas, and kidneys. All teams are present, and the organs are removed in a coordinated effort in order to preserve all organ function. The heart team makes the initial incision from the sternal notch to the symphysis pubis. The sternum is cracked and retracted for complete visualization. The heart is examined to assess for any damage that could not be previously detected. The heart team then steps back and the liver team steps in. The liver is examined visually. Dissection begins by removing the adhesions and muscles holding the liver in place. The liver is extremely vascular, and all blood vessels must be dissected and tied. The major vessels that supply the liver are left intact until the last minute in order to prevent ischemic damage. Dissection of the liver can take approximately two to four hours. If the pancreas is also being removed, it is dissected at the same time as the liver. Once the liver team is finished, the kidney team steps in and minimally frees up the kidneys.

Once all the organs are anatomically freed up, all the surgical teams step back in around the table. The aorta is clamped and all organs are flushed with a cold electrolyte solution. The solution is specific to each organ and causes immediate cellular standstill, decreasing the risk of warm ischemic damage. The heart is the first organ to be physically removed. It is placed in a sterile basin, examined, rinsed, and quickly

TABLE 2–6. PRINCIPLES OF DONOR MANAGEMENT

Nursing Diagnosis	Predisposing Factors	Signs and Symptoms	Nursing Interventions
Potential fluid volume deficit	Minimal fluid replacement due to head trauma and risk of increased intracranial pressure Administration of osmotic diuretics (e.g., mannitol) Administration of steroids Pituitary gland injury resulting in decreased release of antidiuretic hormone (ADH)	Decreased urine output Decreased blood pressure Increased heart rate Decreased CVP Initial decrease in urine output followed by an increase in urine output with fluid replacement	Increase I.V. fluid replacement with initial bolus of fluids (500–1000 cc over 1–2 hr) to maintain CVP 8 to 12 mm Hg Maintain fluid balance with cc for cc plus 100 cc replacement per hour. Monitor accurate I & O Administer Pitressin as ordered.
Potential alteration in electrolyte balance	Diabetes insipidus secondary to decreased ADH release	Increased urine output Increased glucose level Decreased serum potassium level Increased serum sodium level	Monitor serum potassium and sodium levels every 2 hr. Replace with appropriate fluids based on laboratory values. Administer insulin as ordered for increased glucose level.
Potential alteration in hemodynamic status	Inadequate neurologic response to maintain hemodynamic status Diabetes insipidus, resulting in increased risk of hypokalemia Altered fluid and electrolyte balance	Tachycardia Frequent premature ventricular contractions Decreased hemoglobin and hematocrit Decreased blood pressure	Monitor ABG's. Adjust ventilatory settings as ordered. Monitor serum potassium levels every 2 hr and prn. Administer potassium bolus as ordered. Maintain systolic blood pressure at 100 mm Hg. Administer vasopressors as ordered (dopamine is the vasopressor of choice).
Potential for infection	Compromised total body system due to brain death status Immobility Ventilator dependence	Elevated temperature Increased WBC (these signs may also be secondary to neurologic injury and must be closely evaluated) Cloudy, foul-smelling urine	Monitor temperature every 2 hr. Provide adequate pulmonary hygiene. Use aseptic technique for all invasive procedures. Maintain patent, aseptic urinary catheter system. Obtain blood, urine, and sputum cultures as ordered.

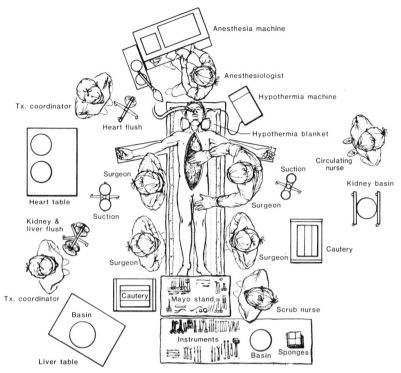

FIGURE 2–2. Positioning of equipment and personnel for surgery involving multiple organ donation. (Reprinted with permission from *AORN Journal*, Vol. 44, No. 6 [December 1986, p. 940]. Copyright © AORN Inc., 10170 East Mississippi Avenue, Denver, CO 80231.)

placed in a sterile container for transport. A limited preservation time of four to six hours currently forces the team to return immediately to its transplant center for implantation of the heart.

Lung removal is done in conjunction with removal of the heart. The lungs are placed in a sterile container with a cold solution for transport. The preservation time for lungs is currently six hours.

The liver is the next organ to be removed. It is placed in a sterile basin where any additional fat or adhesions may be dissected. It is then either placed in a sterile container or triple-bagged in sterile bowel bags with a cold solution around it. The preservation time for a liver is 8 to 12 hours. The liver team also immediately returns to its transplant center to implant the liver into the recipient.

If the pancreas is removed instead of the liver, it would be done after the heart is taken. The pancreas is placed in a cold sterile basin and then packaged in a sterile container with the cold solution surrounding it. The preservation time for the pancreas is approximately 12 hours.

If both the liver and the pancreas are to be removed, there are two surgical methods that can be used, depending on whether the pancreas is being removed whole or as a segment. For a segmental dissection the pancreas is flushed through the splenic artery and dissected at the isthmus. This allows the body and tail of the pancreas to be separated and removed. Inferior to the pancreas are the portal and splenic veins, which are dissected and used to reanastomose the pancreas in the recipient. The liver is flushed through the inferior mesenteric or superior mesenteric veins. The liver is then removed with the portal vein and celiac artery.

If the whole pancreas is to be removed, it is done in continuity with part of the duodenum. The flush to both the liver and the pancreas is the same as in the segmental procedure. The major difference is in the vasculature that is taken with each organ. The portal vein and a patch of aorta with the celiac and superior mesenteric artery are dissected and removed with the pancreas. The hepatic artery and the portal vein above the ligament to the liver are dissected with the liver. In both surgical procedures, once the organs are removed, they are packaged in sterile containers with the appropriate preservation solution for transport.

It must be noted that in cases in which the preservation time is limited, the recipient must be in surgery so that when the organ arrives it can be immediately implanted. Research is actively being conducted to find means of increasing preservation time for all organs so that transplant can occur under optimal conditions. Dr. Folkert Belzer of the University of Wisconsin in Madison has recently developed a preservation solution for livers. The solution has been tested in selected programs throughout the United States and found to increase preservation time effectively up to 24 hours. It has been approved by the Food and Drug Administration and is marketed under the trade name Viaspan.

The kidneys are the final solid organs to be removed. They are removed in an en bloc procedure and are dissected in a sterile basin. Once separated, the kidneys can be preserved in one of two ways. Most often the kidneys are placed in a sterile container, packed in ice, and then refrigerated until transplantation. Infrequently, a machine is used to flush a cold plasma solution through the kidneys to control their metabolic activity until transplant. The maximum preservation time for both methods is 72 hours, although, ideally, they are transplanted within 24–36 hours. Kidney recipients are often not identified at the time of procurement. Tissue from the donor is sent to the regional tissue-typing laboratory, where specific tissue-typing and crossmatching are done. This usually takes approximately eight hours and identifies the most appropriate recipient. The transplant center with which the recipient is listed is then notified, and the transplant is usually performed.

Once all the organs are removed, the kidney surgeons close the abdomen and chest cavity. (If, however, rib bone donation is to occur, the chest remains open.) All care and respect are given to the donor so that there is no disfigurement. If the family has consented to the donation of tissues, these procurement teams become involved at this time. Tissue procurement can take approximately another three hours of operating time.

The eyes are usually the first tissue to be removed. The eyes must be removed within eight hours after oxygenation has stopped. In most cases the entire eye is enucleated, although some technicians are trained to remove only the corneas. The technicians bring all the necessary equipment to the donor hospital. If the donor is not an organ donor and is not in the operating room, the technician can do the enucleation in the patient room or the morgue if necessary. The face is draped sterilely, the eyelid pulled back with special ophthalmologic equipment, and the muscles surrounding the sclera sterilely incised to free the eyeball. The eye is then placed in a sterile container with an antibiotic solution and transported to the local eye bank, where the cornea is microscopically removed and examined. The cornea is then placed in a preservation medium and transplanted within two to three days. A plastic prosthesis with a cotton ball is inserted into the donor so that the eye cavity will retain its natural shape. No external incisions are made.

Bone is recovered within 24 hours after oxygenation has ceased. If the donor was not an organ donor, the body should be refrigerated in the morgue until the procurement team arrives. The bones of the upper and lower extremities, every other rib, every other vertebra, and the iliac crest can be removed. This procedure can be done either in the morgue or sterilely in the operating room. Multiple incisions are made to remove the bone. Once the bone is recovered, wooden dowels are used to replace the bone so that the body retains its natural form. The incisions are then sutured closed. The bone team comes prepared with the necessary equipment and prosthetics. If the procedure is done in the operating room, the team will need the assistance of a circulating nurse. Once the bone is removed, it is packaged and brought back to the bone bank, where it is either secondarily sterilized, if removed in the morgue, or frozen intact, if removed in the operating room. Bone has a preservation time of two to five years.

Skin is the final tissue to be removed. It is used in the treatment of severely burned patients. Skin can be procured in the operating room or in the morgue, and is removed with a surgical dermatome, which the team brings. Only 8 to 10 one-thousandths of an inch is removed from the large body surface areas. This is similar to the peeling of skin after a sunburn. Areas from where skin is procured include the abdomen, back, buttocks, and thighs. No skin is removed from any area that would be seen during an open-casket service. The skin is preserved in an antibiotic solution for a period of time and then placed in a $-70°C$ freezer until it is used. The preservation time is approximately two years.

In conclusion, nurses play a key role in organ procurement by working with donor families and by participating in the medical management of potential donors. The system for procuring and distributing organs in the United States is evolving rapidly, and the government continues to work with transplant groups to develop a national transplant system. Improvements in transplantation, medically and organizationally, offer hope to patients with end-stage organ and tissue disease.

References

A.C.T. Newsline (1988). American Council on Transplantation.

Batten, H.L. & Prottas, J.M. (1987, Summer). Kind strangers: The families of organ donors. Health Affairs, 35–47.

The Gallup Organization, Inc. (1987). The U.S. public's attitudes toward organ transplants/ organ donations. A Gallup survey.

Malecki, M. & Hoffman, M. (1987). Getting to yes: How nurses' attitudes affect their success in obtaining consent for organ and tissue donations. Dialysis and Transplantation, 16(5), 276–278.

Organ Transplantation Issues and Recommendations (1986). Dept. of Health and Human Services.

Report of the Ad Hoc Committee of the Harvard Medical School (1968). Journal of the American Medical Association, 205(6), 337–340.

Report of the Medical Consultants on the Diagnosis of Death to the President's Commission for the Study of Ethical Problems in Medicine and Biomedical and Behavioral Research (1981). Journal of the American Medical Association, 246(19), 2184–2186.

3

The Immunology of Transplant Rejection

Marilyn Rossman Bartucci and Mary Cusella Seller

Progress has been made in the art and science of organ transplantation since the first kidney transplant in 1954. The advances made in surgical techniques, tissue typing and matching, understanding the immune system, preventing and treating rejection, and organ procurement and preservation techniques have dramatically increased the demand for organs for transplantation. In 1987 there were almost 9,000 kidney transplants, 1,512 heart transplants, 1,182 liver transplants, 127 pancreas transplants, and 43 heart/lung transplants performed in the United States (American Council on Transplantation, 1988).

The most dramatic advances have been made in the biochemical and immunologic aspects of transplantation. In most instances the body can be selectively prevented from recognizing the transplanted organ as being foreign, while its ability to mount an immune response to infection is preserved. Greater potency and specificity and less toxicity have been the objectives in developing immunosuppressive therapies. These therapies are detailed in Chapter 4.

NORMAL IMMUNE RESPONSE

A thorough understanding of the immunology of rejection requires a review of the normal immune response. The immune response includes all the physiologic mechanisms that enable recognition of foreign material entering the body, as well as the metabolism, neutralization, and elimination of the foreign material. Those mechanisms that have implications for transplantation are discussed in this chapter.

Immunologic responses have three functions: defense, homeostasis, and surveillance. Response to infection is the defense function most commonly attributed to the immune system. If the cellular elements of defense are successful, the host will eliminate the pathogen. When these elements are hyperactive, allergy or hypersensitivity may occur. Conversely, when these elements are hypoactive, there may be increased susceptibility to repeated infections, as seen in the immune deficiency disorders or in drug-induced immune deficiency, such as in organ transplant recipients or cancer patients receiving chemotherapy.

The immune system preserves the internal environment by maintaining homeostasis. This is accomplished by immunocompetent cells that act as scavengers, degrading and removing damaged or dead cells from the body. When these mechanisms are unduly enhanced, autoimmune diseases result.

The surveillance mechanism consists of mobile and stationary immune system cells that detect and remove abnormal cells that constantly arise within the body. These abnormal cells, or mutants, can occur spontaneously or may be induced by certain viruses and chemicals. Failure of this mechanism is suspected to be responsible for the development of malignant disease.

Immune responses are not always beneficial, as in the case of organ transplant rejection; nor are they associated solely with resistance to infection. A breakdown in any one of the complex pathways in the immune response can lead to disease. There are three general types of immunologically mediated diseases classified according to the nature of the antigen. Antigens are substances that are capable of eliciting the immune response, specifically directed at the inducing substance and not at other, unrelated substances. These antigens include atopic disease and reactions to environmental allergens, like tree and grass pollens. Allogeneic antigens or alloantigens include organ transplants, blood transfusions, and erythroblastosis fetalis. Autologous antigens include autoimmune diseases, like systemic lupus erythematosus (Bellanti, 1985). For the purposes of this chapter, the alloantigens related to organ transplantation are discussed in greater depth.

FACTORS THAT MODIFY IMMUNE MECHANISMS

The external and internal defense forces do not function at the same level of efficiency in all people. Such factors as genetic control, age, metabolic and hormonal influences, and environmental and nutritional status markedly influence the level of a person's natural resistance.

Genetic Control

The whole of the immune response is under genetic control. Marked differences exist in the susceptibility of different species to infective agents. Additionally, the major histocompatibility complex (MHC) controls both immune responsiveness and the expression of histocompatibility antigens on cells. The ability of the immune system to recognize tissue from a different individual of the same species as foreign is determined by these tissue antigens. This is discussed later in the chapter.

Age Factors

Age influences on immunity and infectious diseases are severer at the extremes of life. In the very young, these influences appear to be associated with immaturity of the immune system. In the elderly there is evidence that a hypofunctional state of the immune system exists. This state is presumed to be a result of deficiencies of nonspecific immunity, such as thin integument and a poor inflammatory response. In addition, decreased immunoglobulin concentrations and cell-mediated immunity in the elderly may be associated with the known higher incidence of autoimmune phenomenon and malignancy in this age group.

Metabolic and Hormonal Factors

Metabolic and hormonal modifications of natural resistance are readily recognized. Insulin deficiency affects the integrity of cell membranes, rendering diabetics more susceptible to staphylococcal, streptococcal, and fungal diseases. In both hypoadrenal and hypothyroid states there is an increased susceptibility to infection. For the transplant recipient, treatment with corticosteroids reduces the inflammatory response and depresses phagocytosis (or produces an inhibitory effect on phagocytosis). This increases susceptibility to bacterial infection and certain viral diseases such as herpes.

Environmental and Nutritional Factors

The correlation between increased rate of infectious diseases and poor nutrition and living conditions is well established. An increased susceptibility to infections may be related to diminished resistance caused by malnutrition and to a greater exposure to pathogens. Protein-calorie malnutrition increases the incidence of bacterial, fungal, and viral infections because phagocytic cells of the malnourished person function at only 10 to 30 per cent efficiency compared with those of the well nourished. Those who suffer from end-stage organ disease are often malnourished, and this may increase the incidence of infection after transplantation.

INTERNAL NONSPECIFIC DEFENSE MECHANISMS

Cells of the immune response are formed, mature, and then are dispersed from the bone marrow. At this point they are reclassified as cells of the phagocytic, lymphoid, or other systems, according to the functions they acquire or express outside the bone marrow.

The mononuclear phagocytes are produced from a stem cell in the bone marrow. They undergo proliferation and maturation and then are delivered to the blood. After they are in the blood for one to two days the monocytes migrate to the main site of their action in the tissues, where they differentiate into macrophages. Macrophages serve at least three distinct functions in host defense. They secrete biologically active molecules, remove excess antigen and present antigen to induce the immune response.

Tissue macrophages are named according to their anatomical location. Histiocytes are found in connective tissue; Kupffer's cells, in the liver; alveolar macrophages, in the lungs; and microglial cells, in the nervous system. Both free and fixed macrophages are found in the spleen, lymph nodes, and other organs. Unlike blood monocytes, which have a half-life of only a few hours, tissue macrophages have a long life span, extending for many months or years. The tissue macrophage is an abler phagocyte and more destructive of its phagocytosed cells. When exposed to foreign cells or pathogens it is capable of an even greater phagocytic capacity and cytocidal behavior than a normal macrophage. This heightened responsiveness is induced by the T lymphocytes because a chemotaxin from T cells attracts the macrophages. Two internal nonspecific defense mechanisms are operational in organ transplant rejection. These mechanisms are phagocytosis and inflammation.

Phagocytosis

When a foreign substance or antigen enters the body, phagocytosis is set in motion. The primary role of phagocytosis is to localize an antigen, destroy it, inactivate it, and "process" it for handling by other components of the immune system.

Once an antigen has been introduced, the phagocytes are drawn to the area of antigen invasion by a process called chemotaxis. A chemical is released by the antigen itself or by the tissue it has injured. This chemical, the chemotactic factor, stimulates the body's initial efforts to search and destroy. The next step is phagocytosis, the process by which a particle is ingested by a cell. This process occurs in two steps, the attachment phase and the ingestion phase. During the attachment phase firm contact is established between the cell and the particle. This contact is largely dependent on the surface properties of the particle to be ingested. Molecular factors that promote attachment of phagocytes to the object they engulf are called opsonins. Virtually any substance that improves phagocytosis is an opsonin. The best opsonin is antibody against the subject cell (antigen).

The ingestion process includes the engulfment of the particle. The phagocyte extends its cell membrane to form a vacuole that surrounds and encloses the antigen. The membrane then pinches off from the cell surface and internalizes the antigen, where it is digested by lysosomal enzymes contained within the phagocyte.

The fate of the ingested antigen depends on its interaction with the phagocyte. The antigen may either be completely destroyed or remain as fragments within the phagocyte. Occasionally both the antigen and the phagocyte die. The necrotic debris that results becomes purulent matter, or pus. Another outcome of the interaction between the antigen and phagocyte can be survival of the antigen. If the phagocyte lives, it may be responsible for the spread of disease as it travels through the body carrying a live organism. If the phagocyte dies, the antigen is released and may encounter other specific immunologic defense mechanisms.

Inflammation

Inflammation is a complex series of events that develops when the body is injured. Although there is a tendency to consider this response harmful, inflammation is a protective mechanism by which the body attempts to either return to the preinjury condition or repair itself after injury.

The clinical signs of inflammation include swelling, redness, heat, pain, and altered function. The response depends on intact blood vessels and on the circulating cells and fluids within these channels. The acute inflammatory response begins with dilatation of blood vessels and an outpouring of leukocytes and fluids. This results in redness (erythema), caused by blood vessel dilatation; swelling (edema), caused by escape of fluids into soft tissues; and firmness (induration), caused by accumulation of fluids and cells.

If the inflammatory response is not completely successful in restoring the injured tissue to its original state, or if repair of the tissue is not accomplished, chronic inflammation may result. This is characterized by the continued presence of lymphocytes, monocytes, and plasma cells.

Depending on the severity of the inflammatory response, fever may result. This occurs because many microorganisms and certain white blood cells produce pyrogenic materials that act on the hypothalamus to increase temperature. Although there is a tendency to consider fever harmful to the body, it can be beneficial. An elevation in body temperature can result in the inhibition or death of a variety of microorganisms. It has frequently been observed that patients who are unable to mount a febrile response or who have subnormal temperatures carry a poorer prognosis than those who mount a normal febrile response.

Other systemic effects of inflammation can be increased production of white blood cells, decreased serum white blood cell count, and increased sedimentation rate. An increased production of white blood cells can occur with cell injury, but it is a nonspecific phenomenon. The white blood cell differential count, however, can provide more specific information. A decreased white blood cell count may be found in viral infections, typhoid fever, and toxic reactions that depress the bone marrow. An increase in the sedimentation rate occurs during the acute inflammatory state of infection. This is thought to be caused by an increase in the protein fibrinogen, essential to the healing process.

THE LYMPHOID SYSTEM

The immune system is organized around several special tissues collectively designated lymphoid or immune tissues. These tissues are distributed throughout the entire body and can be subdivided into central and peripheral lymphoid tissues (Fig. 3–1). The lymphoid cells of the immune system differ from other cells in their ability to react specifically with an antigen and to produce specific cell products. The lymphoid cells include plasma cells and lymphocytes. The lymphocytes include a population of cells with different immune functions. Approximately 30% of the total white blood cell count is made up of lymphocytes. The lymphocyte is responsible for the primary recognition of antigen. Specific immunologic defense mechanisms recognize antigens as nonself and respond in a matter unique to each antigen's composition. There are two mechanisms that mediate specific immune responses: (1) that mediated by a cell product of the lymphoid tissues, antibody (humoral immunity), and (2) that mediated by specifically sensitized lymphocytes themselves (cell-mediated immunity). These two mechanisms are responsible for organ transplant rejection. A schematic representation of the activation of immunocompetent cells for humoral and cell-mediated immune responses is shown in Figure 3–2.

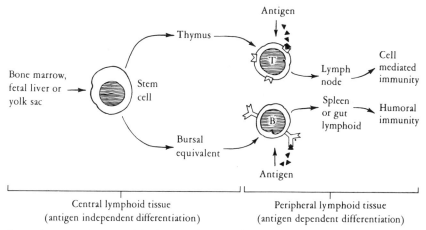

FIGURE 3–1. Development of the lymphoid system. (From Bellanti, J.A. (1985). Immunology: Basic Processes (2nd ed.) Philadelphia: W.B. Saunders, p. 33.)

Humoral Immunity

Humoral immunity is mediated by the mature B lymphocytes, or B cells. B cells tend to remain fixed in tissues, predominating over T cells in the bone marrow and gut-associated lymphoid tissues. They are responsible for the production of antibody, a serum protein known as immunoglobulin. B cells are not generally antibody-secreting cells, but once stimulated by an antigen, they differentiate into plasma cells that do secrete antibody.

Once an antigen enters the lymphoid tissue, it may encounter the B cell specific for that antigen. The B cell has the ability to recognize the antigen because it possesses a receptor site specific for that antigen on its cell membrane. After this encounter, the B cell enlarges, divides, and differentiates into a plasma cell. The mature plasma cell produces and secretes antigen-specific immunoglobulins and antibody. Each plasma cell produces only one type of antibody. Some B cells never encounter the antigen for which they are programmed, and in this case the person will remain susceptible to the organism carrying that particular antigen.

It is currently accepted that triggering a humoral response to almost all antigens requires the cooperation of B cells, macrophages, and T cells. The theory that a B cell requires more than one signal to be activated is based on this concept. The need for macrophages and helper T cells to assist the B cell is well established, but the precise mechanism is not known. It is believed that the first step involves antigen processing by the macrophage. During antigen processing the macrophage releases interleukin-1, a lymphokine that appears to assist in the differentiation

HUMORAL IMMUNE RESPONSE

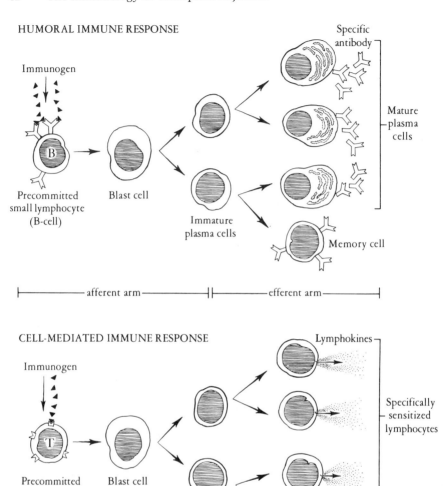

FIGURE 3–2. Schematic representation of the activation of immunocompetent cells for humoral and cell-mediated immune responses. (From Bellanti, J.A. (1985). Immunology: Basic Processes (2nd ed.). Philadelphia: W.B. Saunders, p. 125.)

of inducer T cells, which in turn release interleukin-2. This second lymphokine promotes the maturation of helper T cells.

On initial exposure to an antigen there is a delay before antibody can be found in the blood. During this delay antigen is recognized by the B cell. The B cell then divides and differentiates into a plasma cell, which forms antibody specific to the antigen. The antibody does not reach a high level or persist unless a second dose of antigen is given. During the secondary antibody response any remaining antibody is rapidly removed by combination with the antigen. The result is a decrease in detectable antibody in the blood. Within one to two days a rapid rise in the level of antibody occurs in amounts 10 to 50 times higher than the primary response. This secondary response is maintained at a high level, falling only slowly over a period of months. Once a person has responded to an antigen, the immune system retains a memory of the antigen. Therefore, subsequent exposure to the same antigen stimulates the B cell memory cells. Even after an interval of months to years the immune system may mount a secondary response through rapid mobilization of antibody-secreting cells within one to two days.

One of the most complex and powerful results of antigen–antibody binding is activation of complement. The complement system acts as an amplifier of the humoral system. It consists of at least 20 proteins that circulate in the plasma in an active form. Recent research has shown that complement plays a broader role in the immune response process than previously thought. Complement participates in inflammation, immune tissue injury, and modulation of the immune response. The coating of bacteria or other immune complexes with components of complement facilitates opsonization, ingestion of the bacteria by phagocytic cells. In addition, several of the products of complement proteins serve as chemotactic factors that attract phagocytes to the site of the reaction. This is the inflammatory function of complement. Still other complement fragments are released when certain complement components are activated. These molecules release histamine from mast cells that are chemoattractants for polymorphonuclear leukocytes. Histamine increases vascular permeability and enhances smooth muscle contraction. The late-acting proteins of the complement cascade form the complex, which attacks and causes death of target cells. This activity may be directed against viruses, bacteria, fungi, parasites, virus-infected cells, tumor cells, and the cells of transplanted organs.

Cell-Mediated Immunity

Cell-mediated immunity is the second major mechanism that underlies specific immune responses. The active component of cellular immunity is a lymphocyte that is derived from stem cells maturing in the thymus gland. These cells are T lymphocytes, or T cells. This arm of the immune system is carried out by specifically sensitized lymphocytes or by specific cell products that are formed on interaction of an antigen with a sensitized lymphocyte. These specific cell products are called lymphokines, and include migration inhibition factor, cytotoxin, interferon, and interleukin-2 (a T cell growth factor). The lymphokines have three main functions: (1) recruitment of uncommitted lymphocytes, (2) retention of these cells and phagocytes at the inflammatory site, and (3) activation of the retained cells so they can take part in the inflammatory response (Weir, 1977).

Until recently cell-mediated immune reactions were thought to be carried out only by T cells, independent of antibody. It is currently proposed that these reactions may also be carried out by a variety of cell types, humoral substances, or combinations of both. The major functions of the T cells are (a) mediation of cytolytic reactions, (b) mediation of cutaneous delayed hypersensitivity reactions, and (c) regulation of the immune response.

In the cytolytic reaction T cells function to kill other cells. This process provides protection against most viral, fungal, and slow-acting bacterial infections. By this reaction some regulation of tumor cells also occurs. The cutaneous delayed hypersensitivity reaction is a localized immune reaction to a previously encountered antigen. This is accomplished through the release of lymphokines. Migration inhibition factor is the lymphokine that participates in delayed hypersensitivity by causing the macrophages to stick together, thereby limiting their movement from the site of inflammation. Regulation of the immune response by the T cells can be either positive or negative (Graziano & Bell, 1985). The subpopulations of T cells act to either suppress or enhance the immune response.

Approximately 65 per cent to 80 per cent of all lymphocytes in the blood are the T type. These cells, which have a longer life span than B cells, are the major recirculating cell type in the lymph nodes. There are several types of T cells. Helper T cells assist with triggering the immune response. These cells assist B cells in the synthesis of immunoglobulins to the T cell–dependent antigens. These antigens are more complex than those that activate B cells directly. Suppressor T cells retard immune responses by restricting B cell antibody production. Cytotoxic T cells are able to kill other cells that are recognized as nonself, like tumor cells and cells of transplanted organs. In transplantation the grafted organ would quickly be destroyed by an immunocompetent T cell; however, immunosuppressive medications suppress cytotoxic function.

When T cell function is suppressed by age, medications, poor nutrition, serious infections, or other disease processes, the risk of cancer increases. This is due to the loss of immune surveillance activity by the T cells (Barrett, 1980; Gurevich, 1985; Virella, Goust, Fudenberg & Patrick, 1986).

A small number of circulating lymphocytes that contain no known T cell or B cell surface markers are called null cells. A number of cell lines are included under this term, and among them a natural killer cell has been identified. These cells have been extensively studied in mice and have been shown to participate in immune reactions without requiring prior sensitization for their generation (Bellanti, 1985; Graziano & Bell, 1985; Groenwald, 1980; Sell, 1980). Natural killer cells may act directly as cytotoxic cells or produce cytotoxicity through combination with antibody-coated target cells. Although the role of natural killer cells in humans is yet undefined, they are thought to be involved in transplant rejection, nonspecific killing of viruses, and immune surveillance of malignant diseases (Bellanti, 1985).

The mononuclear phagocytes make up a second set of cell types that are active in cellular immunity. These cells "process" and "present" antigen for T cell activation and antibody production by B cells. Their actions are mediated in part by the production of interleukin-1. Most important, they destroy foreign organisms either by phagocytosis or by their direct cytotoxic effect on target cells.

Like the antigen–antibody reactions in humoral immunity, cell-mediated reactions occur in three stages. After initial processing by the phagocytes, antigens travel to the regional lymph node, draining the area of antigen invasion. The first stage is initiated by the binding of antigen with an antigen receptor on the surface of the T cell. In the second stage a variety of morphologic and biochemical changes have been demonstrated in vitro, including DNA, RNA, and protein synthesis. The third stage consists of the generation of helper, suppressor, cytotoxic, and memory T cells. In addition, the T cells that release the mediators are generated.

The third stage is the most complex. Initially, macrophages activate the small number of helper T cells that possess receptors for the antigen. In response to antigen contact, helper T cells release lymphokines that activate macrophages and recruit other lymphocytes and monocytes-macrophages to participate in the reaction. Activated macrophages produce monokines, which are necessary for T cell activation and induction of inflammation. A reaction that initially involves a small number of sensitized cells can be amplified and expanded to include a large number of cells that were not sensitized to the antigen that initiated the reaction.

Lymphokines have recently been shown to mediate other lymphocyte functions. Interferon, an important lymphokine, acts nonspecifically to inhibit viral replication, stimulate phagocytic action of macrophages, and stimulate the killing activity of sensitized lymphocytes. Gamma interferon has also been shown to promote the killer function of the natural killer cells.

Like the humoral immune response, the cell-mediated immune response results in the formation of long-lived memory T cells. With the production of memory cells, a subsequent exposure to antigen will evoke a more rapid and intense cell-mediated immune response.

IMPLICATIONS FOR TRANSPLANTATION

Immune responses are genetically controlled by a series of linked genes known as the major histocompatibility complex (MHC). If tissue from one person is transplanted to a second, genetically different person, a characteristic reaction, allograft rejection, is observed. Rejection occurs when the donor contains a specificity not present in the recipient.

The human MHC is called human leukocyte antigen (HLA) because the serologically defined markers were first found on lymphocytes. The HLA gene complex is located on chromosome number 6. Each chromosome contains four loci, HLA-A, B, C, and D. Each person has two antigens on each of the four loci. These transplantation antigens are usually inherited according to codominant mendelian rules (Table 3–1). That is, each person inherits one chromosome from each parent and thus one antigen from each of the four loci from each parent. A parent, then, will share exactly half of the antigens with an offspring, and siblings may share all, some, or none of these antigens.

HLA antigens have been divided into three classes. Class I antigens include the HLA-A, -B, and -C antigens. They are expressed on all nucleated cells, being particularly abundant on the surface of lymphocytes, skin cells, and other organs except for the nervous system and the striated muscles. Class I antigens determine tissue transplantation antigens and cellular immune cytotoxicity. The Class II antigens, HLA-D and -DR, are expressed by only two groups of leukocytes, the B cells and the cells of the monocyte-macrophage family. T cells do not express these antigens except under specific circumstances. Class II antigens control the induction of immune responses (help, augmentation, and suppression). Class III antigens include complement components and some red blood cell antigens.

In humans more than 150 antigens have been recognized in the HLA system: 24 on the A locus, 52 on the B locus, 11 on the C locus, and 61 on the D locus. Because of the millions of combinations of antigens, the chance of two unrelated persons having an identical combination of histocompatibility genes is less than 1 in 20 million. Any cell surface protein configuration different from a person's own, then, is an antigen and capable of provoking the immunologic defensive response.

In addition to the implications for organ transplantation, some HLA phenotypes have been found to determine the genetic susceptibility to certain diseases (Table 3–2). For example, the HLA-B27 specificity may be linked to an immune response–type gene that influences the response to an infectious agent or degree of inflammation in rheumatoid diseases. It is suspected that HLA-B8 and -Bw15 are associated with lupus erythematosus, and HLA-B13, with pemphigus. Thus certain people must have an inherited tendency to produce an immunopathologic response

TABLE 3–1. HAPLOTYPE INHERITANCE OF HLA ANTIGENS*

| | A Series Specificities | | | B Series Specificities | | | | | Phenotype | Genotype | Haplotype Designation |
	A1	A3	A9	Aw19	B5	B7	B12	B13			
Father	+		+		+		+		A1, A9; B5, B12	A1, B5; A9, B12	a/b
Mother		+		+		+		+	A3, Aw19, B7, B13	A3, B7; Aw19, B13	c/d
Sib 1	+	+			+	+			A1, A3; B5, B7	A1, B5; A3, B7	a/c
Sib 2			+	+			+	+	A9, Aw19; B12, B13	A9, B12; Aw19, B13	b/d
Sib 3	+	+			+	+			A1, A3; B5, B7	A1, B5; A3, B7	a/c

*In this series the father's haplotypes are a = A1, B5 and b = A9, B12; the haplotypes represent the transmission of that HLA gene segment to the offspring. The + signs indicate positive reactions (lysis) of the test lymphocytes with the specific antiserum. (From Bellanti, J. A. (1985). *Immunology: Basic Processes.* (2nd ed.) Philadelphia: W. B. Saunders, p. 65.)

TABLE 3–2. HLA AND DISEASE ASSOCIATIONS

DISEASE TYPE	HLA ALLELE
Rheumatologic Diseases	
Ankylosing spondylitis	B27
Reiter's syndrome	B27
Acute anterior uveitis	B27
Juvenile arthritis	B27, Dw5, or Dw8
Rheumatoid arthritis	Dw4(DR4)
Autoimmune/Endocrine Diseases	
Chronic hepatitis	Dw3(DR3)
" "	B8
Celiac disease	Dw3(DR3)
Graves' disease	Dw3(DR3)
Hashimoto's thyroiditis	Dw5(DR5)
Idiopathic Addison's disease	Dw3(DR3)
Juvenile-onset diabetes mellitus	Dw4(DR4)
" " " "	Dw3(DR3)
Congenital adrenal hyperplasia	B47
(21-hydroxylase deficiency)	
" " "	B5
Myasthenia gravis	B8
" "	Dw3(DR3)
Multiple sclerosis	Dw2(DR2)
Systemic lupus erythematosus	Dw3(DR3)
Malignant Disorders	
Chronic myelocytic leukemia (CML)	A2
Chronic lymphocytic leukemia (CLL)	B18
Acute lymphoblastic leukemia (ALL)	A2
Hodgkin's disease	A1, A11, B8, B15

Modified from Bellanti, J. A. (1985). *Immunology: Basic Processes.* (2nd ed.) Philadelphia: W. B. Saunders, p. 72.

to infectious or inflammatory stimuli. Other diseases associated with specific HLA antigens are multiple sclerosis (DR2) and diabetes mellitus (DR3 and DR4) (Sell, 1980; Virella, Goust, Fudenberg & Patrick, 1986).

Although immunosuppression has prolonged human graft survival, tissue matching of donor and recipient combined with less vigorous immunosuppression is the most advantageous approach to organ transplantation. Extensive serologic testing has been used pretransplant. It is thought, to the extent that the MHC antigens on the transplanted organ are the same as those of the recipient, in general, that a less vigorous immune response may result. In addition, these tests permit a prediction of the potential recipient's response to a specific donor organ before transplantation. These tests include the mixed lymphocyte culture (MLC), lymphocyte crossmatching, and determination of percentage of reactive antibody (PRA).

The MLC is based on the fact that the degree of histocompatibility difference between two genetically different persons can be determined by culturing a mixture of their lymphocytes. This can be either a two-way test or a one-way test. The two-way test measures the interaction of the living lymphocytes. In the one-way test the lymphocytes of the potential organ donor are either killed by radiation or treated with an antimetabolite, mitomycin C, to prevent them from responding. In this way an estimation of the response of a potential recipient (living cells) to a potential donor (treated cells) can be made. The MLC is primarily the result of HLA-D differences between donor and recipient. A low response of the recipient's cells to the potential donor's cells is predictive of a successful transplant. This test is particularly helpful, prospectively, in live donor transplants. It is not helpful in a prospective manner for cadaveric transplants because the test takes approximately seven days to complete, and currently vital organs cannot be preserved for that length of time. However, the results may be useful retrospectively, to assist in the determination of immunosuppression regimens for specific recipient organ pairs post transplant. Retrospective studies have shown that low response of recipient lymphocytes to cadaveric donor lymphocytes is associated with better allograft survival (Bellanti, 1985).

Transplantation across a current positive T cell crossmatch is prohibited because hyperacute rejection will occur. A positive T cell crossmatch occurs when the recipient has demonstrable circulating antibodies against the donor's T cell antigens. These circulating cytotoxic antibodies are routinely tested for, before transplantation, by incubating donor lymphoid cells in recipient serum in the presence of complement. After a period of incubation a marker of cell death is added to the cell suspension and the proportion of dead cells is counted. The presence of significant numbers of dead cells indicates a positive crossmatch (Bellanti, 1985). Because of immune memory, it was once thought that any past positive T cell crossmatch was a contraindication to transplantation with that recipient-organ pair, despite a negative current T cell crossmatch. It has since been discovered that not all HLA antibodies activate the complement cascade with comparable efficiency. In addition, cyclosporine offers added protection against a subliminal state of presensitization.

In the late 1970s and early 1980s the significance of a positive B cell crossmatch was controversial. Established investigators had shown that it could be associated with either enhanced graft outcome, early graft loss, or no effect on graft survival. The need to distinguish harmful from benign B cell sensitization became apparent. It has recently been suggested that certain antibodies may not prevent successful transplantation. These include anti–B cell antibodies, particularly those reacting at 4° C. or "cold" B cell antibodies (Bellanti, 1985).

Finally, the serologic technique using lymphocytotoxic antibodies obtained from multiparous females or from recipients of multiple transfusions that provided the HLA antigens has led to the PRA. Now one can determine a person's reaction to a panel of potential donor antigens and calculate the percentage of circulating cytotoxic antibodies present against the panel of antigens. This information is invaluable in assisting with matching recipient organ pairs for the best chance of success.

The Immunobiology of Rejection

Rejection is the process by which the immune system of the host recognizes, becomes sensitized against, and attempts to eliminate the foreign antigens of the donor organ. Some degree of rejection occurs with every transplant, but how clinically significant the rejection becomes is very individual. The function of immunosuppression is to control the host's natural response and to prevent clinically significant rejection.

Primary rejection is the prototype. Here, the host encounters the histocompatibility antigens on the surface of the cells of the transplant for the first time. Then, locally or within regional lymph nodes, macrophages "process" antigenic material and "present" it to B and T cells for sensitization. This sensitization of lymphocytes is facilitated by the antigen-stimulated release of interleukins. Sensitized lymphocytes can then enter the peripheral circulation directly or by way of the lymphatics. On arrival in the transplanted organ and encountering specific antigens of the organ, sensitized lymphoid cells initiate immune injury. The immune injury may be mediated by either the humoral or the cellular limb of the immune response in a variety of ways. Injury can occur (a) directly, by cytotoxic T cells or the natural killer cells; (b) indirectly, by the soluble T cell mediators, the lymphokines; (c) by B cell–mediated antibody; or (d) by antibody-dependent cellular cytotoxicity attack on the target organ. This process of primary rejection is the classic model and often becomes clinically evident after the first week post transplantation.

Another type of rejection is hyperacute rejection. Here, the recipient has been sensitized to the histocompatibility antigens of the transplanted organ by previous transfusions, pregnancy, or previous transplantation. Circulating cytotoxic antibodies to the HLA antigens of the graft can be found in the serum of recipients who hyperacutely reject their organs. On completion of the vascular anastomosis there is prompt deposition of antibody along the vascular endothelium with activation of the complement and coagulation systems. This results in fibrin deposition, polymorphonuclear leukocyte infiltration, platelet thrombosis, and prompt coagulative necrosis, with graft loss within hours after transplantation.

Acute rejection describes the clinical situation associated with the abrupt onset of signs and symptoms of rejection. The graft is tender and heavily infiltrated with mononuclear and inflammatory cells. This type of rejection, however, often resolves with immunosuppressive therapy. Both cellular and humoral immune responses are responsible for this type of rejection.

Chronic rejection occurs after an extended period of time following transplantation and is characterized by gradual loss of organ function. Sensitized B cells initiate the humoral immune process, resulting in the production of antibodies against the transplanted tissue. These antibodies activate complement, which attracts platelets. Aggregates of immunoglobulins, complement factors, platelets, and fibrin adhere to the blood vessel endothelium of the transplanted organ, leading to stenosis and occlusion. The compromised arterial circulation provokes ischemia and eventual graft loss. This type of rejection is indolent and unresponsive to currently available immunosuppressive therapy.

Consequences of Immune Response Suppression

Immunosuppressive therapy provides one of the rare opportunities in clinical medicine to be too successful. Because most immunosuppression regimens are nonspecific assaults on immune responsiveness, successful efforts to prevent normal graft rejection must invariably be accompanied by depression of host immune responses. Fortunately, in most instances, alterations in immune competence do not result in major complications. Future advances in organ transplantation will include some form of specific or selective alteration in immune responsiveness of the recipient-organ pair. One way for this to occur is through immunologic tolerance, that is, the induction of a state of immunologic unresponsiveness to a specific antigen but not to others. These states have been achieved in animal experiments by the induction of blocking antibodies, by a noncytotoxic form of specific antibody, and by the establishment of tolerance in the recipient through high- or low-dose antigen administration. The future of organ transplantation rests on some form of more specific control of the immune response.

References

American Council on Transplantation (1988). Alexandria, VA.

Barrett, J.T. (1980). *Basic Immunology and Its Medical Application.* (2nd ed.) St. Louis: C.V. Mosby.

Bellanti, J.A. (1985). *Immunology: Basic Processes.* (2nd ed.) Philadelphia: W.B. Saunders.

Bellanti, J.A. (1985). *Textbook of Immunology.* (3rd ed.) St. Louis: C.V. Mosby.

Graziano, F. & Bell, C. (1985). The normal immune response and what can go wrong. *Medical Clinics of North America, 69*, 439–451.

Groenwald, S. (1980). Physiology of the immune system. *Heart & Lung, 9*, 645–650.

Gurevich, I. (1985). The competent internal immune system. *Nursing Clinics of North America, 20*(1), 151–161.

Sell, S. (1980). *Immunology, Immunopathology and Immunity.* (3rd ed.) Philadelphia: Harper & Row.

Virella, G., Gouse, J.M., Fudenberg, H., & Patrick, C. (Eds.). (1986). *Introduction to Medical Immunology.* New York: Marcel Dekker.

Weir, D.M. (1977). *Immunology: An Outline for Students of Medicine and Biology.* (4th ed.) New York: Churchill Livingstone.

4

Immunosuppression

Betty Crandall

The purpose of the human immune response is to protect against foreignness, specifically from pathogens that cause disease. A competent immune system is essential for life. However, that same invaluable response spells disaster in the form of rejection for the transplant recipient if it is not controlled with medications. The success of transplantation depends on the ability to surgically place a foreign organ or tissue and then alter the recipient's immune response so that rejection does not occur. This chapter discusses the medications used to achieve that altered immune state, their actions and adverse effects, and the nursing implications of their administration.

Rejection is a normal physiologic reaction of the immune system to a transplanted (foreign) organ. The immunology of transplant rejection is described in detail in Chapter 3. If unchecked, rejection results in destruction of the graft. To prevent irreversible rejection of transplanted organs, immunosuppressive medications are administered. Even with the availability of several effective immunosuppressive agents, rejection continues to be a major problem in transplantation. It remains the primary reason for graft loss.

Because immunosuppressive medications alter the person's immune response, they can potentially interfere with the ability to mount an effective response to invading pathogens. The person may be rendered immunodeficient, unable to ward off infections. Thus all immunosuppressants must be considered double-edged swords, capable of both great good and great harm. The goal of immunosuppression is to adequately suppress the immune response to prevent rejection of the transplanted organ while maintaining sufficient immunity to prevent overwhelming infection. In addition, many of the medications used to achieve immunosuppression have other adverse effects. One also hopes to minimize these untoward effects.

The history of transplantation, discussed in Chapter 1, must include the history of immunosuppression. The two are intricately intertwined. Much of the progress in transplantation resulted from advancements in the knowledge of immunology, from the development of new immunosuppressive agents, and from more effective application of those agents already in use. The first attempts at achieving immunosuppression, between 1959 and 1962, involved total-body irradiation (Hamilton, 1984). Chemical immunosuppression, involving the use of 6-mercaptopurine (6-MP), was first used successfully in 1960–61. Shortly thereafter, in 1962, a 6-MP derivative, azathioprine, was found to be even more effective as an immunosuppressant in kidney transplantation. Reports from Starzl, Marchioro, and Waddell (1963) urged the use of combination therapy with the corticosteroids and azathioprine. That combination therapy continued to be the foundation of long-term immunosuppression to prevent rejection until the late 1970s, when cyclosporine was discovered. Other agents, such as the various antilymphocyte and antithymocyte preparations, were important adjuncts to the regimen to treat rejection but were not reasonable maintenance therapy. Calne, White, Thiru, Evans, McMaster, and co-workers (1978) described the first clinical use of cylosporine, a drug that was to revolutionize transplantation. In 1983 cyclosporine became generally available. It is now widely used alone and in various combinations with azathioprine and corticosteroids, with or without prophylactic antilymphocyte preparations. Most recently a monoclonal antibody, orthoclone (OKT3), has emerged as a highly effective agent for treating acute allograft rejection. Although great progress has been made in immunosuppressive therapy, much work remains to be done. We still do not have an agent that can selectively interfere with the ability to react to a foreign organ while preserving the recipient's ability to mount a response to infection. That is the ultimate goal of immunosuppressive therapy.

This chapter presents the immunosuppressive techniques used in clinical organ transplantation today. The five major immunosuppressive agents in use (corticosteroids, azathioprine, cyclosporine, antithymocyte preparations, and OKT3) are discussed in greater detail, and their pharmacology, mechanism of action, adverse effects, and commonly used regimens are presented. Particular aspects related to the administration of each medication are detailed with a focus on nursing implications. Brief mention is made of total lymphoid irradiation and thoracic duct drainage, techniques no longer frequently used but of importance historically. Two major adverse effects of all immunosuppressive agents, infection and malignancy, are discussed. The chapter ends with a look to the future of immunosuppressive therapy in clinical organ transplantation.

CORTICOSTEROIDS

It has been known since the 1920s that adrenocorticosteroids have an effect on the immune system. Steroids were first used successfully in kidney transplantation at the Peter Bent Brigham Hospital in 1960 when cortisone was used to reverse a rejection episode. The patient, who was the recipient of a living-related donor kidney, had initially been immunosuppressed by total-body irradiation (d'Apice, 1984). After the discovery and release of azathioprine in the early 1960s, steroids and azathioprine were used in combination as maintenance therapy. Reports by Starzl (1963) and others led to the acceptance of this regimen as standard immunosuppressive therapy from the early 1960s until the early 1980s.

Corticosteroids continue to be a major part of the immunosuppressive regimen used in most centers, both for maintenance therapy and to treat rejection. A few kidney transplant centers, primarily in Europe, and at least one heart transplant center, in Utah, attempt to discontinue administration of steroids soon after transplant and to use azathioprine, cyclosporine, or both as maintenance therapy (Gilbert, Eiswirth, Renlud, Menlove, DeWitt, Freedman, Herrick, Gay, & Bristow, 1987). Although most clinicians attempt to minimize the doses, few have been routinely able to completely discontinue steroids.

Pharmacology and Action

The pharmacology of steroids and the way in which they alter the immune system are complex, incompletely understood, and diverse. Corticosteroids do appear to particularly affect T cells, causing their death as well as altering their functions. The sensitivity of T cells to antigens is diminished, the proliferative response of sensitized T cells is decreased, and the production of lymphokines is reduced. The end result is an impairment of the cellular immune response (Smith, 1986). However, these actions may not be the primary reason for the effectiveness of steroids in preventing and treating acute rejection. Steroids are potent anti-inflammatory agents. As such, they inhibit capillary dilatation, infiltration of leukocytes, fibrin deposition, and phagocytic activity at the site of inflammation—in this case the transplanted organ (Bass, 1986). These anti-inflammatory effects may be the most important in transplantation. Perhaps, by preventing the end results of inflammation in the organ, the steroids protect it from permanent damage from rejection.

Adverse Effects

Steroids have multiple and quite nonspecific actions. As a result, numerous adverse effects are seen when these drugs are administered.

Most side effects are dose-related, and all patients will not experience all side effects. The adverse effects most commonly seen are summarized in Table 4–1.

One of the most worrisome side effects of corticosteroid therapy is the increased susceptibility to infection. The infection may be bacterial, fungal, viral, or protozoal. Those in high-risk categories, such as the elderly and diabetics, and those in a poor nutritional state are especially vulnerable. High-dose steroid therapy and multiple episodes of rejection treated with steroids place the patient at great risk. The infectious complications of transplantation are discussed in detail in Chapter 5.

With the many complications of steroid therapy, it is easy to see why steroids often become medications that patients both respect for their ability to prevent and treat rejection and hate for their side effects. An important part of nursing care is to educate patients about potential adverse effects and how to help minimize them.

Common Regimens

The number of currently used regimens for steroid therapy in transplant recipients is nearly as large as the number of transplant programs. In addition, regimens change continuously. For that reason, only a few general comments are made about how steroids are administered.

Most transplant recipients initially receive intravenous steroids either immediately preoperatively, or intraoperatively. This is usually in the form of methylprednisolone; dosages vary. When the patient is able to tolerate oral medications, conversion to oral prednisone or prednisolone occurs (see Table 4–2 for dose equivalencies). Doses of steroids tend to be high (0.5–2.0 mg/kg/day) in the immediate postoperative period and are rapidly tapered. Most physicians attempt to reduce the dose of steroids to 0.15 to 0.20 mg/kg/day by one year after transplant.

Most patients take their maintenance corticosteroids once daily, although some programs recommend a twice-daily regimen. Many physicians attempt to convert children to an every-other-day dosing schedule in hopes of encouraging growth and reducing some of the side effects. This may have a beneficial effect but also may be less immunosuppressive (d'Apice, 1984). When converting to an alternate-day regimen, one must be especially alert to evidence of rejection.

Increased doses of steroids are most often used as the first-line treatment for rejection. Either intravenous methylprednisolone, or oral prednisone or prednisolone may be used. When patients are being treated for rejection with high-dose steroids, one must take precautions to prevent infection and the other adverse effects that are commonly seen in the immediate postoperative period when steroid doses tend to be high.

AZATHIOPRINE

The use of azathioprine (Imuran) as an immunosuppressive agent developed from work using 6-MP as an anticancer drug. In the late 1950s Dameshek and Schwartz at the New England Medical Center looked for alternatives to irradiation to create an immunosuppressed state in their bone marrow transplant recipients. They postulated that anticancer drugs such as 6-MP or methotrexate might serve as adequate immunosuppressive agents. Their laboratory work captured the attention of Calne in London, who found 6-MP to be successful in prolonging kidney allograft survival in dogs. Calne subsequently went to Boston for a period of research and was provided with derivatives of 6-MP, including azathioprine, for his research work. Azathioprine proved to be more successful and less toxic than 6-MP in experiments with dog transplants. In 1961 Imuran became available for human use. The first extended successes with kidney allografts were obtained in April 1963 in Boston. Shortly thereafter combination therapy with azathioprine and steroids became the standard (Hamilton, 1984).

When cyclosporine first became available in the late 1970s and early 1980s, it was substituted for azathioprine. Most centers used cyclosporine and steroids in combination as standard therapy and reserved azathioprine for those patients who were showing toxicity to cyclosporine or were being converted off the drug. More recently triple-drug regimens, including steroids, azathioprine, and cyclosporine, have become popular as have quadruple, sequential therapy regimens. The benefits of such regimens are discussed at the end of this chapter.

Pharmacology and Action

Azathioprine belongs to a class of drugs known as antimetabolites. It interferes with the purine synthesis necessary for antibody production and for the synthesis of nucleic acids (ribonucleic acid and deoxyribonucleic acid) in rapidly dividing cells. As such, it is valuable in preventing acute rejection in transplant recipients by interfering with the stimulation and proliferation of T cells, which are rapidly dividing in response to antigen presentation.

Azathioprine is rapidly absorbed from the gut but must be metabolized in the liver before it becomes active. The full immunosuppressive effect is seen 12 to 48 hours after administration of an oral dose.

TABLE 4-1. ADVERSE EFFECTS OF STEROID THERAPY

Adverse Effects/Toxicity	Predisposing Factors	Signs and Symptoms	Nursing Implications	Patient Education
Increased susceptibility to infection	High doses of immunosuppressive agents Multiple episodes of rejection treated	Fever Pain, tenderness over affected area Leukocytosis or leukopenia Cough; infiltrate on chest x-ray	Monitor temperature. Monitor white blood cell count. Maintain sterile technique with dressing changes and procedures. Practice good handwashing technique. Monitor surgical site. Administer antibiotics, antivirals, and antifungals as ordered.	Notify doctor of elevated temperature. Avoid people with infections. Report signs and symptoms of infection immediately.
Bone disease: aseptic necrosis, osteoporosis	High doses of steroids Postmenopausal female Prolonged bed rest, inactivity Poor calcium absorption	Pain in weight-bearing joints Pathologic fractures	Monitor mobility. Monitor for pain on ambulation. Provide diet adequate in calcium and vitamin D.	Avoid excessive weight gain. Exercise to tolerance. Avoid high-impact exercise. Provide diet adequate in calcium and vitamin D content. Joint replacement may be necessary.
Weight gain; obesity	High dose of steroids Poor eating habits before transplantation	Excessive weight gain	Provide well-balanced diet; avoid excessive caloric intake for needs. Provide low-calorie snacks.	Provide diet instruction related to control of weight.
Salt and water retention; hypertension	Preexisting hypertension Excessive salt intake High doses of steroids	Elevated BP Edema Weight gain (rapid)	Monitor daily weights. Monitor BP. Provide diet low in salt. Administer antihypertensives as ordered.	Monitor BP and weight. Diet low in salt. Take antihypertensives as ordered.
Hyperglycemia, steroid-induced; diabetes mellitus	Overweight High doses of steroids Family history of diabetes	Elevated blood glucose level Polydipsia Polyuria	Monitor intake and output. Monitor blood glucose level. Administer insulin or oral agents as ordered. Provide diet low in concentrated sweets.	Follow diet to control weight. Take insulin or oral agents as ordered. Monitor blood glucose level. Restrict consumption of concentrated sweets.
Acne	High doses of steroids Adolescence	Rash or pimples on face and trunk	Encourage good personal hygiene. Administer specific agents recommended by dermatologist.	Observe good hygiene practices.

Clinical manifestation	Contributing factors	Signs and symptoms	Nursing interventions	Patient education
Hirsutism	High doses of steroids Use of other androgens Concomitant use of cyclosporine	Excessive hair growth on face, trunk, extremities	Administer depilatories as ordered.	Understand reasons for excessive hair growth. Learn safe bleaching techniques and safe use of depilatories.
Sensitivity to ultraviolet rays of sun	Use of other immunosuppressives Excessive sun exposure Previous x-ray therapy	Sunburn Skin malignancies	Encourage ↓ sun exposure and use of sunscreens on daily basis. Examine skin on regular basis.	Use creams and lotions with SPF >15. Avoid excessive sun exposure. Examine skin for skin lesions.
Cataracts; glaucoma	High doses of steroids	Decreased visual acuity	Administer medications if ordered.	Have ophthalmologic examinations regularly.
Gastritis; gastrointestinal ulceration	High doses of steroids Excessive caffeine intake Excessive anxiety Past history of such disorders	Dysphagia Abdominal pain Hematemesis Dark, tarry stools	Administer medications if ordered. Administer antacids and H_2 blockers as ordered. Monitor for signs and symptoms. Administer steroids with food.	Report signs and symptoms of gastritis or ulceration immediately. Take antacids and H_2 blockers as ordered. Take steroids with foods.
Growth retardation (children, adolescents)	High doses of steroids Preexisting growth abnormalities	Failure to achieve normal height and weight for age	Administer steroids on alternate-day regimen as ordered.	Follow-up visits with pediatrician and perhaps endocrinologist are necessary.
Mood swings; depression; nervousness	Preexisting symptoms High doses of steroids	Patient or family reports excessive crying, tearfulness Ringing of hands Inability to sleep	Provide relaxing environment, particularly at night. Allow time for discussion of fears and anxieties and for questions. Encourage family to visit. Recommend counseling if indicated.	Practice relaxation techniques.
Night sweats		Patient reports damp bed linen	Change linen as necessary. Provide blankets to avoid chilling. Provide reassurance that this is probably due to medication.	Understand reasons for occurrence.
Cushingoid appearance	Altered utilization of fats, carbohydrates, and insulin	Fat deposition along face, neck, trunk		Understand reasons for changes in appearance. Follow diet to control weight.

BP, blood pressure; H_2 = histamine$_2$.

TABLE 4–2. DOSAGE EQUIVALENCIES OF STEROID PREPARATIONS

Steroid Preparation	Prednisone Equivalent
Methylprednisolone	4/5:1
Prednisolone	1:1
Hydrocortisone	1:4

Adverse Effects

Most of the adverse effects of azathioprine are clearly dose-related and reflect the action of azathioprine on rapidly dividing cells. Bone marrow suppression (including leukopenia, thrombocytopenia, and anemia) is the most frequently seen and most serious side effect of azathioprine therapy. The degree of marrow suppression is directly related, in most instances, to the dose of Imuran and usually responds well to dose reduction. The dose of azathioprine administered is usually titrated to keep the white blood cell count between 5000 and 7000 cells per cubic millimeter.

As with any immunosuppressive agent, susceptibility to infection and risk of malignancy are adverse effects of azathioprine therapy as well. Malignancy is discussed at the end of this chapter. Infectious complications of transplantation are discussed in detail in Chapter 5. Other side effects of Imuran are alopecia and hepatotoxicity. Abnormalities of liver function are frequently seen in transplant recipients. Determining whether such abnormalities represent drug toxicity, a viral process, or some other metabolic problem can be difficult. Determining whether Imuran is the offending agent is especially difficult. When liver dysfunction becomes evident, or if the patient has underlying liver disease, some physicians substitute another derivative of 6-MP, cyclophosphamide (Cytoxan), for azathioprine (Bass, 1986). There is disagreement as to whether cyclophosphamide is as effective an immunosuppressant and as to whether it increases the risk of malignancy. Cytoxan is usually given at one-half the Imuran dose. It should be administered in the morning and the patient instructed to drink plenty of fluids because hemorrhagic cystitis may occur with Cytoxan. The adverse effects of Imuran are summarized in Table 4–3.

Common Regimens

Azathioprine is usually administered at a dose of 2 to 3 mg/kg/day, with the dose being adjusted to keep the white blood cell count between 5000 and 7000. Currently, in both kidney and heart transplantation, triple therapy with cyclosporine, steroids, and azathioprine is becoming

TABLE 4-3. ADVERSE EFFECTS OF AZATHIOPRINE

Adverse Effects/Toxicity	Predisposing Factors	Signs and Symptoms	Nursing Implications	Patient Education
Increased susceptibility to infection	High doses of immunosuppressive agents Multiple episodes of rejection treated	Fever Pain, tenderness over affected area Leukocytosis or leukopenia Cough; infiltrate on chest x-ray	Monitor temperature. Monitor WBC. Maintain isolation as indicated. Maintain sterile technique with dressing changes and procedures. Practice good handwashing technique. Monitor surgical site. Administer antibiotics, antifungals, and antivirals as ordered.	Notify doctor of elevated temperature. Avoid people with infections. Report signs and symptoms of infection immediately.
Sensitivity to ultraviolet rays of sun	Use of other immunosuppressives Excessive sun exposure	Sunburn Skin malignancies	Discourage sun exposure; use sunscreens on daily basis. Examine skin on regular basis.	Use creams and lotions with SPF > 15. Avoid excessive sun exposure. Watch for lesions on skin.
Bone marrow suppression: leukopenia, anemia, thrombocytopenia	High doses of azathioprine Use of antilymphocyte preparations	Decreased WBC, platelet count, hemoglobin, hematocrit	Monitor WBC, platelet count, hemoglobin, hematocrit.	Avoid changing dose of azathioprine without physician order. Continue to have lab work checked as ordered.
Alopecia	High doses of azathioprine	Hair loss	Reassure patient that this is most likely a temporary problem.	Condition often is temporary, occurring most often early after transplant, when doses are high.
Hepatotoxicity	High doses of azathioprine Viral hepatitis Concomitant use of cyclosporine	Elevated bilirubin, alkaline phosphatase, SGOT, and SGPT levels Jaundice Bilirubinuria (dark-colored urine)	Monitor liver function tests. Monitor color of urine. Monitor color of skin and sclera.	Continue to have lab work checked as ordered. Notify doctor of change in color of skin or sclera.
Increased risk of malignancy	High doses of multiple agents	Related to type and location of malignancy	Monitor for signs and symptoms of malignancy.	Regular check-ups are important. Watch for evidence of malignancy (examine skin, breast, etc.).

*WBC, white blood cell count.

61

the norm. Azathioprine is used less frequently in liver transplantation, probably because of the fear of hepatotoxicity (Crandall, 1987). When azathioprine is used in triple-therapy regimen, the dose is usually not as high as when it is used with steroids alone. The dose of Imuran is generally not tapered over time, as is the practice with steroids. Rather, the white blood cell count is closely monitored and the dose adjusted if marrow toxicity becomes evident.

CYCLOSPORINE

Cyclosporine (Sandimmune), a potent immunosuppressive agent, was first used clinically by Calne in 1978 (Calne et al., 1978) and only released for general use in the United States in 1983. This naturally occurring substance is the metabolite of a strain of Fungi Imperfecti, Tolypocladium Inflatum. Cyclosporine was first isolated from soil samples by the microbiology department at Sandoz Pharmaceuticals in Basel, Switzerland. Jean Borel at Sandoz then demonstrated that it had potent immunosuppressive properties. Many experiments in numerous species were performed over the next several years, and in 1978 Calne, in Cambridge, began clinical trials with the drug. Multiple trials in Europe, Canada, and the United States documented the efficacy and safety of cyclosporine, and it was released by the Food and Drug Administration (FDA) in 1983 for general use. Since that time transplantation has been revolutionized. Graft survival has dramatically improved. Extrarenal transplantation, specifically heart, heart/lung, and liver, has become an accepted and successful treatment modality for patients with end-stage disease of those organs. The numbers of transplant centers and transplants performed have increased almost beyond belief. Cyclosporine is now used in nearly all transplant programs, although specific protocols for its use vary widely.

Pharmacology and Action

Cyclosporine is a cyclic endecapeptide that is able to suppress the immune response without significant myelotoxicity (Hess, Colombani, & Esa, 1986). Available data suggest that the primary action of cyclosporine is to inhibit cytotoxic T cell generation in response to transplantation antigens (Hess et al., 1986). Specifically, cyclosporine appears to interfere with the production and release of interleukin-2 (IL-2) by helper T cells and with the ability of precursor cytotoxic T cells to respond to IL-2 (Hess et al., 1986). These actions prevent the activation and proliferation of cytotoxic T cells, which actively attack the transplanted organ during rejection. In addition, cyclosporine inhibits the generation of interleukin-1 (IL-1) by macrophages. IL-1 is the second signal, in addition to antigen, necessary to activate helper T cells (Kahan, 1985). Because of its specific action, cyclosporine does not interfere as greatly as many other immunosuppressive agents with the ability to prevent infection, especially bacterial infection. Figure 4–1 shows diagrammatically the current understanding of the mechanism of action of cyclosporine.

Cyclosporine is metabolized in the liver. It is excreted in bile and reabsorbed from bile by way of the enterohepatic circulation to be further metabolized. Bile is also the main excretion route of the metabolites (Maurer, 1985). In liver transplant recipients this is particularly important to remember. During the time that such patients have external drainage of bile by way of a T tube or other biliary stent, adequate absorption of oral cyclosporine will not occur. The cyclosporine is excreted in bile on the first pass through the liver and not adequately absorbed and metab-

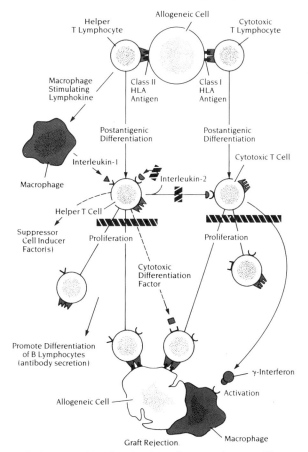

FIGURE 4–1. Cyclosporine (Sandimmune) mechanism of action. (Courtesy of Sandoz Pharmaceuticals.)

TABLE 4-4. ADVERSE EFFECTS OF CYCLOSPORINE

Adverse Effects/ Toxicity	Predisposing Factors	Signs and Symptoms	Nursing Implications	Patient Education
Increased susceptibility to infection, especially viral infection	High doses of immunosuppressive agents Multiple episodes of rejection treated	Fever Pain, tenderness over affected area Leukocytosis or leukopenia Cough Infiltrate on chest x-ray	Monitor temperature. Monitor white blood cell count. Monitor surgical site. Practice good handwashing technique. Maintain isolation as indicated. Maintain sterile technique with dressing changes and procedures. Administer antibiotics, antivirals, antifungals as ordered.	Notify doctor of elevated temperature. Avoid people with infections. Report signs and symptoms of infection immediately.
Increased risk of malignancy	High doses of multiple agents Excessive sun exposure	Related to type and location of malignancy	Monitor for signs and symptoms of malignancy.	Regular follow-up visits are necessary Watch for evidence of malignancy (examine skin, breast, etc.).
Nephrotoxicity	High doses of cyclosporine Dehydration Preexisting kidney failure	Elevated BUN, creatinine levels Hypertension Decreased urine output Increased weight Edema	Monitor BUN and creatinine levels. Monitor BP. Monitor daily weight. Maintain accurate intake/ output records. Monitor cyclosporine level.	Lab work needed as ordered. Notify doctor of increased weight or decreased urine output.

Hypertension	High doses of cyclosporine Kidney dysfunction	Elevated BP	Monitor BP. Administer antihypertensives as ordered.	Monitor BP at home (if able). Regular follow-up visits are necessary.
Hirsutism	High doses of cyclosporine Use of other androgens Concomitant steroid administration	Excessive hair growth on face, trunk, and extremities (particularly evident on females)	Monitor for excessive or abnormal hair growth. Administer depilatories as ordered.	Learn safe bleaching techniques and safe use of depilatories. Understand reason for excessive hair growth.
Tremors, paresthesias, occasionally seizures	High doses of cyclosporine Preexisting seizure disorder Hypertension	Fine motor tremors, especially noted in hands Numbness Seizure activity	Monitor for tremors and seizure activity. Inquire about paresthesias. Monitor cyclosporine level.	Report development or worsening of tremors, paresthesias, or seizures.
Gingival hyperplasia	High doses of cyclosporine	Growth of gums over teeth Oral bleeding	Monitor condition of oral cavity. Provide good mouth care.	Observe good mouth care. Routine dental follow-ups are necessary.
Hepatotoxicity	High doses of cyclosporine Concomitant use of azathioprine Viral hepatitis	Elevated bilirubin, alkaline phosphatase, SGOT, and SGPT levels Jaundice Bilirubinuria (dark-colored urine)	Monitor liver function tests. Monitor color of urine, skin, and sclera.	Continue to have lab work checked as ordered. Notify doctor of change in color of skin, urine, or sclera.

BUN, blood urea nitrogen; BP, blood pressure.

olized. Continued administration of intravenous cyclosporine is usually necessary to assure adequate levels.

Adverse Effects

The addition of cyclosporine to the immunosuppressive regimen of transplant centers has not been without problems. Many adverse effects are associated with cyclosporine therapy, the most serious of which is nephrotoxicity. This is especially troublesome for those in the field of kidney transplantation, but it presents difficulties for those involved with heart, liver, pancreas, and bone marrow transplantation as well. In kidney transplantation, management of the patient is made more difficult because in the presence of kidney dysfunction, one must differentiate between acute tubular necrosis, allograft rejection, and cyclosporine toxicity. In all patients the development of renal insufficiency or even failure complicates the patient's recovery and may result in a less than optimal outcome. Fortunately, the nephrotoxicity seen with cyclosporine is often dose-related and usually responds well to reduction of the dose. At times, however, kidney dysfunction progresses and necessitates the discontinuation of the drug. Careful monitoring of cyclosporine levels and of the parameters of kidney function with early reduction of the dose of cyclosporine will help to avoid much of the nephrotoxicity. Clinicians also hold out much hope for the development of analogs of cyclosporin A, which will be equally immunosuppressive but less nephrotoxic.

Once again, as was mentioned with both steroids and azathioprine, an increased risk of malignancy and increased susceptibility to infection are adverse effects. With cyclosporine therapy the risk of infectious complications is primarily with viral infections. Because of the specificity of its action on the immune response, cyclosporine preserves the ability to mount a response to bacterial infections. T cells are, however, necessary to ward off viral infections, and cyclosporine's interference with T cell function prevents full immunologic competence against viral infections. Other adverse effects associated with the use of cyclosporine are summarized in Table 4–4. Most are bothersome rather than a major threat. Many respond well to the usual dose reduction planned by most clinicians.

Monitoring of Cyclosporine Levels

Much discussion has centered on the need to monitor the levels of cyclosporine in the blood of patients receiving the drug, and on the best method of performing that monitoring. Monitoring has been advocated both as a method of assuring adequate levels of cyclosporine to prevent graft rejection and as a method of preventing toxicity. Two methods are available for measuring levels: radioimmunoassay (RIA) and high-performance liquid chromatography (HPLC) (Steinmuller, 1986).

HPLC measures the parent compound only, whereas the RIA method measures the parent compound and some of its metabolites. This occurs because there is crossreactivity with some of the metabolites when using the RIA method (Steinmuller, 1986). HPLC assays require expensive equipment and are labor-intensive, whereas the RIA method is much less expensive and easier to perform. The immunologic and nephrotoxic effects of the cyclosporine metabolites are not entirely known. For that reason the HPLC method, which measures only the parent compound, may be preferable.

Both the RIA and HPLC assays can be used on whole blood, plasma, and serum. A large percentage of cyclosporine accumulates in the red blood cells; therefore, levels measured in whole blood specimens will be higher than those measured in serum or plasma specimens. The ratio of whole blood to plasma levels is generally about 2:1; however, this varies considerably with the patient's hematocrit. The distribution of cyclosporine between the red blood cells and the serum also changes if the blood is kept at room temperature after being drawn (Steinmuller, 1986).

There is no general consensus about whether HPLC or RIA is the better method to use or about which component of blood to measure. What is clear is that one must consistently measure levels in the same manner and carefully control all variables such as the timing of blood drawing, the amount of time that elapses between when the blood is drawn and when the test is performed, and whether the blood is refrigerated or kept at room temperature.

Most clinicians monitor trough levels. This involves drawing the blood for cyclosporine level just before administering the dose. Monitoring appears to be most useful in the early posttransplant period and less valuable months or years post transplant. Some centers do not routinely monitor levels or do so infrequently. They rely on clinical examination and other laboratory tests to diagnose toxicity. Rejection is diagnosed by tests of organ function of the specific organ transplanted or by biopsy.

Common Regimens

Despite the fact that cyclosporine has gained widespread acceptance as a primary immunosuppressant in all types of solid organ transplants, there is still controversy about the optimal way to incorporate the drug into immunosuppressive protocols (Crandall, 1987). Land (1987), in summarizing the various approaches that have been published, concludes that "there is general consensus about the fact that there is not general consensus regarding the optimal use of cyclosporine in the context of clinical organ transplantation" (p. 130). In extrarenal transplantation there is a tendency to begin cyclosporine at the time of transplant, whereas in kidney transplantation the tendency is to delay starting cyclosporine therapy for a few days to allow for the diagnosis or resolution of postoperative acute tubular necrosis. In liver transplantation the use of intravenous cyclosporine is necessary, as explained previously. Most clinicians who are involved in the transplantation of organs other than the liver attempt to avoid the use of intravenous cyclosporine because of its greater risk of producing nephrotoxicity.

In general, the recipients of organ transplants other than those of the kidney can expect to remain on cyclosporine for life. In contrast, some programs attempt to convert kidney transplant recipients off cyclosporine at a specified time post transplant, usually 3, 6, or 12 months postoperatively. The rationale for planned conversion is to avoid the effects of long-term nephrotoxicity on the transplanted kidney. With all patients there is an attempt to taper the dose of cyclosporine over the first few months after surgery.

The usual immunosuppressive regimens specific to each type of transplant are addressed in the individual chapters about those organs. The use of triple and quadruple regimens is discussed at the conclusion of this chapter.

ANTITHYMOCYTE AND ANTILYMPHOCYTE PREPARATIONS

Near the turn of the century it was observed that leukocytes could be destroyed by xenotypic antisera. However, not until the early 1960s was it demonstrated that antilymphocyte serum (ALS) could interrupt the immune response and delay the progression of allograft rejection (Jaffers & Cosimi, 1984). Starzl, Marchioro, Porter, Iwasaki, & Cerilli (1967) were the first to report a major clinical trial using ALS in kidney transplant recipients. Since then there have been numerous controlled and uncontrolled clinical trials in which polyclonal or heterologous antilymphocyte antibodies have been administered to kidney allograft recipients either prophylactically to prevent rejection or to treat an established rejection episode (Jaffers & Cosimi, 1984). After many years of trials the clinical value of such antilymphocyte sera has been clearly established.

There are many antilymphocyte and antithymocyte preparations, both sera and globulins, available for use today. Earlier it was a common practice for each transplant center to make its own serum or globulin.

Now there are several commercial products available. In the United States two products predominate: Atgam, produced by Upjohn, and Minnesota ALG. Both are horse sera. Only Atgam is FDA-approved, although the safety and efficacy of Minnesota ALG have been clearly demonstrated. Other antilymphocyte sera or globulins are available but are less widely used. These sera or globulins may be produced in horses, rabbits, or goats.

Preparation

The sequence of events in the production of an antilymphocyte preparation is shown in Figure 4–2. An animal, usually a horse, rabbit, or goat, is immunized with human lymphocytes (or thymocytes). The animal produces antibody to the human cells. That antibody can be extracted from the animal's serum. The serum from several animals is pooled, purified, tested for microbes, and prepared for distribution. If an antilymphocyte globulin is to be produced, rather than a serum, the globulin molecules are extracted from the animal serum.

Pharmacology and Action

It is clear that the administration of an antilymphocyte preparation depletes the patient's circulating T cells. This inhibits that person's

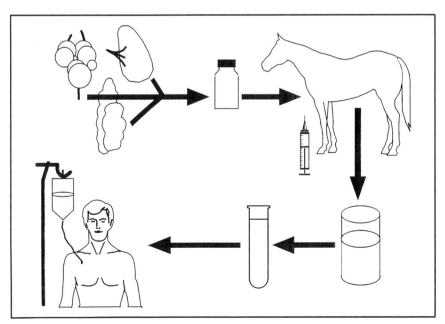

FIGURE 4–2. Production of antilymphocyte globulin. (By permission of Ortho Pharmaceutical Corp.)

ability to reject a transplanted organ. Antilymphocyte preparations have also been shown to reduce the proliferative function of T cells (Jaffers & Cosimi, 1984). The reduction in proliferative function persists even after the medication has been stopped. Some investigators have proposed that this continued immunosuppressive effect results from the generation of nonspecific suppressor T cells (Jaffers & Cosimi, 1984). Nonetheless, antilymphocyte preparations have been very effective at reversing rejection episodes. They are also extensively used as part of a quadruple regimen to prevent rejection in the first few days after transplantation, particularly kidney transplantation. Many programs use such preparations before beginning cyclosporine in order to assure adequate immunosuppression.

Administration and Monitoring of Effectiveness

Antilymphocyte preparations may be administered intravenously or intramuscularly. When administered intramuscularly, local inflammatory reactions with pain, swelling, redness, and often temporary disability are common. For this reason many clinicians favor the intravenous route. Because of the severe irritating nature of the preparation and the chance of phlebitis, administration through a central catheter or through the patient's arteriovenous fistula is recommended.

Before the administration of the first dose, preexisting immunity to the foreign (animal) protein should be evaluated by skin-testing the recipient. An intradermal injection of a 1:1000 dilution of the preparation is used. A positive skin test indicates preexisting immunity and the likelihood of an anaphylactoid reaction. The drug should probably be avoided in such a patient. Another antilymphocyte preparation may be tested.

The usual dose of an antilymphocyte preparation is 10 to 15 mg/kg/day. This is diluted 1 to 2 mg/ml in a saline solution and administered over four to six hours. Dextrose solutions should not be used to dilute the medication. The duration of therapy depends on center preference and whether the drug is used prophylactically or to treat rejection, but 7 to 14 days is typical.

One method for monitoring the effectiveness of therapy is to determine whether the preparation has resulted in reversal of rejection. This can be done by assessing clinical parameters or by obtaining a biopsy. During therapy, however, the adequacy of treatment is most often monitored by determining the reduction in circulating T cells accomplished by giving the drug. The goal is to reduce the T cell level to about 10 per cent of pretreatment levels (Jaffers & Cosimi, 1984).

Adverse Effects

The incidence and severity of adverse effects seen with antilymphocyte and antithymocyte preparations vary with the particular preparation used. Patients also show great variability in their responses to such drugs. Fever and chills occur almost universally, especially with the administration of the first dose. Subsequent infusions of the same preparation may not cause such a reaction. This observation has led some to postulate that the symptoms result from the release of endogenous pyrogens during the massive T cell lysis that occurs with the initial infusion. To ameliorate these symptoms it is recommended that patients be medicated with acetaminophen and diphenhydramine before the first dose. True anaphylactic reactions are rare but possible, and patients must be carefully monitored. Epinephrine and diphenhydramine should always be readily available at the patient's bedside during administration.

Leukopenia, thrombocytopenia, and, occasionally, anemia may be adverse effects of antilymphocyte therapy. Although the desired antibodies are directed only against human lymphocytes, there may be antibodies present to platelets, red blood cells, or other white blood cells. The patient's counts must be closely monitored and the dose adjusted if such problems develop.

Serum sickness resulting from the development of antibody to the animal protein has occurred in some patients. Such a hypersensitivity reaction usually develops late in the course of therapy. Symptoms include fever, joint pains, and sometimes a worsening of kidney function resulting from transient immune complex deposition in the kidney. When this occurs the drug is usually discontinued, although retreatment at a later date with the same drug may be safely accomplished if the skin test is negative.

Common adverse effects of antilymphocyte and antithymocyte preparations are summarized in Table 4–5. Opportunistic infection and an increased incidence of malignancy are seen in highly immunosuppressed patients who receive antilymphocyte preparations. Infection with cytomegalovirus and herpes simplex has been a particular problem in patients treated with these preparations.

MONOCLONAL ANTIBODIES (ORTHOCLONE OKT3)

Antilymphocyte preparations proved to be a valuable addition to the immunosuppressive protocols of many institutions. However, several problems became evident. Because of the manner of production, polyclonal antilymphocyte or antithymocyte preparations demonstrate batch-to-batch variability in both immunosuppressive potency and toxicity (Jaffers

TABLE 4-5. ADVERSE EFFECTS OF ANTITHYMOCYTE OR ANTILYMPHOCYTE PREPARATIONS

Adverse Effects / Toxicity	Predisposing Factors	Signs and Symptoms	Nursing Implications	Patient Education
Local inflammatory reactions	Infiltration at an I.V. site I.M. route of administration	Pain, redness, swelling, perhaps temporary disability	Monitor I.V. site for any evidence of infiltration. Stop infusion at once if this occurs. Apply cold compresses initially for 24 hours. Apply warm compresses after 24 hours. Ambulate patient if lower extremity is affected. Arrange for physical therapy consult.	I.V. site needs to be monitored. Arm must be kept immobilized while medication is infusing.
Anaphylactic reactions	Presensitization to the animal protein Positive skin test	Dyspnea Wheezing Fever Hypotension	True anaphylaxis is rare. Closely monitor patient during first dose. Keep epinephrine at bedside.	Reactions to the medication are possible.
Fever, chills	Occur most often with first dose		Closely monitor temperature. Premedicate with acetaminophen and diphenhydramine as ordered.	Febrile reactions to medications are possible.
Bone marrow suppression	Concomitant use of azathioprine High doses or prolonged use of these preparations	Leukopenia Thrombocytopenia Anemia	Monitor WBC, platelet count, hemoglobin, and hematocrit.	Low WBC predisposes to infection. Isolation may be reinstituted.
Serum sickness	Formation of antibody to the animal protein	Fever Joint pain Elevated BUN and creatinine levels	Monitor temperature. Monitor BUN and creatinine levels.	Late reactions to medication are possible.

I.V., intravenous; I.M. intramuscular; WBC, white blood cell count; BUN, blood urea nitrogen.

72

& Cosimi, 1984). Not even the most meticulously prepared and extensively tested of the preparations can be considered a standardized agent (Cosimi & Delmonico, 1986). In addition, antilymphocyte preparations fall short of being perfectly specific immunosuppressive agents because they cause pan–T cell and some B cell depletion.

The science of immunology advanced to the point that it was known that there were functionally distinct subpopulations of T cells. In addition, it was determined that each of these types of lymphocytes had cell surface antigens that were distinctive. Hybridoma techniques evolved to the point that it was possible to produce antibodies to the specific cell surface antigens found on a type of T cell. Thus it was possible to produce an extremely specific antibody directed against a particular cell type. Cloning techniques allowed that antibody molecule to be indefinitely replicated, solving the problem of batch-to-batch variability. This set the stage for the development of monoclonal antibodies.

Early work by Kung, Goldstein, Reinherz, and Schlossman (1979) led to the development of OKT3, a pan–T cell monoclonal antibody. It was first tested in humans at the Massachusetts General Hospital (Cosimi, Burton, Colvin, Goldstein, Delmonico, et al., 1981). Subsequently a multicenter randomized trial demonstrated the safety and efficacy of using OKT3 to treat acute kidney allograft rejection (Ortho Multicenter Transplant Study Group, 1985). In that study OKT3 was compared with steroid therapy and found to be more effective at reversing acute rejection. Later trials evaluated the effectiveness of OKT3 as rescue therapy when all other therapeutic interventions had failed or were contraindicated. After extensive laboratory and clinical work, Orthoclone OKT3 was released by the FDA in June 1986 for general use in treating acute kidney allograft rejection. OKT3 has been widely used to treat acute rejection in other types of organ transplants. However, official FDA approval is still pending for heart and liver allograft rejection as an indication for the use of OKT3. Other monoclonal antibodies have been developed and used to treat acute kidney allograft rejection. Monoclonal anti-T12 antibody has been used to treat a limited number of patients (Kirkman, Araujo, Busch, Carpenter, Milford, et al., 1983). The results of its use to date have not been as promising as those of OKT3. Still to come are clinical trials of more specific monoclonals directed at T cell subsets.

For the purposes of this chapter, the discussion of monoclonal antibody therapy in clinical transplantation is limited to OKT3. It is with this drug that most of the clinical experience has been gained to date.

Preparation

The production of monoclonal antibodies is based on technology that combines two previously recognized observations into a single effort.

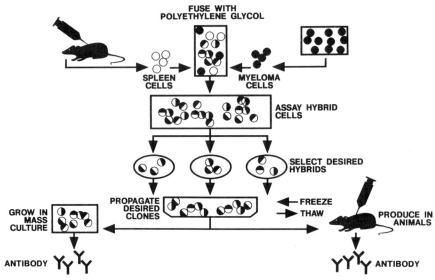

FIGURE 4–3. Production of OKT3. (By permission of Ortho Pharmaceutical Corp.)

Lymphocytes, specifically B cells from the spleen of an animal that has been immunized, when cultured in vitro, produce antibodies to the cells with which the animal was immunized. These antibody-producing cells, however, have a very short life span. In contrast, myeloma cells can be grown indefinitely in culture but do not produce a specific antibody. By fusing these two types of cells one can develop a hybridoma that has the characteristics of both. That is, the cells will grow indefinitely or immortally in culture and will produce a specific desired antibody (Jaffers & Cosimi, 1984). This technology is the basis for the production of monoclonal antibodies such as OKT3.

The steps in the production of OKT3 are shown in Figure 4–3. Lymphocytes from the spleens of mice previously immunized with human T cells are isolated, fused with mouse myeloma cells to obtain hybridomas, and selected to retain only those clones that secrete the desired antibody. The selected hybridomas then undergo clonal expansion either in vivo or in vitro (Cosimi & Delmonico, 1986). A number of monoclonal antibodies directed against cell surface antigens have been developed by this method.

PHARMACOLOGY AND ACTION

OKT3 is a monoclonal antibody directed against the T3 antigen, an antigen located on the cell surface of mature peripheral T cells. When

OKT3 was developed, researchers thought that it would be effective in much the same way as antilymphocyte preparations. That is, it was thought that OKT3 would remove T cells from circulation through the formation of antigen–antibody complexes. It was postulated that OKT3 would be more useful than previous preparations because it would have no batch-to-batch variability and would be free of impurities.

Since then there is good evidence that OKT3 may not only remove T cells from circulation, but also, at least in part, block their ability to recognize foreignness. This mechanism of action of OKT3 is shown diagrammatically in Figure 4–4. Note that the T3 antigen complex to which OKT3 is directed is located immediately adjacent to the antigen recognition structure on the cell surface. It has been shown that the two comodulate. That is, during OKT3 therapy the T3 antigen complex and the antigen recognition structure modulate off the cell surface. T cells can be detected in the circulation using other pan–T cell markers, but they lack a T3 antigen and cannot recognize foreign antigens, a process necessary to begin or continue a rejection reaction. The T cells are, in a sense, rendered impotent. When OKT3 therapy is discontinued, the T3 antigen complex and the antigen recognition structure reappear on the cell surface.

Administration

OKT3 is administered intravenously after being drawn through a 0.22-μm filter to remove any particulate matter. The usual adult dose is 5 mg given daily for 7 to 14 days. Young or physically smaller children

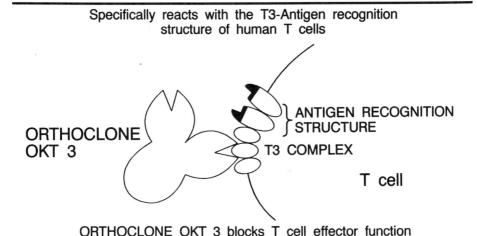

FIGURE 4–4. OKT3 mechanism of action. (By permission of Ortho Pharmaceutical Corp.)

are usually given half the dose, or 2.5 mg daily. The drug should be given as a bolus injection (I.V. push), not added to fluids or administered by way of a continuous infusion. Careful attention must be given to the patient's fluid status and to adequate premedication before administering the first dose. These are discussed in detail in the next section on adverse effects.

Adverse Effects

Table 4–6 summarizes the adverse effects associated with the administration of OKT3, most of which occur with the first few doses. Patients almost universally exhibit pyrexia with fevers to 39° or 40° C., rigors, and a general malaise, described by many as similar to the effects experienced during a severe episode of the flu. Diarrhea commonly occurs with the second or third dose. Some patients report a severe headache, nausea, vomiting, dyspnea, and wheezing. The symptoms seen with the administration of the first few doses of OKT3 are believed to be due to the release of intracellular mediators from T cells when opsonization occurs in the reticuloendothelial system. This process would be expected to be the severest with the first few doses of OKT3, when large numbers of T cells exhibiting the T3 marker are in circulation. As the T3 marker modulates off the cell surface, the number of cells to be opsonized drops dramatically, and thus fewer mediators are released to cause adverse reactions. In practice, adverse reactions are seldom seen after the third or fourth dose.

In a few patients these adverse reactions have included life-threatening respiratory difficulties, including frank pulmonary edema. In all cases such patients were found, retrospectively, to be grossly fluid overloaded before therapy was initiated. No such serious respiratory problems have been evident in patients who were euvolemic at the time of the first dose of OKT3 and were premedicated with an appropriate dose of corticosteroids. Because of these findings, careful attention must be paid to the patient's fluid status at the time OKT3 is to be given. Fluid overload must be corrected before instituting therapy with OKT3. Table 4–7 summarizes the evaluation and management relative to fluid status recommended before OKT3 administration.

Experience in using OKT3 has also led to a regimen of concomitant drug administration to ameliorate many of the adverse effects. This regimen is summarized in Table 4–7. The administration of steroids, acetaminophen, and diphenhydramine before the first dose of OKT3 does reduce the severity of reactions seen. Other adverse effects can be treated symptomatically with appropriate medications. Adverse reactions seldom persist for more than three to four days after drug administration.

TABLE 4–6. ADVERSE EFFECTS OF ORTHOCLONE OKT3

Adverse Effects / Toxicity	Predisposing Factors	Signs and Symptoms	Nursing Implications	Patient Education
Respiratory distress with first-dose administration	Fluid overload Pulmonary congestion	Wheezing Dyspnea Chest tightness	Assure that patient's weight is within 3% of lowest weight recorded for past week. Assure that chest x-ray within 24 hours shows no infiltrate or pulmonary congestion. Assure that patient has no clinical signs of fluid overload. Closely monitor respiratory status. Administer steroids as ordered before first dose.	Understand reasons for monitoring fluid status. Watch for possible adverse effects.
Pyrexia; rigors; malaise	Usually occur only with first few doses	Fever Chills Flu-like symptoms	Administer steroids, acetaminophen, and diphenhydramine as ordered. Cooling blanket on bed before first-dose administration.	Watch for expected adverse effects.
Headache			Administer pain medication as ordered. Provide relaxing, quiet, darkened environment.	Watch for expected adverse effects.
Diarrhea		Loose, watery stools	Administer antispasmodics as ordered. Assure adequate hydration. Quantitate amount of diarrhea. Make sure bedside commode is readily available.	Adequate fluid intake must be maintained.

TABLE 4–7. INTERVENTIONS TO AMELIORATE ADVERSE REACTIONS SEEN WITH FIRST DOSE OF OKT3

Evaluation of fluid status before administration of OKT3. All criteria should be met before administration of first dose.	Physical examination demonstrates no clinical evidence of fluid overload. Chest x-ray within 24 hours is clear of infiltrates and fluid. Weight is at baseline or no more than 3% above lowest weight within previous week.
Correction of fluid overload	Fluid may be removed by diuresis, dialysis, or ultrafiltration to meet the criteria above.
Medication to reduce severity of first-dose reactions	Methylprednisolone 1 mg/kg I.V. 1–6 hours before first dose of OKT3 Acetaminophen 1.2 g ⎱ p.o. 30 minutes Diphenhydramine 50 mg ⎰ before first dose

Common Regimens

Most of the clinical work with OKT3 to date has centered on its use as an agent to reverse a documented acute rejection episode. It has been very effective in that role. Several centers are currently studying the use of OKT3 prophylactically to prevent early acute rejection. Some centers are using OKT3 rather than antilymphocyte preparations as part of a quadruple-drug regimen. Such regimens are discussed later in this chapter.

Retreatment and Development of Antibody

As with any animal protein, OKT3 has the potential to stimulate the production of antibody when it is administered to humans. In the initial trials at Massachusetts General Hospital, Jaffers and colleagues (1986) found that 75 per cent of patients developed antibody to OKT3. It was feared that this would severely limit the use of OKT3, preventing treatment a second time if rejection should recur or if a second transplant was required. It was also feared that treatment for any person would be limited to the use of one mouse monoclonal antibody. More recently Shield (1987) has reported a much lower incidence of antibody formation, about 40 per cent of patients, when full-dose Imuran was administered during OKT3 therapy. Equally important is the finding that most of that antibody is anti-idiotypic and not directed generally against mouse protein. Thus even those patients who do develop antibody with a course of OKT3 could theoretically be treated with another idiotype (another form of a mouse monoclonal). Antibody formation may not be as much a limiting factor as was first feared.

TOTAL-LYMPHOID IRRADIATION

Total-lymphoid irradiation involves radiating the thoracicoabdominal lymphoid structures of the body with low-dose radiation before transplantation. This is done to reduce lymphocyte production in order to prevent rejection of the transplanted organ (Hooper, Sweeney, & Pierce, 1984). Total-lymphoid irradiation is seldom used today except in bone marrow transplantation. Problems with overimmunosuppression and the development of life-threatening infection limit its use. In addition, improved immunosuppressive agents have decreased the need for such a nonspecific method of suppressing the immune response.

THORACIC DUCT DRAINAGE

Like total-lymphoid irradiation, thoracic duct drainage is performed to deplete the potential transplant recipient's body of lymphocytes. It involves draining the lymphatic system through an indwelling catheter in the right or left thoracic lymph duct. The fluid that is drained undergoes pheresis to remove the lymphocytes and is then returned to the patient (Taylor, 1981). Thoracic duct drainage is a cumbersome procedure and places the patient at extraordinary risk of overwhelming infection. In addition, one must time the transplant so that recipients are lymphocyte-depleted when they receive the organ. Such timing is difficult to achieve when one must depend on cadaver organ donors. For these reasons and with the advent of better immunosuppressive agents, thoracic duct drainage is now of only historic interest.

ADVERSE EFFECTS OF ALL IMMUNOSUPPRESSIVE AGENTS

Previous sections of this chapter have included discussion of adverse effects specific to each of the immunosuppressive agents in current use in transplantation. Two major adverse effects deserve particular attention because they are common to all agents and because of the high rate of morbidity and mortality associated with them. These two are infection and malignancy.

Potential for Infection

All transplant recipients are chemically immunosuppressed after transplantation; thus they are at increased risk for developing infection.

The perfect immunosuppressant has not yet been discovered or developed. Such an agent would suppress the body's ability to mount an immune response to the transplanted organ while preserving its ability to respond to microorganisms that threaten infection. Until such an agent is developed, transplant recipients must live in a state of increased susceptibility to infection. The infectious complications of transplantation are discussed in Chapter 5.

Altered Immune Response: Potential for Altered Cellular Development (Malignancy)

It is now well recognized that there is an association between the development of malignancies and the immunosuppressive agents used in transplantation. The first reports of this association were made independently in 1969 by two groups: McKhann (1969), and Penn, Hammond, Brettschneider, & Starzl (1969). Since that time numerous reports from transplant centers around the world have documented an increased incidence of malignancy in transplant recipients. Hanto and Simmons (1986), in summarizing a number of reports, state that the reported incidence ranges from 1 per cent to 16 per cent at different centers, averaging 4 per cent. This is the same reported incidence of cancer in those with genetically determined immunodeficiency diseases, and is also a far greater incidence than that in the general population matched for age. In transplant recipients the most frequent neoplasms are nonmelanotic skin and lip cancers followed by lymphoproliferative diseases. Transplant patients do not normally develop the common solid tumors that are more prevalent in the general population and that usually occur more frequently with advanced age (Hanto & Simmons, 1986).

Various authors have proposed several theories for the increased incidence of cancer in patients who are immunodeficient. These include impaired immune surveillance mechanisms, chronic antigen stimulation, oncogenic viruses, and the direct oncogenic effects of immunosuppressive drugs (Hanto & Simmons, 1986; Sheil, 1984). Evidence has been presented supporting each of these theories. The final determination of the reasons for the increased incidence of malignancy is yet to be made. Perhaps all play a role, depending on the type of cancer that develops.

As mentioned, skin and lip cancers are the most common malignancies seen in the transplant population. Of these, squamous cell and basal cell carcinomas are most common (Hanto & Simmons, 1986). Although these malignancies account for only a small percentage of patient deaths, they do result in significant morbidity, often necessitating disfiguring surgery. There is a clear relation between the amount of exposure to ultraviolet light and the development of skin and lip cancers. For example, the incidence in Australia and New Zealand is several times higher than that in northern climates, where sun exposure is less. The incidence of skin cancer after transplantation also increases with time (Hanto & Simmons, 1986). Management of skin and lip cancers usually involves local excision, cryosurgery, local irradiation, or topical chemotherapy. Early detection, diagnosis, and treatment improve results. For this reason all patients should be taught regular skin examination and early reporting of any symptoms such as lesions that do not heal or that increase in size or become ulcerated. Skin examination by health professionals must be an integral part of posttransplant care. Prevention is also vital. Patients must be advised to avoid exposure to the sun and to use creams or lotions with a sun protection factor of at least 15 when they will be exposed to the sun.

Lymphoproliferative disorders constitute the second most common type of malignancy seen in transplant recipients. The overall incidence varies, depending on the type of organ transplanted and the center reporting. Incidences of 1 per cent to 33.3 per cent have been reported (Hanto & Simmons, 1986). Many of these diseases have been clearly linked to the Epstein-Barr virus (EBV). There was early concern that cyclosporine therapy would lead to a higher incidence of lymphoproliferative diseases because early series using the drug did show an increased incidence. However, this fear has not been realized. It has become evident that the amount (or degree) of immunosuppression, rather than the particular agents used, is the most important predisposing factor in the development of lymphoproliferative diseases (Hanto & Simmons, 1986). Therapy for this group of malignancies usually includes a reduction in immunosuppressive therapy and standard chemotherapy or radiation therapy. Some success has been achieved using acyclovir to treat some of the tumors that were EBV-induced (Hanto, Frizzera, Gajl-Peczalska, Balfour, Simmons, & Najarian, 1985). For many patients, reduction in immunosuppressive therapy results in regression of the disease, especially if it is in a premalignant stage.

Certainly any health professional who provides care to transplant recipients must remain alert to the development of malignancy in this patient population. Prevention through reduced exposure to the sun, avoidance of carcinogens, cessation of smoking, and minimization of immunosuppression to the greatest possible extent must be emphasized. Patients, too, need to remain attentive to any evidence of the development of cancer. They must be educated to recognize and report the signs and symptoms that may warn of malignancy. Routine physical examinations are vital, with surveillance for any indications of tumor development. Annual gynecologic examinations and Papanicolaou smears are recommended for all female patients, as are monthly breast self-examinations. Many centers suggest an annual chest x-ray.

FUTURE TRENDS IN IMMUNOSUPPRESSIVE MANAGEMENT

The field of transplantation is rapidly changing. One major aspect of that change is the immunosuppressive management of the transplant recipient. Earlier sections of this chapter have described the history of immunosuppressive management and outlined current practice. Emphasis has been placed on current understanding of the immune response and the ways in which one may interfere with that normal physiologic response in order to prevent or treat graft rejection. Scientific investigation constantly adds to the understanding of immunology and the body's reaction to a transplanted organ. From that understanding will come new immunosuppressive agents as well as improved methods of using currently available agents to achieve long-term graft and patient survival.

Triple- and Quadruple-Drug Regimens

The current trend is to use multiple immunosuppressive agents in combination in regimens referred to as triple- or quadruple-drug therapy. Triple-drug regimens call for the use of steroids, azathioprine, and cyclosporine, all in doses lower than one would expect with traditional double-drug regimens (either steroids and azathioprine or steroids and cyclosporine). The goal of triple-drug therapy is to provide adequate immunosuppression to prevent graft rejection while avoiding the toxicity associated with giving higher doses of any one agent. Such regimens became popular because of the significant nephrotoxicity associated with the use of high doses of cyclosporine. Quadruple-drug regimens usually call for induction therapy with steroids, azathioprine, and either antithymocyte or antilymphocyte preparations or OKT3. Cyclosporine is added to the regimen after the transplanted kidney begins to function or, in the case of extrarenal transplantation, after initial postoperative kidney function is established (Crandall, 1987). The impetus for the development of quadruple-drug regimens came primarily from those involved in kidney transplantation, where early postoperative cyclosporine toxicity confused the clinical picture and may have adversely affected long-term outcomes. Quadruple-drug therapy allows one to safely delay the administration of cyclosporine because adequate immunosuppression is assured by covering the patient with an effective polyclonal or monoclonal antibody preparation.

The rationale for using several immunosuppressive agents in combination is that each of the agents acts in a slightly different way to alter the immune response. Thus it was postulated that the immune response could be better suppressed if several agents with presumed different mechanisms of action were used. In fact, there is some evidence that not only is an additive effect involved, but also a synergistic effect. As previously stated, the other advantage of using several agents is that one can reduce the dose of any one agent used, and thus, it is hoped, avoid toxicity.

Multiple reports in the literature relate early success with triple and quadruple regimens (Dierhoi, Sollinger, Kalayoglu, & Belzer, 1987; Schweizer, Rovelli, Roper, & Bartus, 1987). Most reports have discussed their use in kidney transplantation. Many heart transplant centers are, however, beginning to use triple therapy because of the increased incidence of nephrotoxicity and hypertension in this patient population. The use of triple therapy in liver transplantation has not been as common to date, possibly because of the fear of azathioprine hepatotoxicity. The reported results of triple- and quadruple-drug therapy are quite promising; however, one must remember that most centers are now reporting results at only one year. Judgment about the safety and efficacy of such regimens cannot be made until long-term results are available. The dangers of overtreatment with immunosuppressants, with the development of chronic infectious states and malignancy, are real (Crandall, 1987).

New Agents

As scientists and clinicians together learn more about the incredibly complex immune response, better ways of altering it to successfully transplant vital organs are developed. The problem today is not that of controlling rejection, for it is possible to do that in nearly all circumstances with current agents. The problem is to control rejection while keeping the patient healthy (Burdick, Williams & Solez, 1986). Certainly cyclosporine and OKT3 have allowed us to more closely approach that goal; however, neither drug is the perfect immunosuppressive agent. It is quite possible that new agents will be available in the 1990s. Cyclosporin G, a relative of cyclosporin A, is being used in continuing laboratory trials and will soon be available for clinical trials. Work on developing a second idiotype of a pan–T cell monoclonal related to OKT3 is ongoing. Other, even more specific monoclonals are being investigated. The hope for transplantation lies in the development of more specific and less toxic agents to alter the immune response to a transplanted organ.

References

Bass, M. (1986). Common complications of immunosuppression in the renal transplant patient. *ANNA Journal, 13,* 196–199.

Burdick, J., Williams, G.M., & Solez, K. (1986). Kidney transplant rejection: Overview and update. In G.M. Williams, J.F. Burdick, & K. Solez (Eds.). *Transplant Rejection: Diagnosis and Treatment* (pp. 481–487). New York: Marcel Dekker, Inc.

Calne, R.Y., White, D.J.G., Thiru, S., Evans, D.B., McMaster, P., Dunn, D.C., Craddock, G.N., Pentlow, B.D., & Rolles, K. (1978). Cyclosporin A in patients receiving renal allografts from cadaver donors. *Lancet, 2,* 1323–1327.

Cosimi, A.B. & Delmonico, F.L. (1986). Antilymphocyte antibody immunosuppressive therapy. In G.M. Williams, J.F. Burdick, & K. Solez (Eds.). *Kidney Transplant Rejection: Diagnosis and Treatment* (pp. 335–351). New York: Marcel Dekker, Inc.

Cosimi, A.B., Burton, R.C., Colvin, R.B., Goldstein, G., Delmonico, F.L., La Quaglia, M.P., Tolkoff-Rubin, N., Rubin, R.H., Herrin, J.T., & Russell, P.S. (1981). Treatment of acute renal allograft rejection with OKT3 monoclonal antibody. *Transplantation, 32,* 535–539.

Crandall, B.C. (1987). Immunosuppressive protocols: Triple and quadruple drug therapy. *ANNA Journal, 14,* 322–323.

d'Apice, A.J.F. (1984). Non-specific immunosuppression: Azathioprine and steroids. In P.J. Morris (Ed.). *Kidney Transplantation: Principles and Practice* (2nd ed.) (pp. 239–259). Orlando: Grune & Stratton.

DeVecchi, A., Tarantino, A., Montagnino, G., Egidi, F., Vegeto, A., Berardinelli, L., & Ponticelli, C. (1987). A controlled prospective trial of triple therapy with low-dose azathioprine, cyclosporine, and methylprednisolone in renal transplantation. *Transplantation Proceedings, 19,* 1933–1934.

Dierhoi, M.H., Sollinger, H.W., Kalayoglu, M., & Belzer, F.O. (1987). Quadruple therapy for cadaver renal transplantation. *Transplantation Proceedings, 19,* 1917–1919.

Gilbert, E.M., Eiswirth, C.C., Renlund, D.G., Menlove, R.L., Dewitt, C.W., Freedman, L.A., Herrick, C.M., Gay, W.A., & Bristow, M.R. (1987). Use of Orthoclone OKT3 monoclonal antibody in cardiac transplantation: Early experience with rejection prophylaxis and treatment of refractory rejection. *Transplantation Proceedings, 19,* (2, Supplement 1), 45–53.

Hamilton, D. (1984). Kidney transplantation: A history. In P.J. Morris (Ed.). *Kidney Transplantation: Principles and Practice,* (2nd ed.) (pp. 1–13). Orlando: Grune & Stratton.

Hanto, D.W., Frizzera, G., Gajl-Peczalska, K.J., Balfour, H.H., Jr., Simmons, R.L., & Najarian, J.S. (1985). Acyclovir therapy of Epstein-Barr virus (EBV)-induced posttransplant lymphoproliferative diseases. *Transplantation Proceedings, 17,* 89–92.

Hanto, D.W. & Simmons, R.L. (1986). Cancer in recipients of organ allografts. In G.M. Williams, J.F. Burdick, & K. Solez (Eds.). *Kidney Transplant Rejection: Diagnosis and Treatment* (pp. 459–480). New York: Marcel Dekker, Inc.

Hess, A.D., Colombani, P.M., & Esa, A. (1986). Cyclosporine: Immunobiologic aspects in transplantation. In G.M. Williams, J.F. Burdick, & K. Solez (Eds.). *Kidney Transplant Rejection: Diagnosis and Treatment* (pp. 353–382). New York: Marcel Dekker, Inc.

Hopper, S.A., Sweeney, J.T., Pierce, P. (1984). The patient receiving a renal transplant. In L.E. Lancaster (Ed.). *The Patient with End Stage Renal Disease* (2nd ed.) (pp. 235–276). New York: John Wiley & Sons.

Jaffers, G.J., Cosimi, A.B. (1984). Antilymphocyte globulin and monoclonal antibodies. In P.J. Morris (Ed.). *Kidney Transplantation: Principles and Practice* (p. 281–299). (2nd ed.) Orlando: Grune & Stratton.

Jaffers, G.J., Fuller, T.C., Cosimi, A.B., Russell, P.S., Winn, H.J., & Colvin, R.B. (1986). Monoclonal antibody therapy: Anti-idiotypic and non anti-idiotypic antibodies to OKT3 arising despite intense immunosuppression. *Transplantation, 41,* 572–578.

Kahan, B.D. (1985). Cyclosporine: The agent and its actions. In B.D. Kahan (Ed.). *Cyclosporine: Diagnosis and Management of Associated Renal Injury* (pp. 5–18). Orlando: Grune & Stratton.

Kirkman, R.L., Araujo, J.L., Busch, G.J., Carpenter, C.B., Milford, E. L., Reinherz, E.L., Schossman, S.F., Strom, T., & Tilney, N.L. (1983). Treatment of acute renal allograft rejection with monoclonal anti-T12 antibody. *Transplantation, 36,* 620–626.

Kung, P.C., Goldstein, G., Reinherz, E.L., & Schlossman, S.F. (1979). Monoclonal antibodies defining distinctive human T-cell surface antigens. *Science, 206,* 347–349.

Land, W. (1987). Optimal use of cyclosporine in clinical organ transplantation. *Transplantation Proceedings, 19,* 130–135.

Lundgren, G., Albrahtsen D, Brynger, H., Flatmark, A., Frodin, I., Gabel, H., Persson, N., & Groth, C.G. (1987). Improved early course after cadaveric renal transplantation by reducing the cyclosporine dose and adding azathioprine. *Transplantation Proceedings,* *19,* 2074–2079.

Mauer, G. (1985). Metabolism of cyclosporine. *Transplantation Proceedings,* 17 (4, Supplement 1), 19–26.

McKhann, C.F. (1969). Primary malignancy in patients undergoing immunosuppression for renal transplantation. *Transplantation, 8,* 209–212.

Ortho Multicenter Transplant Study Group. (1985). A randomized clinical trial of OKT3 monoclonal antibody for acute rejection of cadaveric renal transplants. *New England Journal of Medicine, 313,* 337–342.

Penn, I., Hammond, W., Brettschneider, L., & Starzl, T. (1969). Malignant lymphomas in transplantation patients. *Transplantation Proceedings, 1,* 106–112.

Schweizer, R.T., Rovelli, M., Roper, L., & Bartus, S.A. (1987). A flexible immunosuppression protocol for organ transplantation using cyclosporine, azathioprine, and prednisone. *Transplantation Proceedings, 19,* 1944–1946.

Sheil, A.G.R. (1984). Cancer in dialysis and transplant patients. In P.J. Morris (Ed.). *Kidney Transplantation: Principles and Practice* (2nd ed.) (pp. 491–507). Orlando: Grune & Stratton.

Shield, C.F. III (1987, March). Reuse of monoclonal antibodies. In Monoclonal Antibodies in Transplantation: State of the Art 1987. Symposium conducted at Montefiore Hospital, New York, N.Y.

Smith, S.L. (1986). Immunosuppressive drugs used in clinical practice. *Critical Care Quarterly, 9,* 19–24.

Starzl, T.E., Marchioro, T.L., Porter, K.A., Iwasaki, Y., & Cerilli, G.J. (1967). The use of heterologous antilymphoid agents in canine renal and liver homotransplantation and in human renal homotransplantation. *Surgery, Gynecology, & Obstetrics, 124,* 301–318.

Starzl, T.E., Marchioro, T.L., & Waddell, W.R. (1963). The reversal of rejection in human renal homografts with subsequent development of homograft tolerance. *Surgery, Gynecology, & Obstetrics, 117,* 385–395.

Steinmuller, D.R. (1986). Usefulness of cyclosporine levels one to six months posttransplant. In R.M. Ferguson & B.G. Sommer (Eds.). *The Clinical Management of the Renal Transplant Recipient with Cyclosporine* (pp. 158–164). Orlando: Grune & Stratton.

Taylor, J. (1981). Thoracic duct drainage. *AANNT Journal, 8* (1), 42–47.

RECENT DEVELOPMENT: FK 506

by Sandra M. Staschak and Karen Zamberlan

A new and potent experimental antirejection drug known as FK 506 has demonstrated stunning success in the prevention of rejection among adults and children receiving liver transplantation. It also shows promise for patients who undergo kidney, heart, and lung transplants. This drug is currently being researched at the University of Pittsburgh (Starzl, Fung, McCauley, Jain, Alessiani, et al., 1989; Starzl, Fung, Venkataramman, Todo, Demetris, & Jain, 1989). FK 506, a macrolide antibiotic produced from a strain of soil fungus, *Streptomyces tsukubaensis*, was discovered in 1984 by the Fujisawa Pharmaceutical Company during a search for naturally occurring immunosuppressive agents (Thomson, 1989). Offered initially as compassionate rescue therapy for patients with cyclosporine nephrotoxicity, chronic rejection despite cyclosporine immunosuppression, or both, FK 506 proved so successful that it is now being used for primary transplant immunosuppression.

Phase I human clinical trials with FK 506 began in February, 1989 after three years of animal studies proved the drug efficacious. As of December, 1989, a total of 200 adults and children have been treated with this new therapy.

FK 506 shares many of the properties of cyclosporine as an immunosuppressive agent but is structurally quite different from cyclosporine and has been noted to have fewer side effects. Immunosuppression by FK 506 may be mediated through the inhibition of interleukin-2 release (Warty, Diven, Cadoff, Todo, Starzl, & Sanghvi, 1988). FK 506 is insoluble in water but dissolves readily in organic solvents. It is reported to be stable for many months at room temperature as a white crystalline powder, but its stability in solution is unknown (Tanaka, Kuroda, Marusawa, Hashimoto, Hatanaka, et al., 1987).

Animal studies using FK 506 to prolong heart, kidney, and liver allograft survival have shown this drug to have marked immunosuppressive qualities (Morris, Hoyt, Murphy, & Shorthouse, 1989; Todo, Murase, Ueda, Podesta, ChapChap, et al., 1989; & Yokota, Takashima, Sato, Osakabe, Nakayama, et al., 1989). Synergistic effects have been demonstrated when FK 506 and cyclosporine were administered together; however, clinical trials have not shown this to be a viable combination. In rats, intramuscular doses as low as 0.1 mg/kg/day and 0.3 mg/kg/day have extended the survival of heart and skin allografts.

Ongoing trials in adult and pediatric heart, renal, and liver transplants are presently being conducted with FK 506 immunosuppression. One outstanding feature of these trials is that FK 506 does not appear to be as nephrotoxic in therapeutic doses and that it does not cause hypertension.

Overall the drug has proved to be remarkably free from major side effects. Headache, nausea, vomiting, hyperkalemia, tingling and burning of the hands and feet, and insomnia were noted. The headaches, nausea, and vomiting have occurred with the intravenous (IV) administration and have been seen primarily in those patients who still have a cyclosporine blood level. Once the IV dose was stopped, these symptoms diminished. Hyperkalemia due to low aldosterone and renin has also occurred; treatment with potassium-restricted diets and/or Florinef can be initiated.

FK 506 is administered via an IV pump into a central or peripheral line. The dosing schedule has been variable and may be as frequent as every 12 hours and as infrequent as every third day. During the initial dose of FK 506 a physician should be available to provide emergency care should it be necessary, although this has never been required. Nursing actions require vital signs to be taken every 15 minutes during the initial two-hour infusion. Thereafter, vital signs are taken hourly. Once the patient is out of the intensive care environment, vital signs are monitored every four hours.

The dosage of FK 506 is adjusted on the basis of the liver chemistries, FK 506 blood levels, and how well the patient tolerates the drug. An initial intravenous dose of 0.15 mg/kg will be administered in the immediate perioperative period. Additional dosages of 0.075 mg/kg will be given IV every 12 hours until the patient is able to take the drug orally. The oral dose of 0.15 mg/kg will be given every 12 hours in capsule form. The usual maximum dose that may be given is 0.30 mg/kg every 12 hours orally. Steroids, at lower doses, are part of the immunosuppressive protocol.

The oral dose of FK 506 is provided in clear gelatin capsules. The capsules can be opened and the white powder mixed in a small amount of food or fluid (orange juice, yogurt, or apple sauce).

It is recommended that cyclosporine be discontinued for a minimum of 24 hours prior to starting the first IV dose of FK 506. The synergistic side effects that have occurred in these patients include hypertensive episodes and a body rash.

Therapeutic blood levels for FK 506 have not been established. Presently, ranges that are expected to prevent rejection are 0.5 to 2.0 ng/ml of serum by ELISA. Blood levels should be drawn one hour before the dose is administered, with usually a minimum of 0.7 ml of blood necessary to perform the test in the FK 506 laboratory.

Future developments and applications of FK 506 may be found outside of organ transplantation. Since FK 506 is a potent immunosuppressive agent with little toxicity, autoimmune diseases may be targeted for FK 506 trials. Arita and associates (1989) reported their experience with rats and suggest that FK 506 may effectively reduce the manifestations of collagen arthritis. Clinical trials are currently under way in this area.

REFERENCES

Arita, C., Hotokebuchi, T., Miyahara, H., Arai, K., Sugioka, Y., Takagishi, K., & Kaibara, N. (1989). Effect of FK 506 (FR 900506) on collagen arthritis in rats: A preliminary report. *Transplantation Proceedings, 21*, 1056–1058.

Morris, R.E., Hoyt, E.G., Murphy, M.P., & Shorthouse, R. (1989). Immunopharmacology of FK 506. *Transplantation Proceedings, 21*, 1042–1044.

Starzl, T.E., Fung, J., McCauley, J., Jain, A., Alessiani, M., Staschak, S., Mieles, L., Van Thiel, D., Todo, S., Shapiro, R., & Kang, Y. (1989). Clinical trials of FK 506. *IV Congress of the European Society for Organ Transplantation.* Barcelona, Spain.

Starzl, T.E., Fung, J., Venkataramman, R., Todo, S., Demetris, A., & Jain, A. (1989). FK 506 for liver, kidney, and pancreas transplantation. *Lancet, 2*(8617), 1000–1004.

Tanaka, H., Kuroda, A., Marusawa, H., Hashimoto, M., Hatanaka, H., Kino, T., Goto, T., & Okuhara, M. (1987). Physiochemical properties of FK 506, a novel immunosuppressant isolated from *Streptomyces tsukubaensis. Transplantation Proceedings, XIX*, 11–16.

Thomson, A.W. (1989). FK 506—how much potential? *Immunology Today, 10*, 6–9.

Todo, S., Murase, N., Ueda, Y., Podesta, L., ChapChap, P., Kahn, D., Okuda, K., Imventarza, O., Casavilla, A., Demetris, J., Makowka, L., & Starzl, T.E. (1988). Effect of FK 506 in experimental organ transplantation. *Transplantation Proceedings, XX*, 215–219.

Warty, V., Diven, W., Cadoff, E., Todo, S., Starzl, T.E., & Sanghvi, A. (1988). FK 506: A novel immunosuppressive agent. *Transplantation, 46*(3), 453–455.

Yokota, K., Takishima, T., Sato, K., Osakabe, T., Nakayama, Y., Uchilda, H., Aso, K., Masaki, Y., Ohbu, M., & Okudaira, M. (1989). Comparative studies of FK 506 and cyclosporine in canine orthotopic hepatic allograft survival. *Transplantation Proceedings, 21*, 1066–1068.

5

Infectious Disease and Transplantation

Marya Weil and Mary Rovelli

An important aspect of the nursing care of a transplant patient revolves around prevention of infection, prompt recognition of infection, and thorough follow-up with appropriate interventions. To help in planning care, this chapter discusses the factors that predispose transplant patients to infection. The most common opportunistic infections that threaten this patient population, with incidence, morbidity and mortality, and treatment, are covered. An additional section is devoted to nursing issues that affect care, and to nursing diagnoses and care plans as they relate to the transplant patient and infectious disease.

PREDISPOSITION TO INFECTION

A transplant patient is at increased risk for infection by virtue of compromised defense mechanisms from previous chronic illness (uremia, liver or heart failure, malnutrition, diabetes, and other systemic illness), surgery, and subsequent medication regimens essential to the survival of the transplanted organ. The role of the immune system in transplantation and the mode of action and effects of various immunosuppressive medications are covered in other chapters. In short, however, all of the medications alter the external (skin, mucous membranes, and tears) and internal (phagocytic/inflammatory system, cell-mediated system, and humoral system) defense mechanisms (Gurevich, 1985).

Increased immunosuppression for the treatment of a rejection episode and the role it plays in infections are not always clear. Because immunosuppression affects cellular immunity, and especially the function of polymorphonuclear leukocytes, the level of immunosuppression often relates to the incidence of infection (Ristuccia, 1985). Several studies have confirmed this relation, although other studies have demonstrated no correlation with the level of immunosuppression and the frequency of certain pulmonary infections (Axelrod, 1980; Gentry & Zeluff, 1986; Simpson, Stinson, Egger, & Remington, 1981). And despite the fact that most pulmonary infections occur within the first three months after the organ transplant, astute observation for pneumonia is important at all times, not only after a recent period of heavy immunosuppression (Vij, Dumler & Toledo-Pereyra, 1980).

Overall, researchers are reporting a decreased incidence of infectious complications in patients treated with cyclosporine as compared with those treated with conventional immunosuppressants (steroids and azathioprine). Presumably this is due to the effect of cyclosporine on only the T cell population of the white blood cell and the fact that, generally, less steroids are needed to control rejection in this group of patients (Hofflin, Potasman, Baldwin, Oyer, & Stinson, 1987; Shaffer, Hammer & Monaco, 1987).

Because of chronic illness, the patient may already be nutritionally depleted. It is well known that nutritional deficits contribute to the process of infection, and may also aggravate the general immunosuppressed state (Munda, Alexander, First, Gartside, & Fidler, 1978). The use of steroids further disturbs carbohydrate, fat, and protein metabolism. Steroid-induced diabetes may occur because of the alterations in pancreatic secretions and necrosis of pancreatic tissue. All this may be further upset if infection should develop and increase caloric requirements (Doenges, Jeffries & Moorhouse, 1984).

Patients who have alterations in the function of the respiratory tract, such as chronic obstructive airway diseases and changes in the amount and quality of mucus and the function of cilia, as occurs in people who smoke or have only recently quit smoking, can predispose a patient to pneumonia (Ristuccia, 1985; U.S. Department of Health and Human Services, 1981). A particular concern for heart-lung and lung transplant patients are changes related to denervation of the lung. Additionally, a "reimplantation response" consisting of alveolar edema may predispose these patients to pulmonary infections (Brooks, Hofflin, Jamieson, Stinson, & Remington, 1985). Heart and liver transplant patients tend to have more serious pneumonias of a nonviral nature than do kidney transplant patients (Dummer, Hardy, Poorsatter, & Ho, 1983). This may be due to greater overall immunosuppression in heart and liver transplant recipients.

Most nosocomial infections involve the urinary tract (Axnick, 1983; Underwood, 1983). In an immunocompromised host, urinary tract infections are a potential problem. But even more important is the development of gram-negative septicemia after such infections in these patients.

A transplant patient is prone to develop a wound infection (Rubin,

1988). An abscess deep to the transplanted organ drains with difficulty, and this may become the source of repeated septicemia (Peterson & Andersen, 1986). The incidence of wound infections varies greatly from one report to another, but meticulous surgical technique in organ procurement and subsequent transplant surgery prevents wound infection (Rubin, 1988). Bacterial wound infections are a potential complication in any surgery, but for an immunocompromised patient the consequences may be greater (Tolkoff-Rubin & Rubin, 1988). The most common site of infection is the transplant site. Therefore, heart and heart-lung transplant recipients are at greater risk for pulmonary complications (Dummer et al., 1983).

In liver transplantation, besides the usual risk and threat of infection, there is the unusual need to keep the patient in bed for 48 hours postoperatively to allow stabilization of the vascular anastomoses. There may also be prolonged anesthesia effects in liver transplant patients, as well as extensive subdiaphragmatic manipulation, which is not usually seen in other organ transplant procedures. The patient is usually intubated and mechanically ventilated during the first 48 hours postoperatively. All this adds to the increased risk of infection (Smith, 1985).

After liver transplantation, infection can also arise from the biliary tract, which requires a T tube to provide drainage and a biliary anastomosis stent. This anastomosis is prone to breakdown, obstruction, and infection. There can be abscess formation, peritonitis, cirrhosis, and bacteremia. Obstruction and cholangitis can result from "biliary sludging," that is, the shedding of the epithelial lining of the donor bile ducts. Infection can ascend by way of the T tube from skin flora, duodenal flora, and a contaminated drainage system. The T tube is important for postoperative cholangiography, but it must be handled respectfully, lest graft sepsis and cholangitis occur. Absence of infection in the T tube is the desired outcome, allowing bile to be manufactured and excreted normally (Smith, 1985).

Patients with end-stage kidney disease often have gastrointestinal (GI) symptoms related to their uremia. Upper GI complaints include esophagitis, heartburn, and dysphagia. Common lower GI disturbances include chronic diarrhea, but more commonly chronic constipation and bowel obstruction; paralytic ileus; enterocolitis; and melena. After kidney transplantation any of these can be serious complications. Bowel perforation can lead to gram-negative sepsis or to peritoneal infection, two of the most lethal GI complications (Wetzel, 1987).

DETECTING INFECTION IN THE IMMUNOCOMPROMISED HOST

Because the signs and symptoms of infection are subtle and may even be absent in patients who are receiving corticosteroids, health care professionals must be particularly astute in their physical assessment. In addition to performing frequent lung auscultation, they must be alert for the subtler signs of infection. These include tachycardia, tachypnea, cough, confusion, and pain (Gurevich & Tafuro, 1985). Although tachycardia is a sign of infection in most patients, those who are receiving beta-blocker therapy for control of blood pressure may not respond with an increased heart rate, even when they have profound hypoxia or high fever (Govani & Hayes, 1982).

Fever is often the only sign of infection in an immunosuppressed patient, and even low-grade fevers require further assessment (Cunha, 1985). The investigation of fever includes a careful physical examination, including auscultation of the heart and lungs and examination of the skin, mouth, wound, and vaginal and perianal areas for potential sources of infection. Additionally, urine, sputum, and blood samples and specimens taken from the pharynx, wound, and any other area that appears to be infected should be sent for culture. The patient should also have a chest x-ray (Reheis, 1985).

Other organ- or disease-specific signs of infection, such as dysuria, signs of pneumonia, local pain and tenderness, and rigors may or may not be present. The timing of the infection post transplant is also helpful in establishing a diagnosis because opportunistic infections tend to occur at specific times (Fig. 5–1).

Infections of the lungs and central nervous system (CNS) are particularly dangerous to an immunosuppressed patient, and efforts must be taken to diagnose and treat these infections in a timely manner. Because identification of the organisms may be elusive, but of the utmost importance, diagnosis of these infections is discussed in detail.

Septic shock may develop in transplant patients. Patients who are receiving corticosteroid therapy and who develop septic shock need to receive additional steroid therapy, despite the presence of sepsis, to prevent an addisonian crisis. Symptoms of an addisonian crisis include low blood pressure and vasomotor collapse. Treatment includes administration of colloids such as albumin, corticosteroids, and, possibly, vasopressors (Luckman & Creason-Sorensen, 1987).

Pulmonary Infections

Diagnosis

A pervasive theme in the literature regarding diagnosis of pulmonary infections has been the need for aggressive diagnostic action, including invasive procedures (Peterson & Andersen, 1986; Ristuccia, 1985; Simpson et al., 1981). Initial laboratory studies include a complete blood count with white blood cell differential, blood and sputum cultures, and measurement of arterial blood gases. A chest x-ray must be performed. If

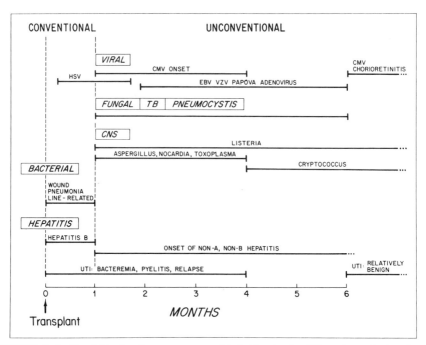

FIGURE 5–1. Timetable for the occurrence of infection in the kidney transplant patient. (From Rubin, Wolfson, Casimi, & Tolkoff-Rubin (1981), p. 406.)

these measures do not yield a diagnosis, then more invasive procedures, including transtracheal aspiration, fiberoptic bronchoscopy, and, often, an open-lung biopsy, must be performed (Ristuccia, 1985). Even if a sputum culture indicates infection, a transbronchial and/or open-lung biopsy may be performed to confirm the diagnosis and thereby direct specific therapy (Weiland, Ferguson, Peterson, Snover, Simmons, & Najarian, 1983).

Although an open-lung biopsy is the most definitive invasive procedure, other radiographic and radionuclide tests may be helpful in establishing the diagnosis (Ristuccia, 1985). A computed tomography (CT) scan as well as nuclear imaging scans may help to localize an infection (Gentry & Zeluff, 1986). Gallium lung scans have been helpful in making the diagnosis of pneumocystis pneumonia in the absence of chest x-ray infiltrates. Identification of the agent causing the pneumonia is extremely valuable in determining the treatment of choice. Thus the patient is spared the use of antimicrobial agents that may be toxic and increase susceptibility to suprainfections.

Treatment

Treatment of pulmonary infections is aimed at antimicrobial eradication of the causative organism. Because immunocompromised patients can rapidly develop overwhelming sepsis, treatment is often initiated with empiric therapy based on "clinical judgment," that is, the experience of the physician caring for the patient (Peterson & Andersen, 1986). In fact, when the diagnosis is particularly elusive, the patient may receive multiple-drug therapy to cover the most likely causes.

Beyond the antimicrobial treatment, other interventions may be required. These include surgical excision of the lung lesion, particularly for Aspergillus infection (Weiland et al., 1983). Reduction in immunosuppressive therapy is also important although some diseases (e.g., bacterial pneumonia) may not require changes in immunosuppression (Marshall, Foster & Winn, 1981; Munda et al., 1978).

Central Nervous System Infections

A CNS infection often develops after an episode of bacteremia and the causative organisms are often the same (Smith, 1980). Infections of the CNS can lead to encephalitis, meningitis, and brain abscesses. Early diagnosis of CNS infections, particularly those of bacterial origin, is important for successful treatment.

Almost all CNS infections present with fever and some form of deficit, depending on the site of infection. CNS deficit varies from headache to changes in the level of consciousness, including coma, to obvious seizures (Masur & Jones, 1980; Smith, 1980; Weiland et al., 1983). Behavior that is inappropriate is often a warning sign that a CNS infection is present (Masur & Jones, 1980). Fever associated with nuchal rigidity also indicates meningitis, although patients who are receiving corticosteroids may have meningitis without nuchal rigidity.

The presenting symptoms help to identify the area of CNS involvement. For instance, nuchal rigidity indicates inflammation of the meninges, whereas other deficits, such as focal seizures and difficulty with speech or memory, indicate involvement of areas of the brain. Careful attention to specific symptoms will aid in the diagnosis and in the identification of causative organisms.

Although many CNS findings are nonspecific, some may indicate a particular infection. For example, herpes simplex encephalitis frequently causes the general symptoms previously mentioned. Specific symptoms of gustatory and olfactory hallucinations, indicating dysfunction of the temporal lobe, are also suggestive of encephalitis caused by herpes simplex (Smith, 1980). Other types of infection may not have such specific symptoms. Evaluation of concomitant infections may help to establish the diagnosis.

Diagnosis

Physical assessment and evaluation of the patient often provide preliminary information that indicates the location of the infection and a potential differential diagnosis. Because CNS infections tend to occur after episodes of bacteremia, it is important to evaluate blood cultures and sensitivities (Smith, 1980). A lumbar puncture to obtain a sample of cerebrospinal fluid, and a CT scan of the head are two important diagnostic tools in the patient evaluation (Peterson & Andersen, 1986). As in other infections, body fluids from potential sources of infection should be cultured with sensitivity analysis. Magnetic resonance imaging may also help to determine the diagnosis. If the diagnosis cannot be established with these methodologies, a brain biopsy may be required (C.T. Poor, personal communication, March 1988; Smith, 1980).

CAUSATIVE ORGANISMS

Viral Infections

Cytomegalovirus

Cytomegalovirus (CMV) infection infects anywhere from 37 per cent to 80 per cent of the general public. In a healthy immunocompetent person the disease may appear as a form of infectious mononucleosis or as current symptoms of a self-limiting respiratory illness, or it may go unrecognized. In the past its most ominous and potentially devastating effect has been on the developing fetus in a woman with concurrent infection (Gold & Nankervis, 1982).

However, in any immunocompromised patient—be it from acquired immunodeficiency syndrome (AIDS), immunosuppressive therapy required by organ or bone marrow transplantation, or the stress of surgery and prolonged illness (Schulman, 1987)—this virus has gained new notoriety. Heart transplant recipients seem particularly prone to severe CMV infection with an unexplained high incidence of 70 per cent to 100 per cent (Schulman, 1987).

CMV is acquired by direct, intimate contact. Children spread it by respiratory and oral routes. Blood transfusions and donor organs have also been identified as sources of CMV infections (Chou, 1986; Chou, Kim & Norman, 1987).

The infection may be primary or recurrent. In primary disease a patient who is seronegative before the transplant becomes seropositive after the transplant. Primary infections post transplant tend to be severer than recurrent infections (Bia, Andiman, Gaudio, Kliger, Siegel, et al., 1985; Weir, Irwin, Maters, Genemans, Shen, et al., 1987).

In recurrent disease a patient with a previous positive titer will demonstrate a fourfold or greater rise in CMV titer post transplant. This may be due to either a previously dormant strain that has reactivated as a result of immunosuppression or a new strain introduced by any of the routes above (Bia et al., 1985; Rubin et al., 1985; Weir et al., 1987). The documentation of CMV-specific IgM antibody may help to identify recent or concurrent infection (Gold & Nankervis, 1982; Wreghitt, Gray & Chandler, 1986). During active infection the virus can be cultured from various body sites, body fluids such as blood and urine, bronchial washings, and liver and kidney biopsies (Gold & Nankervis, 1982).

CMV infection should be suspected by the clinical presentation and confirmed by serology and viral cultures. Because CMV is so common in the general population, pretransplant CMV titers are useful to document prior unrecognized infection. CMV infection should be suspected in any transplant patient who:

1. receives a transplant from a CMV-positive donor,
2. was CMV antibody–negative pretransplant,
3. is less than 90 days post transplant,
4. has been treated for a rejection episode, and/or
5. has prolonged, unexplained fever and vague symptoms.

Manifestations of CMV infection include prolonged cyclical episodic fever (most common), leukopenia, thrombocytopenia, hepatitis, pneumonia, CNS disturbances (i.e., headache, lethargy, stupor, coma), renal insufficiency, arthritis, arthralgia, GI bleeding, pancreatitis, retinitis, and superinfection (with bacteria, fungi, protozoa, or other viruses) (Smiley, Wlodaver, Grossman, Barker, Perloff, Tustin, Starr, Plotkin, & Friedman, 1985).

Schumann (1987) describes three typical clinical pictures: (1) an illness that is asymptomatic, (2) a self-limiting syndrome, and (3) an unrelenting multisystem disease that may end in death.

Prolonged and episodic fever, arthralgia, fatigue, anorexia, abdominal pain, and diarrhea may be present in the self-limiting syndrome. Hepatic dysfunction may be apparent but may also be due to drug interactions. The syndrome may last for three to four weeks. There may also be some neurologic disturbances and retinitis, but these are usually seen with the severely ill patient. CMV infection may lead to renal dysfunction either by triggering a rejection episode or by causing a glomerulopathy (Weir et al., 1987). CMV has also been found in peptic ulcer disease of kidney transplant patients (Cohen, Komorowski, Kauffman, & Adams, 1985).

Retinitis may be part of this syndrome, and may be difficult to diagnose because it often resembles herpetic, candidal, or toxoplasmic lesions. It should be suspected, however, anytime a transplant patient complains of decreased visual acuity or peripheral blind spots. During the active disease, which can take several months to resolve, there is scarring of the retina and reduced visual acuity. After the infection has subsided vision does not improve (Egbert, Pollard, Gallagher & Marigan, 1980).

The multisystem disease increases in severity week by week. Initially there are several days of spiking fevers, malaise, weakness, nasal stuffiness, and sore throat. Renal function may begin to deteriorate. There also may be orthostatic hypotension, hepatic dysfunction, arterial hypoxemia, and pneumonia.

Worsening of the patient's condition continues with leukopenia, thrombocytopenia, and hypotension. Pulmonary function worsens, and may require ventilatory support. The disease may progress to include nausea, vomiting, and bloody diarrhea. Because CMV is, in itself, immunosuppressive, the already severely deteriorated patient may develop superinfection with other organisms (Schumann, 1987).

Currently there is only one preventive therapy and one treatment therapy specific for CMV. CMV immune globulin may be administered to prevent CMV disease (Hagenbeek, Brummelhuis, Donkers, Dumas, ten Haaft, et al., 1987; Snydman, Werner, Heinze-Lacey, Berardi, et al., 1987). The prophylactic use of CMV immune globulin provides protection for the seronegative kidney transplant recipient who received a seropositive donor kidney. The rate of virologically confirmed CMV-associated syndromes, CMV-associated leukopenia, CMV pneumonia, hepatitis, thrombocytopenia, and other serious and life-threatening opportunistic infections was reduced in patients who received CMV immune globulin prophylactically (Snydman et al., 1987).

Treatment for active CMV infection consists of 9-(1,3-dihydroxy-2-propoxymethyl) guanine (DHPG) (Gancyclovir). Gancyclovir is chemically similar to acyclovir and, like acyclovir, is active against herpes simplex types 1 and 2 and herpes zoster. Gancyclovir is additionally active against CMV (Chachoua, Dieterich, Krasinski, Green, Laubenstein, Wernz, Buhles, & Koretz, 1987; Erice, Jordan, Chace, Fletcher, Chinnock, & Balfour, 1987). Results reported with DHPG have been varied. The Collaborative DHPG Treatment Study Group (1986) reported a clinical response in 43 per cent of their patients with severe combined immunodeficiency, metastatic malignant melanoma, and AIDS. Another study consisting of 10 patients with bone marrow transplants treated for CMV pneumonitis reported a strong virological response, but only one of the patients survived the pneumonia (Shepp, Dandiler, deMiranda, Burnette, Cederberg, Kirk, & Meyers, 1985). In contrast, Keay, Bissett, and Merigan (1987) reported clinical improvement of pneumonitis or retinitis in 70 per cent of the treatment courses. Nonetheless, this treatment is encouraging and further investigations are pending.

Herpes Simplex Types I, II, and Zoster Viruses

Herpes infections most commonly occur as skin infections; however, other body sites such as the eyes and lungs may also be affected. There are three types of herpes infections: herpes simplex type I, herpes simplex type II, and herpes or varicella zoster. Herpes type I is a common infection, affecting 50 per cent or greater of the population. This is the virus that causes cold sores (Pelczar, Chan, & Krieg, 1986). Herpes type II is the virus that has been identified as the agent responsible for primary and recurrent genital herpes (Pelczar et al., 1986). Patients and staff need to know that the presence of a herpes infection does not necessarily mean that the virus was sexually transmitted. This possibility can cause considerable concern among spouses and/or intimate friends.

Most herpes simplex infections are mild; however, some can be severe, covering the face and genitalia (Axelrod, 1980), and may also disseminate. Type 1 and type 2 herpes simplex lesions may occur concurrently (Axelrod, 1980). Although they commonly occur in the perioral and genital areas, they may occur elsewhere, such as on the back or chest (Brooks et al., 1985). Diagnosis is made by the finding of vesicular eruptions on visual examination (Magnussen, 1983). Biopsy or scraping of the lesions is useful for a definitive diagnosis. The treatment of choice is either topical, oral, or intravenous acyclovir, depending on the severity of the infection (Peterson & Andersen, 1986).

Varicella zoster infections occur in organ transplant patients in the form of either varicella, commonly known as chickenpox, or herpes zoster, more commonly known as shingles (Magnussen, 1983). In a patient who has not developed antibodies to this virus the infection manifests as varicella. A patient who has previously been exposed and is partially immune will manifest the disease as herpes zoster (Magnussen, 1983).

Although the frequency of varicella infection may not be increased in organ transplant recipients, it may be severer (Axelrod, 1980). If zoster immune globulin is administered within 72 hours of contact, the severity of the disease may be limited (Wreghitt, 1987). As with the herpes simplex virus, the diagnosis is based on physical examination and laboratory analysis of vesicular scrapings (Magnussen, 1983). The rash that develops in each of these infections is the same as that which occurs in the general population.

Varicella infections may be prevented if patients are able to avoid contact with people who are infected with the virus. If contact has occurred, hyperimmune globulin must be promptly administered. For herpes zoster infection the treatment is aimed at control of pain from the infection and prevention of a secondary infection. If treatment is necessary for infection from this virus, intravenous administration of acyclovir, vidarabine (ara-A), or human interferon may be helpful (Magnussen, 1983; Wreghitt, 1987).

Herpes simplex can cause a pneumonia that presents with symptoms that are similar to those of bacterial pneumonia. Chest x-ray reveals a diffuse process that may be mistaken for bacterial pneumonia (Young, 1980). The clinical course may be rapidly fatal unless appropriate antiviral therapy is instituted, currently with acyclovir.

Herpes simplex and herpes zoster can cause a retinopathy that is similar to that which occurs with CMV. Herpes zoster can also cause an optic neuritis (Newton, 1980).

Encephalitis resulting from herpes infection is usually caused by herpes type 1 in transplant patients and may occur after infection of the mouth, skin, or genitalia (Smith, 1980). In addition to the usual signs of CNS deficit, temporal lobe signs (e.g., gustatory and olfactory hallucinations) may be indicative of herpes encephalitis (Smith, 1980).

Epstein-Barr Virus

Infection in transplant recipients may also result from Epstein-Barr virus (EBV), another type of the herpes virus (Cheeseman, Henle, Rubin, Tolkoff-Rubin, Cosimi, et al., 1980). The incidence of infection with EBV has increased since cyclosporine has been used as an immunosuppressive agent (Wreghitt, 1987). The major concern regarding EBV, however, is not its manifestation as an infection, which is similar to that of CMV (Cheeseman et al., 1980), but the role it plays in the development of lymphoproliferative disorders (Wreghitt, 1987). The relation to and frequency with which lymphomas related to EBV occur have not yet been determined (Dummer et al., 1983).

Nursing Interventions

Nursing care is based on administration of antimicrobial agents as well as on the care of skin lesions when present. Patient comfort is challenging, particularly in those patients with herpes zoster infection. Wound care should be performed with aseptic technique. Nurses must protect themselves from infection when caring for these patients by wearing gowns, masks, and gloves (Gurevich & Tafuro, 1985). These precautions are especially important with varicella infection, since it is highly contagious. The patients should remain in isolation until the lesions have healed or until they are discharged home. Other immunosuppressed patients must be protected from them.

Patient education is an important nursing intervention with skin infections. Patients must be taught how to examine their skin for signs of infection; they also may be responsible for their own dressing changes, especially when discharged home.

Fungal Infections

Candida albicans

Candida albicans causes a variety of infections in the immunosuppressed host; however, most can be prevented with prophylactic oral nystatin or clotrimazole and careful attention to mouth care. The most common sites of candidal infection are the mouth and esophagus, but infection also occurs in the wound, in the respiratory and urinary tracts, and, most serious, in the bloodstream. Clinical pneumonia caused by Candida is relatively rare in transplant recipients (Brooks et al., 1985). However, if Candida is isolated from more than one source, the recipient has an increased risk for developing candidal pneumonia and septicemia (Winearls, Lane & Kurtz, 1984).

Signs and symptoms of candidal infections vary with the site of infection. White, patchy lesions in the mouth, pain, and difficulty swallowing are signs of oral and esophageal infection (Rivers, 1987). Treatment of these infections is important, since localized infection may disseminate in immunosuppressed patients (Brooks et al., 1985).

Systemic candidal infection should be suspected in patients who have Candida identified in more than one area. Patients who are receiving long-term antibiotic therapy are at great risk for developing an associated fungal infection and may be candidates for prophylaxis with an intravenous antifungal agent such as amphotericin B (Warren, 1987). In these patients the diagnosis of systemic candidiasis may not be made in a timely manner because of a concomitant bacterial septicemia (Warren, 1987).

Ocular candidal infections can result in loss of vision. Although removal of the vitreous may be helpful (if the disease has progressed to the stage where this would be necessary), the prognosis for the eye is poor.

Early identification and treatment of Candida are important. Treatment ranges from local application to systemic therapy. Local nystatin or clotrimazole is used both as prophylaxis and in the treatment of oral, esophageal, and vaginal infection. Bladder irrigation with amphotericin B is helpful in the treatment of urinary tract infection. Systemic amphotericin B is necessary for severe localized infections or systemic infection (Peterson & Andersen, 1986).

Although localized infection is relatively common in transplant recipients, systemic infection occurs less commonly and is associated with mortality. Those patients who develop systemic infection are usually more debilitated, have other concurrent infection, and may have multisystem failure.

Aspergillus Infection

Aspergillosis is an insidious fungal infection that presents primarily as a pulmonary or CNS infection. It tends to occur in an epidemic-type pattern, and may be related to hospital construction (Ristuccia, 1985). The route of infection has not been clearly defined, and patients present with a variety of symptoms. The major symptoms include low-grade fever, nonproductive cough, and changes on chest x-ray of a finely nodular infiltrate that may progress to cavitation (Weiland, Ferguson, Peterson, Snovar, Simmons, & Najarian, 1983). Sputum cultures may be positive for *Aspergillus*, although a positive culture may indicate colonization and not active disease. Such a finding necessitates more invasive diagnostic procedures (Weiland et al., 1983). *Aspergillus* infection often develops as a result of an increased dose of corticosteroids as treatment for rejection (Genry & Zeluff, 1986). It is often fatal despite early therapy. Weiland (1983) found that in nine patients with CNS *Aspergillus* infection, eight had a history of recent treatment for infection or rejection.

CNS *Aspergillus* infections are often fatal. For that reason patients with nonspecific CNS deficits, abnormal cerebrospinal fluid analysis findings, and *Aspergillus* in a sputum culture should be treated for CNS *Aspergillus* (Smith, 1980; Weiland et al., 1983). Occasionally intrathecal administration of amphotericin B is required (Smith, 1980). The side effects include headache, nausea, vomiting, and local arachnoiditis, which may be lessened by the administration of corticosteroids (Smith, 1980).

Protozoal Infection

Pneumocystis carinii

Pneumocystis carinii causes pneumonia in immunocompromised patients. Much of the general public has recently become aware of this type of pneumonia because of its prevalence in patients with AIDS. The typical symptoms of pneumocystis pneumonia are fever, malaise, hypoxia, nonproductive cough, shortness of breath, and, rarely, chest pain. One of the most specific symptoms for this type of pneumonia is hypoxia that is disproportionate to both the findings on physical examination and the degree of infiltrate present on chest x-ray (Sterling, Bradley, Khalil, Kerman & Conklin, 1984; Munda et al., 1976). Hypoxia may be significant enough to require intubation and ventilatory support (Sterling et al., 1984). Pneumonia from *Pneumocystis* is now rarely seen in transplant patients if they are treated prophylactically with trimethoprim/sulfamexazole (Septra or Bactrim) (Peterson & Anderson, 1986).

Patients who have pneumocystis pneumonia, and other health care workers involved in their care, may be concerned that this infection means that they have AIDS. The nurse must be alert to this concern and explain the difference between AIDS and therapeutic immunosuppression, and the fact that both types of patients may develop similar diseases.

Bacterial Infection

Nocardia

Nocardia infections are bacterial infections that can manifest as pulmonary, subcutaneous, or disseminated (especially to the central nervous system) infection (Simpson et al., 1981). It is believed that the primary portal of entry and dissemination is the lung (Ristuccia, 1985). Frequently, nocardia infections are detected by the finding of a single nodular abscess on chest x-ray, with patients remaining asymptomatic. Some patients may have fever and a dry cough (Simpson et al., 1981). Additionally, the development of a subcutaneous lesion may precede or follow the diagnosis and treatment (Simpson et al., 1981) of the pneumonia. Simpson et al. (1981) found that subcutaneous nocardial lesions preceded the diagnosis of pulmonary nocardial infection in two patients.

Nocardia infection is not known to be transmitted by person-to-person contact; however, this has been suspected in a few cases involving transmission to an immunocompromised host (Sen & Louria, 1980). The diagnosis may be made by isolation of the bacteria from the sputum, but most often lung tissue is required to establish the diagnosis (Sen & Louria, 1980). The treatment of choice is sulfonamide therapy. Surgical excision of the lesion may also be necessary (Sen and Louria, 1980).

Several other opportunistic infections can occur in an immunocompromised host; however, they occur less frequently than those previously discussed. Also, some infections are endemic to specific areas and therefore are not seen in the majority of transplant centers. The causative organisms for these infections are listed in Table 5–1.

CONCLUSION

Infectious complications have been responsible for significant morbidity and mortality in organ transplant recipients. However, as more is

**TABLE 5–1. OTHER CAUSATIVE ORGANISMS
IN OPPORTUNISTIC INFECTIONS**

ORGANISM	TYPE	BODY SITE USUALLY AFFECTED
Cryptococcus neoformans	Fungus	CNS
Histoplasma	Fungus	Lung
Zygomycosis	Fungus	Eye
Toxoplasma	Protozoa	Lung CNS
Legionella	Bacteria	Lung
Listeria sp.	Bacteria	Lung CNS
Mycobacterium	Bacteria	Lung
Strongyloides stercoralis	Helminth	Lung

CNS, central nervous system.

learned about the immune system, immunosuppression, and the rejection phenomenon, the incidence of serious infections has decreased. Despite these improvements, two of the most important actions necessary to limit opportunistic infections are prevention and a daily comprehensive assessment of the hospitalized patient. In this manner, potential sources of infection are eliminated and actual infections are recognized, diagnosed, and treated at an early stage of illness.

ISSUES IN NURSING CARE

Several issues come to mind when planning nursing care of the transplant patient. The discussion here includes the practice of reverse (protective) isolation and reverse air flow rooms, immunizations in transplant recipients, dental prophylaxis, environmental exposure to infections, AIDS and the prevention of sexually transmitted diseases, and concerns regarding risk of infection to health care workers. Table 5–2 outlines some of these and other issues, using nursing diagnosis and care plans.

Reverse Isolation

Some centers place their transplant recipients in reverse (protective) isolation. Other centers contend that most infections stem from opportunistic organisms, and only use reverse isolation if the patient becomes severely leukopenic (Smith, 1985). In heart transplantation strict protective isolation is advocated for the first 48 hours post transplant (Barnhart & Lower, 1988). Bone marrow transplant patients are placed in laminar airflow rooms for several weeks after the procedure (Thomas & Sargur, 1988).

Immunization of Transplant Recipients

The issue of immunization of organ transplant recipients is one that raises several concerns. Live vaccines should not be given to an immunosuppressed patient because of the risk of enhanced viral replication. Live vaccines include those for measles, mumps, rubella, oral polio, and yellow fever (Reese & Douglas, 1983).

Immune globulins, which contain antibody against a specific disease, can safely be used in immunosuppressed patients. Additional concerns regarding immunizations are those that involve patients who have both minor and major illnesses. Immunizing a patient who has a minor upper respiratory tract infection will not pose a risk; however, vaccination should be delayed if a severe febrile illness is present (Reese & Douglas, 1983).

When possible, potential organ transplant recipients should be immunized before transplantation. If this is accomplished, the patient may receive live vaccine, and the additional question regarding the ability to mount a response to a vaccine while immunosuppressed is obviated (Reese & Douglas, 1983). Because patients are at risk for respiratory infections posttransplantation, influenza and pneumococcal vaccines can be administered before the transplant, but also may be administered post transplant because neither contains live virus.

Dental Prophylaxis

Because dental caries are an occult source of infection, all transplant candidates should be encouraged, if not required, to obtain dental clearance before transplant. After the transplant, dental work (even routine cleaning) should be covered with an antibiotic in accordance with that transplant center's guidelines (Wade & Schimpff, 1988). Dental problems should not be overlooked as a possible source of "fever, unknown origin."

Environmental Exposure to Infections

Transplant patients should be advised to avoid visiting or moving to areas that are endemic for opportunistic infection (Cohen, Galgiani, Potter, & Ogden, 1982). But, since freedom to travel is often a major

TABLE 5–2. TRANSPLANT NURSING CARE PLAN

Nursing Diagnosis	Goal	Interventions
Potential for infection	The patient will remain infection free.	1. Use aseptic technique when changing dressings or inspecting wounds.
		2. Staff with upper respiratory tract infections should not care for these patients.
		3. Infected visitors should not be allowed, even if masks are worn.
		4. Nurses should avoid caring for infected patients and transplant patients simultaneously.
		5. Standing water may become colonized with gram-negative organisms and should be avoided. This includes vases of water for cut flowers (Gurevich & Tafuro, 1985).
		6. Some transplant centers prohibit fresh fruit and vegetables because of spreading infection (Traiger & Bohachick, 1983), but those measures do not appear necessary for most organ transplant patients.
		7. Use of humidifiers should be avoided because they can become contaminated in the same manner as standing water, and the mist will spread infected organisms (Gurevich & Tafuro, 1985).
		8. Identify other potential sources of infection and encourage use of masks, especially when hospital construction is under way.
		9. The transplant patient's room should be cleaned before other patient rooms to prevent cross-contamination.
		10. When necessary to send a transplant patient to other units, such as radiology, notify the department of the patient's immunosuppression. If possible, the transplant patient might be the first to undergo a procedure in that room or would not follow a severely infected patient.
		11. Any deliberate breaks in the skin or mucous membrane (for example, from I.V. lines and catheters) should be treated.

Indication of infection is promptly recognized, reported, and accurate treatment made available.

1. Perform physical assessments carefully, since the signs and symptoms of infection are subtle and may even be absent in patients receiving corticosteroid immunosuppression. (See Chapter 4.)

2. Observe for signs and symptoms of infection and non-healing. In addition to daily or more frequent lung auscultation, the nurse should be alert to subtler signs of infections, such as tachycardia, tachypnea, cough, confusion, and pain.

3. Monitor temperature regularly.

4. Temperature elevations should not be routinely suppressed unless the patient is severely compromised with the fever (Cunha, 1985).

5. Transplant patients should not be routinely given pain medications containing acetaminophen, as this may additionally mask fever.

6. Tachycardia is a sign of infection in most patients, but many transplant patients are receiving beta-blocker therapy for control of blood pressure and may not respond with an increased heart rate (Govani & Hayes, 1982), even with severe hypoxia or high fever.

7. Inspect for breakdown in skin or any mucous membranes

8. Check mouth daily for the white, patchy lesions of *Candida albicans*, and be suspicious of any pain or difficulty swallowing (Rivers, 1987).

9. Cultures must be properly obtained and promptly brought to the microbiology laboratory.

10. Results from specimens processed stat, for example sputum Gram stains, should be brought to the attention of the appropriate physicians for direction of antimicrobial therapy.

Table continued on following page

105

TABLE 5-2. TRANSPLANT NURSING CARE PLAN *Continued*

Nursing Diagnosis	Goal	Interventions
Potential for infection (Continued)	The patient will remain infection free. (Continued)	11. Be vigilant for the presence of multiple infections, such as fungal infection after treatment of bacterial infection. 12. Appropriate antimicrobial agent must be administered as soon as possible. 13. Attention must be paid to the side effects of antimicrobial agents, as they may be nephrotoxic (of concern in renal transplant recipients), or may interfere with immunosuppression. 14. Many antimicrobial medications cause injury to the veins through which they are administered. Use the veins in the hands before arm veins to maximize venous sites (Smith, 1980). Central venous lines are preferred for the administration of sclerosing medications.
Potential for complications and septic shock in transplant patients with septicemia	Prevention of the occurrence of an addisonian crisis.	1. Patients receiving corticosteroid therapy who develop septic shock need to receive additional steroid therapy, despite the presence of sepsis. 2. Symptoms of an addisonian crisis include low blood pressure and vasomotor collapse. 3. Treatment includes administration of colloids such as albumin, corticosteroids and possibly vasopressors (Luckman and Sorensen, 1987).

Potential for bowel perforation and subsequent infection related to steroid therapy	No GI complications are present, and should they develop, interventions will be promptly initiated.	1. Assess and report complaints of esophagitis, heartburn, and dysphagia. 2. Assess and report any complaints of generalized abdominal pain associated with abdominal distention, absence of bowel sounds, guarding, and rebound tenderness. 3. Accurately record date and description of all stools. 4. Assess for presence of frank or occult bleeding in stools or emesis. 5. Report prolonged constipation or diarrhea. 6. Assess and report signs of peritonitis: abdominal pain and increased pulse and respirations, with a decrease in blood pressure, cool and clammy skin, agitation, and anxiety. 7. Teach patient to do all of the above (Wetzel, 1987).
Knowledge deficit regarding self-care, prevention, and for treatment of infection	The patient will be able to identify signs of infection, seek medical attention, and follow up with treatment.	1. Teach patients to identify the subtle signs of infection and to routinely inspect their mouths, skin, and other areas of potential infection. 2. Teach patients how to take antifungal agents, specifically to hold or dissolve in the mouth; not to wash down with liquid. 3. Remind patients to take all oral medications (unless otherwise instructed by physician), even after the symptoms have disappeared (Doenges, Jeffries & Moorhouse, 1984).

benefit to a patient after transplantation, this may be unreasonable to expect. A careful history of where the patient has lived and traveled should be taken when any patient presents with a perplexing infection (Rubin, 1988; Rubin and Greene, 1988).

Animals often harbor parasitic organisms that can infect man. Birds such as parrots, pigeons, and chickens can carry psittacosis. Cats as well as animals such as cattle, pigs, and birds (including poultry) can harbor toxoplasmosis (Ruskin, 1988). Patients should be advised to avoid contact with high-risk animals (Peterson & Andersen, 1986), especially animal excreta and the consumption of raw or poorly cooked meat (Ruskin, 1988).

Transmission of the AIDS virus (human immunodeficiency virus [HIV]) has been reported in the literature in at least three instances (Centers for Disease Control, 1987; Kumar, Pearson, Martin, Leech, Buisseret et al., 1987; Prompt, Reis, Grillo, Kopstein, Kraemer et al., 1985). Five patients were infected with HIV from the donor organ, including one recipient of a living-related graft (Kumar et al., 1987); four died soon after the transplants.

There are several concerns related to AIDS and transplantation. One is whether HIV is more lethal in patients who are immunosuppressed for transplantation. The published reports and informal discussions at national and international transplantation meetings indicate that AIDS may progress more rapidly and lead more quickly to death in this group of patients.

Another concern is the issue of organ transplantation into patients who test positive for HIV antibody but who have not exhibited signs of the disease. Some transplant centers currently transplant HIV antibody–positive patients; others will not, and still others do not test for the presence of antibody to HIV in potential recipients. This topic is still in its infancy; additional data are necessary in order to establish guidelines.

One approach may be in testing not only for antibody against HIV, but also for the presence of the virus. When this test can be performed on a more routine basis, it will be easier to identify patients who have active virus and who will develop AIDS. It would appear now that, in such patients, the immunosuppression needed for an organ transplant would be detrimental.

Patients who have antibody against HIV but do not have virus present might tolerate immunosuppression for an organ transplant and benefit from the transplant. A few liver transplants have been performed in those patients (who were hemophiliacs), but the follow-up period is still too short to predict their ultimate fate. Finally, information presented at the National Symposium on AIDS in 1987 indicated that a few patients who historically tested positive for HIV antibody have now become negative. This will be an important group to study and may provide information of benefit to other patients. The next several years will no doubt provide more information about AIDS and transplantation.

"Safe Sex"

An open, frank discussion of sexual practices with transplant recipients can go a long way in protecting them from sexually transmitted diseases. The safest practice is to avoid the exchange of all body fluids with potentially infected persons. Most medical researchers recommend the use of condoms to reduce the risk of exposure to sexually transmitted diseases such as AIDS, herpes, candidiasis, CMV, EBV, gonorrhea, and syphilis. The local health department should be able to provide patients with public information brochures about "safer" sex practices.

Nursing Concerns Regarding Risks to Self

Nurses who provide care to infected patients are appropriately concerned about the risks to themselves. Because many of the infectious diseases in organ transplantation occur rarely, less is known about them, and the disease may invoke more fear regarding personal susceptibility. However, most of the infections that occur in these patients are opportunistic, and invade an immunocompromised host. People with intact immune systems are not at risk for infection with most of these organisms. Many of the infections, such as *Aspergillus* and legionnaires' disease, normally occur in an epidemic-like manner; no person-to-person infections have been identified (Simpson et al., 1981). CMV infections may be transmitted by person-to-person contact, but the contact is usually intimate, such as occurs when parents care for their infants.

Pregnant women, especially those who are in the first trimester, should be concerned about exposure to CMV infection. Exposure is more likely to come from children in day care settings (siblings) than from patient care, since nurses who care for transplant patients have not been found to have an increased incidence of CMV infection when compared with the general public (Jordan, 1987).

The Centers for Disease Control (1987) have developed clear recommendations that include routine use of barrier precautions to prevent skin and mucous membrane exposure when contact with the body fluids of any patient is expected. All nurses should heed this recommendation when caring for all patients, not just transplant nurses caring for transplant patients.

Infectious organisms surround us. The human body is designed with complex defense mechanisms to protect itself from hostile invasion and to keep malignant organisms under control. The immunosuppression necessary in organ transplantation alters the body's response to the transplanted organ. We must be vigilant lest our deliberate manipulations of the immune system create additional harm.

References

Axelrod, J.L. (1980). Infections complicating uremia and organ transplantation. In M.H. Grieco M.H. (Ed.). *Infections in the Abnormal Host* (pp. 521–545). New York: Yorke Medical Books.

Axnick, K.J. (1983). Infection control considerations in the care of the immunosuppressed patient. In M.A. Roderick (Ed.), *Infection Control in Critical Care,* (pp. 133–192). Rockville, Md.: Aspen Systems Corporation.

Barnhart, G.R. & Lower, R.R. (1988). Cardiac transplantation. In G.J. Cerilli (Ed.). *Organ Transplantation and Replacement* (pp. 493–510). Philadelphia: J.B. Lippincott.

Bia, M.J., Andiman, W., Gaudio, K., Kliger, A., Siegel, N., Smith, D., & Flye, W. (1985). Effect of treatment with cyclosporine versus azathioprine on incidence and severity of cytomegalovirus infection posttransplantation. *Transplantation, 40,* 610–614.

Brooks, R.G., Hofflin, J.M., Jamieson, S.W., Stinson, G.B., & Remington, J.S. (1985). Infectious complications in heart-lung transplant recipients. *American Journal of Medicine 79,* 412–422.

Centers for Disease Control, Morbidity and Mortality Weekly Report (1987). *Human immunodeficiency virus infection transmitted from an organ donor screened for HIV antibody—North Carolina.* (DHHS Publication Publication No. 25–36). Atlanta; U.S. Department of Health and Human Services.

Chachoua, A., Dieterich, D., Krasinski, K., Greene, J., Laubenstein, L., Werne, J., Buhles, W., & Koretz, S. (1987). 9-(1,3-dihydroxy-2-propoxymethyl) Guanine (Gancyclovir) in the treatment of cytomegalovirus gastrointestinal disease with the acquired immunodeficiency syndrome. *Annals of Internal Medicine, 107,* 133–137.

Cheeseman, S.H., Henle, W., Rubin, R.H., Tolkoff-Rubin, N.E., Cosimi, B., Cantell, K., Winkle, S., Herrin, J.T., Black, P.H., Russell, P.S., & Hirsch, M.S. (1980). Epstein-Barr virus infection in renal transplant recipients. *Annals of Internal Medicine, 93,* 39–42.

Chou, S. (1986). Acquisition of donor strains of cytomegalovirus by renal transplant recipients. *The New England Journal of Medicine, 314*(22), 1418–1423.

Chou, S., Kim, D.Y., & Norman, D.J. (1987). Transmission of cytomegalovirus by pretransplant leukocyte transfusions in renal transplant candidates. *Journal of Infectious Diseases, 155,* 565–567.

Cohen, E.B., Komorowski, R.A., Kauffman, H.M. Jr., & Adams, M. (1985). Unexpectedly high incidence of cytomegalovirus infection in apparent peptic ulcers in renal transplant recipients. *Surgery, 97,* 606–612.

Cohen, I.M., Galgiani, J.N., Potter, D., & Ogden, D. (1982). Coccidioidomycosis in renal replacement therapy. *Archives of Internal Medicine, 142,* 489–494.

Collaborative DHPG Treatment Study Group. (1986). Treatment of serious cytomegalovirus infections with 9-(1,3-dihydroxy-2-propoxymethyl) guanine in patients with AIDS and other immunodeficiencies. *The New England Journal of Medicine, 314,* 801–805.

Cunha, B.A. (1985). Significance of fever in the compromised host. *Nursing Clinics of North America, 20,* 163–169.

Doenges, M.E., Jeffries, M.F., & Moorhouse, M.F. (1984). *Nursing Care Plans—Nursing Diagnosis in Planning Patient Care.* Philadelphia: F.A. Davis.

Dummer, J.S., Hardy, A., Poorsattar, A., & Ho, M. (1983). Early infections in kidney, heart, and liver transplant recipients on cyclosporine. *Transplantation, 36,* 259–267.

Egbert, P.R., Pollard, R.B., Gallagher, J.G., & Merigan, T.C. (1980). Cytomegalovirus retinitis in immunosuppressed hosts. *Annals of Internal Medicine, 93,* 664–670.

Erice, A., Jordan, M.C., Chace, B.A., Fletcher, C., Chinnock, B.J., & Balfour, H.H Jr. (1987). Gancyclovir treatment of cytomegalovirus disease in transplant recipients and other immunocompromised hosts. *Journal of the American Medical Association, 257*(22), 3082–3087.

Gentry, L.O. & Zeluff, B.J. (1986). Diagnosis and treatment of infection in cardiac transplant patients. *The Surgical Clinics of North America, 66,* 459–465.

Gold, E. & Nankervis, G.A. (1982). Cytomegalovirus. In A.S. Evans (Ed.). *Viral Infections of Humans—Epidemiology and Control* (pp. 167–186). New York: Plenum.

Govani, L.E. & Hayes, J.E. (1982). *Drugs and Nursing Implications* (4th ed.) East Norwalk, Conn.: Appleton-Century-Crofts.

Gurevich, I. (1985). The competent internal immune system. *Nursing Clinics of North America, 20,* 151–161.

Gurevich, I. & Tafuro, P. (1985). Nursing measures for the prevention of infection in the compromised host. *Nursing Clinics of North America, 20,* 257–261.

Hagenbeek, A., Brummelhuis, H.G.J., Donkers, A., Dumas, A.M., ten Haaft, A:, Schaap, B.J.P., Sizoo, W., Löwenberg, B. (1987). Rapid clearance of cytomegalovirus-specific IgG after repeated intravenous infusions of human immunoglobulins into allogeneic bone marrow transplant recipients. *The Journal of Infectious Diseases, 155,* 897–902.

Hofflin, J.M., Potasman, I., Baldwin, J.C., Oyer, P.E., Stinson, E.B., & Remington, J.S. (1987). Infectious complications in heart transplant recipients receiving cyclosporine and corticosteroids. *Annals of Internal Medicine, 106,* 209–216.

Jordan, M.C. (1987). *Infectious disease in transplantation.* Presented at the meeting of the North American Transplant Coordinators Organization, Philadelphia, Pa.

Keay, S., Bissett, J., & Merigan, T.C. (1987). Gancyclovir treatment of cytomegalovirus infections in iatrogenically immunocompromised patients. *Journal of Infectious Diseases, 156,* 1016–1621.

Kumar, P., Pearson, J.E., Martin, D.H., Leech, S.H., Buissemet, P.D., Bezbak, H. S., Gonzalez, F.M., Royer, J.R., Streicher, H. Z., & Saxinger, W.C. (1987). Transmission of human immunodeficiency virus by the transplantation of a renal allograft, with development of the acquired immunodeficiency syndrome. *Annals of Internal Medicine, 106,* 244–245.

Luckman, J. & Creason-Sorensen, K. (1987). *Medical-Surgical Nursing: A Psychophysiologic Approach.* Philadelphia: W.B. Saunders.

Magnussen, C.R. (1983). Skin and soft tissue infections. In R.E. Reese, R.G. Douglas (Eds.). *A Practical Approach to Infectious Diseases,* (pp. 239–247). Boston: Little, Brown.

Marshall, W., Foster, R.S. Jr., & Winn, W. (1981). Legionnaires' disease in renal transplant patients. *The American Journal of Surgery, 141,* 423–429.

Masur, H. & Jones, T.C. (1980). Protozoal and helminthic infection. In M.H. Grieco (Ed.) *Infection in the Abnormal Host,* (pp. 406–437). New York: Yorke Medical Books.

Munda, R., Alexander, J.W., First, M.R., Gartside, P.S., & Fidler, J.P. (1978). Pulmonary infections in renal transplant recipients. *Annals of Surgery, 187,* 126–133.

Newton, J.C. (1980). Intraocular manifestations of systemic infections. In M.H. Grieco (Ed.). *Infections in the Abnormal Host* (pp. 746–755). New York: Yorke Medical Books.

Pelczar, M.J., Chan, E.C.S., & Krieg, N.R. (1986). *Microbiology* (5th ed) New York: McGraw-Hill.

Peterson, P.K. & Andersen, R.C. (1986). Infection in renal transplant recipients—current approaches to diagnosis, therapy, and prevention. *The American Journal of Medicine, 81*(1A), 2–10.

Prompt, C.A., Reis, M.M., Grillo, F.M., Kopstein, J., Kraemer, E., Manfro, R.C., Maia, M.H., & Comiran, J.B. (1985). Transmission of AIDS virus at renal transplantation. *Lancet, 2,* 672.

Reese, R. & Douglas, R.G. (1983). *A Practical Approach to Infectious Diseases.* Boston: Little, Brown.

Reheis, C.E. (1985). Neutropenia: Causes, complications, treatment, and resulting nursing care. *Nursing Clinics of North America, 20,* 219–225.

Ristuccia, P. (1985). Microbiologic aspects of infection in the compromised host. *Nursing Clinics of North America, 20,* 171–179.

Rivers, R. (1987). Nursing the kidney transplant patient. *RN, 50,* 46–53.

Rubin, R.H. (1988). Infection in the renal and liver transplant patient. In R.H. Rubin, & L.S.

Young (Eds.). *Clinical Approach to Infection in the Compromised Host* (2nd ed.) (pp. 557–621). New York: Plenum Medical Book Co.

Rubin, R.H. & Greene, R. (1988). Etiology and management of the compromised patient with fever and pulmonary infiltrates. In R.H. Rubin, & L.S. Young (Eds.). *Clinical Approach to Infection in the Compromised Host* (2nd ed.) (pp. 131–163). New York: Plenum Medical Book Co.

Rubin, R.H., Tolkoff-Rubin, N.E., Oliver, D., Rota, T.R., Hamilton, J., Betls, R.F., Pass, R.F., Hillis, W., Szmuness, W., Farrell, M.L., & Hirsch, M.S. (1985). Multicenter seroepidemiologic study of the impact of cytomegalovirus infection on renal transplantation. *Transplantation, 40,* 243–249.

Rubin, R.H., Wolfson, J.S., Cosimi, A.B., & Tolkoff-Rubin, N.E. (1981). Infection in the renal transplant recipient. *The American Journal of Medicine, 70,* 405–411.

Ruskin, J. (1988). Parasitic diseases in the compromised host. In R.H. Rubin & L.S. Young (Eds.). *Clinical Approach to Infection in the Compromised Host* (2nd ed.) (pp. 253–304). New York: Plenum Medical Book Co.

Schulman, L.L. (1987). Cytomegalovirus pneumonitis and lobar consolidation. *Chest, 91,* 558–561.

Schumann, D. (1987). Cytomegalic virus infection in renal allograft recipients: Indicators for interventions in the SICU. *Focus on Critical Care, 14,* 40–47.

Sen, P., Louria, D.B. (1980). Higher bacterial and fungal infection. In Grieco, M.H. (Ed.). *Infections in the Abnormal Host,* (pp. 325–351). New York: Yorke Medical Books.

Shaffer, D., Hammer, S.M., & Monaco, A.P. (1987). Infectious complication with the use of cyclosporine versus azathioprine after cadaveric kidney transplantation. *American Journal of Surgery, 153,* 381–386.

Shepp, D.H., Dandiler, P.S., de Miranda, P., Burnette, T.C., Cederberg, D.M., Kirk, L.E., & Meyers, J.D. (1985). Activity of 9-(2-hydroxy-1-(hydroxymethyl) ethoxymethyl) guanine in the treatment of cytomegalovirus pneumonia. *Annals of Internal Medicine, 103,* 368–373.

Simpson, G.L., Stinson, E.B., Egger, M.J., & Remington, J.S. (1981). Nocardial infections in the immunocompromised host: A detailed study in a defined population. *Reviews of Infectious Diseases, 3,* 492–507.

Smiley, M.L., Wlodaver, C.G., Grossman, R.A., Barker, C.F., Perloff, C.J., Tustin, N.B., Starr, S.E., Platkin, S.A., & Friedman, H.M. (1985). The role of pretransplant immunity in protection from cytomegalovirus disease following renal transplantation. *Transplantation, 40,* 157–161.

Smith, L. (1980). Host deficiency states and CNS infections. In M.H. Grieco (Ed.). *Infections in the Abnormal Host* (pp. 623–652). New York: Yorke Medical Books.

Smith, S.L. (1985). Liver transplantation: Implications for critical care nursing. *Heart & Lung, 14,* 617–627.

Snydman, D.R., Werner, B.G., Heinze-Lacey, B., Berardi, V.P., Tilney, N.L., Kirkman, R.L., Milford, E.L., Cho, S.I., Bush, H.L. Jr., Levey, A.S., Strom, T.B., Carpenter, C.B., Levey, R.H., Harmon, W.E., Zimmerman, C.E. II, Shapiro, M.E., Steinman, T., LoGerfo, F., Idelson, B., Schrofer, G.P.J., Levin, M.F., Grady, G.F., & Leszczynski, J. (1987). Use of cytomegalovirus immune globulin to prevent cytomegalovirus disease in renal transplant recipients. *The New England Journal of Medicine, 317,* 1049–1054.

Sterling, R.P., Bradley, B.B., Khalil, K.G., Kerman, R.H., & Conklin, R.H. (1984). Comparison of biopsy-proven *Pneumocystis carinii* pneumonia in acquired immune deficiency syndrome patients and renal allograft recipients. *The Annals of Thoracic Surgery, 38,* 494–499.

Thomas, E.D. & Sargur, M. (1988). Bone marrow transplantation. In G.J. Cerilli (Ed.). *Organ Transplantation and Replacement* (pp. 608–616). Philadelphia: J.B. Lippincott.

Tolkoff-Rubin, N.E., Rubin, R.H. (1988). Infections in the organ transplant recipient. In G.J. Cerilli (Ed.). *Organ Transplant and Replacement* (pp. 445–461). Philadelphia: J.B. Lippincott.

Traiger, G.L. & Bohachick, P. (1983). Liver transplantation: care of the patient in the acute postoperative periods. *Critical Care Nurse, 3,* 96–103.

Underwood, M.A. (1983). Urinary tract infections. In M.A. Roderick (Ed.). *Infection Control in Critical Care* (pp. 115–122). Rockville, Md.: Aspen.

U.S. Department of Health and Human Services. (1981). *The Health Consequences of Smoking: The Changing Cigarette, a Report of the Surgeon General.* Washington, D.C.: Government Printing Office.

Vij, D., Dumler, F., & Toledo-Pereyra, L.H. (1980). Infectious complication in renal transplantation: Approach to the problem of fever, urinary, wound and pulmonary infections. *Dialysis & Transplantation, 9,* 129–134.

Wade, J.C. & Schimpff, S.C. (1988). Epidemiology and prevention of infection in the compromised host. In R.H. Rubin & L.S. Young (Eds.). *Clinical Approach to Infection in the Compromised Host* (2nd ed.) (pp. 5–40). New York: Plenum Medical Book Co.

Warren, R.E. (1987). Bacterial and fungal infections. In S.R. Calne (Ed.). *Liver Transplantation* (pp. 331–363). Orlando: Grune & Stratton.

Weiland, D., Ferguson, R.M., Peterson, P.K., Snover, D.C., Simmons, R.L., & Najarian, J.S. (1983). Aspergillosis in 25 renal transplant patients. *Annals of Surgery, 198,* 622–629.

Weir, M.R., Irwin, B.C., Maters, A.W., Genemans, G., Shen, S.Y., Charache, P. & Williams, G.M. (1987). Incidence of cytomegalovirus disease in cyclosporine-treated renal transplant recipients based on donor/recipient pretransplant immunity. *Transplantation, 43,* 187–193.

Wetzel, D.A. (1987). Gastrointestinal complications following renal transplantation—nursing implications. *Journal of Enterostomal Therapy, 14,* 16 19.

Winearls, C.G., Lane, D.J., & Kurtz, J. (1984). Infectious complications after renal transplantation. In P.J. Morris (Ed.). *Kidney Transplantation: Principles and Practice* (2nd ed.) (pp. 427–467). Orlando: Grune & Stratton.

Wreghitt, T.G. (1987). Viral and *Toxoplasma gondii* infections. In S.R. Calne (Ed.). *Liver Transplantation* (pp. 365–383). Orlando: Grune & Stratton.

Wreghitt, T.G., Gray, J.J., & Chandler, C. (1986). Prognostic value of cytomegalovirus IgM antibody in transplant recipients. *Lancet, 1,* 1157–1158.

Young, L.S. (1980). Diagnosis and treatment of diffuse pneumonias. In M.H. Grieco (Ed.). *Infections in the Abnormal Host,* (pp. 601–622). New York: Yorke Medical Books.

6
Kidney Transplantation

Linda M. Haggerty and Katherine M. Sigardson-Poor

Transplantation is an established therapeutic option for most patients with end-stage renal failure. Experimental kidney transplants were initially performed in the early 1900s. The first reported successful transplants were not performed until the early 1950s, using identical twins (see Chapter 1). Kidney transplants are currently performed worldwide, with an estimated 80,000 persons having received a kidney transplant in the United States alone (Pat O'Connor, personal communication, February 20, 1988).

In 1988 alone, 9123 kidney transplants were performed (7278 from cadaveric donors and 1845 from living related donors) (Staff, 1989). As of April 1989, 14,777 patients were waiting for transplants.

There are many indications for dialysis and transplantation; examples are listed in Table 6–1. Many patients choose transplant over dialysis as therapy for their end-stage renal failure because of the relative normalcy a transplant can bring to their lives, and because of the improved survival time transplant often allows (Fig. 6–1). The longest-surviving transplant recipient has had her graft for more than 33 years. E.H. received a kidney from an identical twin in 1956. The longest-surviving cadaveric recipient is P.M., who received his graft in 1966 (Amy Chang, personal communication, April 4, 1989).

Current success rates average 75 per cent to 85 per cent for cadaver kidney transplants and 90 per cent to 95 per cent for living-related transplants (Monaco, 1985; Sterioff, Engen & Zincke, 1986). Advancements in immunology and immunosuppression have led to significantly decreased morbidity and mortality. The end result is a procedure appreciated for its ability to prolong and promote quality of life.

Kidney transplantation, however, is not a panacea. Although success and significant rehabilitation are likely, there is risk of infection, graft rejection, and even death. Increased understanding of the role and function of the immune system, immunomodulation, and conscientious

114

patient care throughout the transplant process all contribute to the current success of kidney transplantation.

This chapter briefly discusses normal renal function, recipient selection and preparation, the donor and the surgical procedure, and complications. Emphasis is placed on the nursing care during the pretransplant process and the posttransplant period, including short- and long-term needs.

RENAL FUNCTIONS

The kidneys play a vital role in maintaining body homeostasis. Renal excretory functions include metabolization and excretion of metabolic waste products, such as creatinine and blood urea nitrogen (BUN), and control of fluid and electrolyte balance. Regulatory functions include assistance in the control of blood pressure, production of such hormones as erythropoietin factor and growth hormone, production of prostaglan-

TABLE 6–1. INDICATIONS FOR KIDNEY TRANSPLANTATION

Congenital Disorders	**Trauma Requiring Nephrectomy**
Aplasia	**Renal Vascular Diseases**
Hypoplasia	Renal artery occlusion
Horseshoe kidney	Renal vein thrombosis
Metabolic Disorders	**Irreversible Acute Failure**
Hyperoxaluria	Cortical necrosis
Nephrocalcinosis	Hemolytic uremic syndrome
Gout	Acute and subacute
Oxalosis	glomerulonephritis
Fabrey's disease	Anaphylactoid purpura (Henoch-
Amyloidosis	Schönlein syndrome)
Cystinosis	Acute tubular necrosis
Hereditary	**Irreversible Chronic Renal Failure**
Nephropathies	Chronic pyelonephritis
Alport's syndrome	Chronic glomerulonephritis
Polycystic kidney	Diabetic nephropathy
disease	(Kimmelsteil-Wilson syndrome)
Medullary cystic	Goodpasture's disease
disease	Hypocomplementemic nephritis
Toxic Nephropathies	Steroid-resistant nephrotic
Lead nephropathy	syndrome
Analgesic nephropathy	Hypertensive nephrosclerosis
Obstructive Uropathy	**Other**
Acquired	Multiple myeloma
Congenital	Macroglobulinemia
Tumors Requiring	Wegener's disease
Nephrectomy	Scleroderma
Renal carcinoma	Systemic lupus erythematosus
Wilms's tumor	Polyarteritis nodosum
Tuberous sclerosis	(periarteritis nodosa)

From Flye, M.W. (1989). Renal transplantation. In M.W. Flye (Ed.) *Principles of Transplantation* (p. 267). Philadelphia: W.B. Saunders.

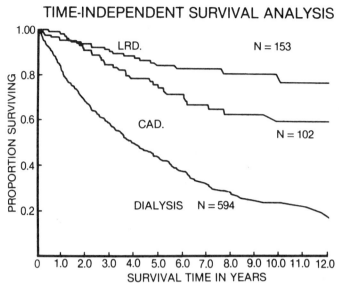

FIGURE 6–1. (From Flye, M.W. (1989). In M.W. Flye (Ed.) *Principles of Transplantation* (p. 266). Philadelphia: W.B. Saunders.)

dins, and activation of vitamin D. Secretory functions include assistance in the removal of various drugs, metabolites, and toxins from blood. Renal dysfunction leads to compromise of these activities and results in a variety of short- and long-term complications. Dialysis can assist with some of the excretory and secretory functions and diminish some of the pathophysiologic changes associated with renal failure. It cannot, however, replace normal renal function and currently offers no means of reestablishing most regulatory functions. Kidney transplantation is, therefore, often considered the best treatment for end-stage renal failure, reestablishing normal renal function and allowing for improved quality of life.

RECIPIENT SELECTION AND PREPARATION

Appropriate recipient selection is important for a successful outcome. Candidacy is determined by a variety of medical and psychosocial factors. A careful evaluation is carried out in an attempt to identify and minimize potential posttransplant complications. A list of commonly performed diagnostic studies is given in Table 6–2. The result of this evaluative process helps to determine a potential recipient's medical candidacy for transplantation. Attempts to assess such psychosocial factors as compliance, the ability to understand the transplant process

TABLE 6–2. KIDNEY TRANSPLANT RECIPIENT EVALUATION

1. **Complete history and physical examination**

2. **Laboratory studies**
   Complete blood count with platelets
   Chemistry profile
   ABO grouping
   HLA tissue-typing
   Viral titers
      Hepatitis B profile
      CMV IgG and IgM
      EBV profile
      Herpes simplex titers
      Toxoplasmosis titers
      Human immunodeficiency virus
   Coagulation profile
   Sickle cell prep (as indicated)

3. **Radiologic studies**
   Posterior/anterior and lateral chest x-ray
   Upper gastrointestinal series (as indicated)
   Lower gastrointestinal series (as indicated and for patients older than 45 years of age)
   Abdominal ultrasonography (to evaluate for gallstones and other organ abnormalities)
   Voiding cystourethrography (to assess for ureterovesical reflux, bladder capacity, and
      neurogenic bladder)

4. **Electrocardiography**

5. **Consultations**
   Dental
   Otorhinolaryngologist
   Cardiologist (as indicated and for patients with diabetes or over 45 years)
   Urologist (as indicated)
   Gynecologist
   Others (as indicated)

and patient responsibilities, as well as rehabilitation potential are important to help guide nursing intervention and determine candidacy.

Patients with a wide variety of causes of chronic renal failure consider the option of transplantation. The most common forms of renal disease include glomerulonephritis, chronic pyelonephritis, interstitial nephritis, and those disorders secondary to such systemic diseases as hypertension and juvenile-onset diabetes mellitus (Briggs, 1988). Certain patients, particularly those over age 55 and those with diabetes, are considered high risk. With advancements in immunosuppressive therapy, especially the use of cyclosporine and a steroid-sparing regimen, these high-risk patients can achieve the same success rates as those patients who are not considered in this category (Cook & Takiff, 1986; Jordan, Novick, Steinmuller, Braun, Buszta, Mintz, Goormastic, & Streem, 1985). Certain patients who do not yet require dialysis, but who are approaching end-stage renal failure, are also considered for transplantation. This approach is considered most advantageous for children, whose physical and mental development is significantly impaired on dialysis, and for patients with diabetes (Belzer, 1984).

Informed consent regarding all aspects of the transplant process must be assured. Patients and families must be provided with complete information regarding the risks, benefits, and procedures of each phase of the process, including patient responsibilities. Financial issues, particularly the cost of medications, must also be openly discussed.

Some patients may require surgical procedures before transplantation. Historically, pretransplant splenectomy was considered a means to modulate the immune system. A splenectomy, theoretically, offered the benefits of reducing lymphoid mass and lessening the leukopenia often associated with azathioprine, thereby decreasing the risk of rejection (Starzl, 1964; Stuart, Reckard, Ketel, & Schulak, 1980). Currently pretransplant splenectomy is seldom performed, and generally only in a severely leukopenic patient who may not be able to tolerate azathioprine therapy.

Other surgical procedures may be considered, depending on the results of the recipient evaluation. For example, a bilateral nephrectomy may be considered in a patient with intractable hypertension secondary to renin activity in the native kidneys. A bilateral or unilateral nephrectomy may be necessary in patients with a renal tumor. Nephrectomy may also be necessary in patients with ureterovesical reflux (causing repeated or chronic urinary tract infection) or infection from polycystic kidneys. Bleeding from polycystic kidneys may also be an indication for nephrectomy. Patients with active ulcer disease may require a highly selective vagotomy and pyeloroplasty, and those with diverticulosis, diverticulitis, or polyps may require colectomy. Additionally, the patient with demonstrated gallstones may undergo a cholecystectomy. However, it is important to weigh the risks of pretransplant surgery with the risks of subsequent immunosuppression.

Pretransplant Blood Transfusions

Blood transfusions are a controversial means of immune modulation. Historically, pretransplant transfusions were avoided because of the risks of infection and antibody formation. However, in 1973, it was found that patients who had received a number of blood transfusions before transplantation realized greater transplant success (Opelz, Sengar, Mickey, & Terasaki, 1973). Then, random blood transfusions were often given to patients awaiting transplantation. The risk of sensitization remained an important disadvantage. Currently the risk for infectious contamination (e.g., hepatitis and human immunodeficiency virus) must also be considered.

Since cyclosporine has been added to the immunosuppressive regimen the controversy regarding blood transfusions has resurfaced. Some authors report no added benefit from random blood transfusions, whereas others continue to report benefit from the random blood transfusions in combination with the use of cyclosporine (Klintman, Brynger, Flatmark, Frodin, Husberg, Thorsby, & Groth, 1985; Opelz, 1985).

The practice of random blood transfusions was expanded to include the concept of donor-specific blood transfusions between the potential living donor and the recipient. Potential recipients may receive one to three separate transfusions from the potential donor with antibody screening performed two weeks after each transfusion. If the antibody screen remains negative, it is thought that a transplant with success rates of 90 per cent to 95 per cent could be carried out between that pair. Unfortunately up to 30 per cent of the recipients did develop antibodies against the donor, thus prohibiting the transplant (Iwaki & Terasaki, 1986). Many of these patients also developed a high level of antibodies in general, making successful transplantation difficult.

Ways of minimizing the sensitization rate have been eagerly sought. Some transplant centers have adopted protocols of donor-specific blood transfusions given concomitantly with azathioprine immunosuppression, with a reported sensitization rate of 5 per cent and an associated low rate of graft loss from rejection (Anderson, Tyler, Sicard, Anderman, Rodey, & Etheredge, 1984). Thus increased numbers of living-related transplants, including those between less well matched donors, have been carried out with success rates reportedly equal to those between human leukocyte antigen (HLA)-identical pairs (Glass, Miller, Sollinger, & Belzer, 1985). Leukopenia and infection, however, are detriments to this protocol. Careful monitoring of the recipient's white blood cell count and infection status is critical in order to avoid complications.

A stored-blood protocol, designed to avoid the use of immuno-suppression while giving donor-specific blood transfusions, has also been carried out, with sensitization rates limited to approximately 10 per cent and an associated high graft survival (Light, Metz, & Oddenino, 1983). Storage reduces the number of T cells in the donor blood, in which most of the HLA-A, HLA-B, and HLA-C antigens are present. Thus a smaller antigen dose stimulates less antibody formation. B cells, however, remain viable, as do the monocytes that contain most of the HLA-DR antigens, whose activity stimulates the suppressor cell system (Light et al., 1983). A crossmatch is again performed after each transfusion. If, at any time, antibodies have developed, the process is discontinued and the transplant with that donor is not pursued. Opelz (1985) reported that random transfusions may be as beneficial as donor-specific blood transfusions. Further research regarding the effects of blood transfusions is required.

DONOR SOURCES

Kidney transplantation is made possible with kidneys from two sources: cadaver and living donors. The identification and maintenance of suitable cadaver donors are discussed in Chapter 2.

The kidneys removed from the cadaver donor are distributed equitably to the most appropriate recipient. HLA tissue-typing and ABO screening are performed. These results are compared with the blood types and antigens of all local patients awaiting transplantation. A national search is also conducted. If a six HLA-antigen match is identified nationally, the kidney will be sent to that recipient's transplant center. On the local level, appropriate potential recipients are identified and a lymphocyte crossmatch is performed. The kidneys are then distributed based mainly on a negative crossmatch and the degree of HLA histocompatibility.

Cadaver donor kidneys present with several disadvantages. First, the supply of cadaver organs is insufficient to meet the growing demand. Patients awaiting transplantation who must rely on a cadaver organ may wait months or even years for a suitable kidney. A small but not insignificant number of patients may die while waiting. Second, the genetic dissimilarity between donor and recipient may increase the risk of acute and chronic rejection. Finally, the prolonged preservation time required during recipient identification may influence short- and long-term graft function.

For these reasons living donor transplants are often considered. The use of living donors, however, is controversial for some transplanting surgeons. Starzl (1985), for example, chooses not to use living donors, citing similar success rates with cadaver donors and electing not to subject a living donor to the slight surgical risk. With a thorough donor workup, however, living donors are often preferred when available. Living-related donors undergo a complete medical and psychological evaluation. The evaluative tests required are summarized in Table 6–3. The goal of the evaluation is to rule out any surgical or long-term health risk to the donor. Living donors, when they meet the strict medical criteria as outlined, have been found not to be at greater risk for health problems after donating than the general population (Vincenti, Amend, Kaysen, Feduska, Birnbaun, Duca, & Salvatierra, 1983; Weiland, Chavers, Simmons, Ascher, & Najarian, 1984).

A psychological evaluation is also critical. It must be determined that the act of donating is a voluntary one. The donor must be informed as to both the process and the risk that the donated organ may fail. Potential donors must be counseled confidentially in order that they have ample opportunity to ask questions and make their own personal decisions. A decision not to donate should be accepted and respected as that

TABLE 6–3. KIDNEY TRANSPLANT LIVING DONOR EVALUATION

1. **Complete history and physical examination**
2. **Laboratory studies**
   Complete blood count with platelets
   Chemistry profile
   ABO grouping
   HLA tissue-typing
   Viral titers
      Hepatitis B surface antigen
      CMV IgG and IgM
      EBV profile
      Human immunodeficiency virus
   Endocrinology studies (for donors with a family history of diabetes), which may
      include:
      Five-hour glucose tolerance test
      Islet cell antibodies
      Glucose infusion stress test
   Urine studies
      24-hour urine for creatinine clearance and protein
      Urinalysis
      Sterile urine culture and sensitivity
3. **Radiologic studies**
   Chest x-ray (posterior/anterior and lateral)
   Intravenous pyelography (to assess for presence of two normal kidneys)
   Renal arteriography (to assess renal vasculature and further rule out renal
      abnormalities)
4. **Electrocardiogram**

   Consults (as indicated, including a complete cardiac evaluation for an older donor)

These tests are performed from least to most invasive, proceeding only when each test is
found to be within normal limits.

---

person's choice. Living donors can be divided into two categories. The first is the living-related donor. Such donors are usually siblings, parents, or children, although more distant relatives may be considered. Donors are assessed for ABO compatibility and the degree of HLA histocompatibility. Ideally, the more closely antigen-matched relative is chosen. Living-unrelated donors may provide another source, albeit controversial. Transplants between living-unrelated donor–recipient pairs have been performed. Success rates are reportedly comparable to those between living-related donors and recipients (Sollinger, Kalayoglu, & Belzer, 1986). Such donors may include spouses, adoptive parents or children, and friends. Careful scrutiny of ethical and motivational issues must be made. Issues, including long-term effects on the donor and recipient and appropriate protocols, must also be carefully addressed in order for this donor pool to be seriously considered.

Living Donor Nephrectomy

After general operative preparation and the induction of general anesthesia the donor is placed in a position (lateral decubitus) such that

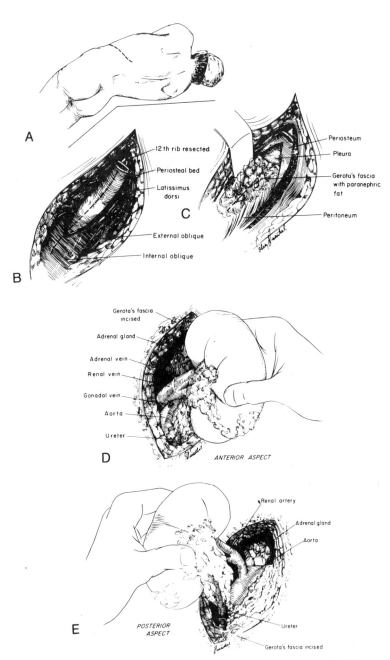

FIGURE 6–2. Incision for living donor nephrectomy. (From Cosimi, A.B. (1988). In Morris, P.J. *Kidney Transplantation: Principles and Practice* (3rd ed.). Philadelphia: W.B. Saunders, p. 100.)

the flank is presented laterally (Fig. 6–2). An incision, approximately at the 11th rib, is made. Often a portion of that rib is removed in order to provide adequate exposure. The kidney is gradually dissected after an incision is made through the muscles to the kidney. Except for the renal hilus, the kidney is dissected free, as are the renal vein and artery. The ureter is then dissected free, with great care taken to preserve the periureteral vascular supply.

Urine output from the dissected kidney is assessed. When determined to be adequate, the vascular supply (i.e., the renal vein and artery) is clamped and divided. The kidney is removed, perfused with a chilled electrolyte solution, and prepared for transplantation into the recipient. The donor's wound is closed, without drains.

THE SURGICAL PROCEDURE

The operative procedure for kidney transplantation has become fairly standardized. Most often the transplanted kidney is placed extraperito-

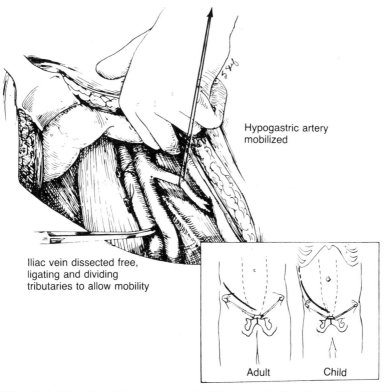

FIGURE 6–3. Incisions for adult recipient and child recipient. (From Lee, H.M. (1988). In Morris, P.J. *Kidney Transplantation: Principles and Practice* (3rd ed.). Philadelphia: W.B. Saunders, p. 217.)

neally in the iliac fossa. Intraperitoneal placement may be indicated in children for whom the transplanted kidney is too large to fit in the extraperitoneal space and in patients with inadequate extraperitoneal vascular accesses or who have received previous transplants. The extraperitoneal procedure is discussed here (Fig. 6–3).

Before any incisions are made, a Foley catheter is placed into the bladder. An antibiotic solution is instilled to distend the bladder and decrease the risk of infection. An oblique or curvilinear incision is then made, extending from the iliac crest to the symphysis pubis. The external oblique muscle, fascia, internal oblique, transverse abdominis muscles, and transverse salis fascia are then incised. The peritoneum is left intact and retracted upward. In the iliac fossa the common iliac, external iliac,

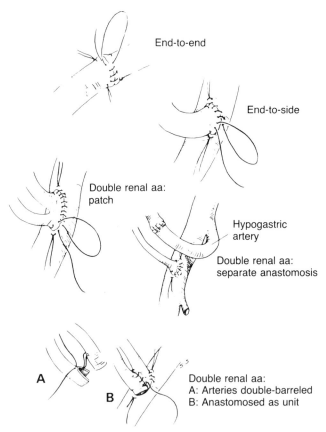

FIGURE 6–4. Some variations of renal artery anastomoses. (From Lee, H.M. (1988). In Morris, P.J. *Kidney Transplantation: Principles and Practice* (3rd ed.). Philadelphia: W.B. Saunders, p. 220.)

hypogastric arteries, and common and external iliac veins are dissected free. Any divided lymphatic vessels are ligated, or tied, to prevent future lymphocele formation.

Efficient revascularization, to prevent prolonged warm ischemia and tissue injury, is critical. Most commonly an end-to-end anastomosis with the donor renal artery and the recipient hypogastric artery or internal iliac artery is performed. An end-to-side anastomosis of the donor renal artery to the recipient external iliac artery may be made. If the donor kidney has multiple renal arteries, these may be anastomosed separately, on a patch of donor artery, or anastomosed together and then to the appropriate recipient vessel (Fig. 6–4).

The kidney is then placed in the iliac fossa, and the iliac vein is

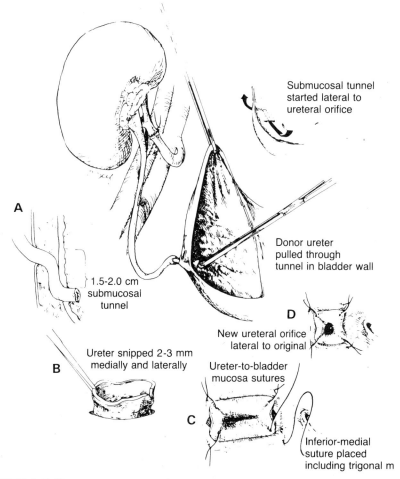

Submucosal tunnel started lateral to ureteral orifice

Donor ureter pulled through tunnel in bladder wall

1.5-2.0 cm submucosal tunnel

New ureteral orifice lateral to original

Ureter snipped 2-3 mm medially and laterally

Ureter-to-bladder mucosa sutures

Inferior-medial suture placed including trigonal m

A

B

C

D

FIGURE 6–5. Ureteroneocystostomy. (From Lee, H.M. (1988). In Morris, P.J. *Kidney Transplantation: Principles and Practice* (3rd ed.). Philadelphia: W.B. Saunders, p. 224.)

clamped until the donor renal vein is anastomosed to the recipient iliac vein. When the clamp is released and blood flow to the kidney is reestablished, the kidney becomes firm and pink, and urine may begin to form. Mannitol or furosemide may be given to promote diuresis.

The donor ureter is then connected to the recipient bladder. This ureteroneocystostomy may be performed as a simple incision and anastomosis, or the ureter may be tunneled into the bladder submucosa before entering the bladder cavity, as shown in Figure 6–5.

NURSING CARE

Nursing care of the kidney transplant recipient is challenging, complex, and rewarding. The successful rehabilitation of the recipient is made possible with careful nursing assessment, diagnosis, intervention, and evaluation of many body systems. Attention must also be paid to discharge teaching and long-term patient care needs.

Immediate Posttransplant Period

Immediately postoperatively maintenance of fluid and electrolyte balance is paramount. As mentioned earlier, renal function with rapid diuresis may begin soon after the blood supply to the kidney is reestablished. This diuresis is due in part to the kidney's ability to filter blood urea nitrogen (BUN), which acts as an osmotic diuretic; operative overhydration; and renal tubular dysfunction, which inhibits the kidney's ability to concentrate urine normally. Urine output during this phase may reach 1 to 2 liters per hour, slowing down as serum BUN and creatinine levels return toward normal. This occurs within several hours or several days. Fluid replacement, often hourly cc for cc replacement with a solution such as dextrose 5% in half-strength normal saline solution, is ordered. Dextrose 1% may be used if the urine output and subsequent replacement are significant, in order to decrease the amount of glucose infused. Electrolyte monitoring to assess for the hypokalemia often associated with rapid diuresis and for the potential hyponatremia resulting from the kidney's decreased concentrating ability is critical. Treatment with potassium supplements or 0.9% normal saline solution infusion or both may be indicated. Intravenous bicarbonate may also be required.

Assessment for dehydration is made by way of central venous pressure (CVP) readings, serum electrolyte levels, and response to a fluid challenge. Dehydration must be avoided, as the potential for subsequent renal hypoperfusion and renal tubular damage exists. Many patients who receive cadaveric kidneys with prolonged preservation time (greater than 24 hours) experience delayed renal function with risk of fluid volume overload. Ischemic damage owing to prolonged preservation or delayed operative anastomosis may cause acute tubular necrosis (ATN). This period of ATN can last for several days to several weeks, with gradually improving renal function. In any case, strict monitoring of fluid and electrolyte balance is critical. Hyperkalemia is a significant risk in the patient with renal dysfunction, and may be treated with furosemide (Lasix), sodium polystyrene sulfonate (Kayexalate), or, in emergent situations, dialysis or glucose and insulin infusion. Serum BUN and creatinine levels will remain elevated until renal function improves and will then return toward normal. Fluid restriction is necessary during the period of ATN in order to prevent fluid overload. Strict measurement of intake and output and accurate daily weights, measured on the same scale, must be recorded. Immediately posttransplant vital signs and CVP readings will be valuable. Further monitoring of fluid status by way of assessment of peripheral edema, changes in urine flow rates, and lung auscultation for pulmonary edema is necessary. Dialysis is often required to stabilize BUN and creatinine levels, remove excess fluid, and help normalize electrolyte levels until ATN resolves. Cardiac monitoring may be necessary to detect arrhythmias associated with electrolyte imbalance.

A decreased urine output in the early postoperative period may suggest several other factors that must be ruled out, such as dehydration, rejection, a technical complication, or an obstruction that impedes urine flow. An accurate diagnosis must be made before ATN can be presumed.

Technical complications such as lymphocele formation, hematoma, iliac vein thrombosis, or other forms of obstruction can also contribute to renal dysfunction or damage and will be discussed below (see Complications below). A common cause of early obstruction is a clot in the Foley catheter. Because the catheter generally remains in the bladder for one to five days, patency must be maintained. A sudden decrease in urine output may require sterile catheter irrigation to dislodge occluding clots.

Various diagnostic tests may be performed to assess for complications. Less invasive procedures are generally performed initially with more invasive procedures following as indicated. Patients who present with oliguria may undergo renal ultrasonography to assess for any fluid collections such as hematoma, lymphocele, or urine leak. Hydronephrosis, with or without a dilated ureter, may indicate obstruction. Abnormalities in the vascular supply to the transplanted kidney may be assessed by Doppler ultrasonography. If necessary, a radionucleotide renal scan is performed to assess blood supply to the kidneys as well as the kidney's ability to concentrate and then excrete the radioisotope iodohippurate sodium iodine 131 (Hippuran-131). Hippuran is injected intravenously, and timed scanning is then performed over the kidney, ureter, and bladder. Abnormal results can include minimal isotope filtering into the kidney, indicating an inadequate vascular supply; isotope slowly being filtered through the kidney into the ureter, demonstrating ATN; isotope being filtered only to a certain point in the urinary tract, suggesting obstruction; or Hippuran filtering outside of the urinary tract, demonstrating urine leakage or extravasation.

Potential for Infection

The potential for infection exists throughout the transplant process, and preventive care is essential. Sterile technique must be adhered to in line and catheter care, dressing changes, and wound care. Assessment for signs of infection (i.e., erythema, tenderness, warmth, and purulence) should be made at least every shift. These classic signs, however, may be masked by prednisone, so observation for other subtle signs is critical. Intravenous lines may be changed or removed when a temperature spike occurs, and the catheter tip should be sent for culture.

Strict pulmonary hygiene must be encouraged. Pulmonary infections can become fulminant and life-threatening. Patients should be encouraged to cough and deep breathe, ambulate, and use an incentive spirometer. Any alterations in the recipient's respiratory status must be evaluated and reported, including tachypnea, dyspnea, hypoxia, and dry or productive cough. Sputum samples for Gram stain, bacterial and fungal culture, acid-fast bacilli, and fungal stain are usually ordered. Repeat cultures may be necessary until the causative organism is isolated and identified and its antimicrobial sensitivities known. A chest x-ray should be taken; this may in fact be the only way to detect early signs of pulmonary infection. Many centers take weekly chest x-rays in order to obtain any early indication of infiltrate. Bronchoscopy or open-lung biopsy may be required in cases of diffuse pulmonary infiltrate and difficulty confirming a diagnosis with obtainable sputum samples. The patients should be monitored for the development of pulmonary edema.

Strict Foley catheter care is essential. Urinary tract infections in the early postoperative period have been associated with recurrence and even allograft dysfunction. The Foley catheter is generally left in place for one to five days. While in place, maintenance of patency and a closed system is critical. When irrigation is required, strict sterile technique must be followed. On removal of the catheter, a bacterial culture of the catheter tip may be obtained, as well as a routine urine culture 24 hours later. Weekly urine cultures are recommended during the hospital stay.

Vital signs should be monitored every six hours. Recipients should be pan-cultured for any temperature spike greater than 38.5° C and with each temperature spike until a causative organism is identified. Because prednisone can mask early fever, other signs of sepsis, such as tachycardia, must be assessed. Strict handwashing before and after patient contact must be performed. Recipients should, ideally, not be assigned to a room with an infected patient, and the nurse caring for a transplant recipient should not simultaneously be caring for an infected patient.

Intermediate Posttransplant Period

Most of the nursing care in the intermediate period involves assessment, diagnosis, intervention, and evaluation of the patient's response to the transplant process. The nursing process focuses on signs and symptoms, prevention and treatment of allograft rejection, infection, and complications of surgery and immunosuppression. Patient education must be an integral part of the process (see Chapter 15).

Evaluation of Fever

Fever is a common occurrence in the intermediate postoperative period and can be indicative of a number of problems. A careful and systematic evaluation is essential in order to arrive at the proper diagnosis and then implement appropriate care (Table 6–4).

TABLE 6–4. EVALUATION OF FEVER IN A KIDNEY TRANSPLANT PATIENT

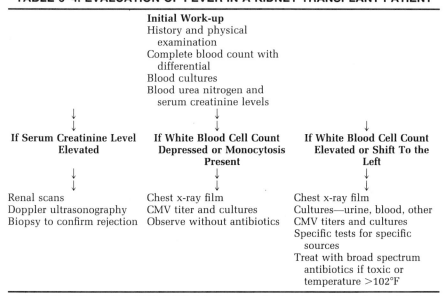

If Serum Creatinine Level Elevated	If White Blood Cell Count Depressed or Monocytosis Present	If White Blood Cell Count Elevated or Shift To the Left
Renal scans	Chest x-ray film	Chest x-ray film
Doppler ultrasonography	CMV titer and cultures	Cultures—urine, blood, other
Biopsy to confirm rejection	Observe without antibiotics	CMV titers and cultures
		Specific tests for specific sources
		Treat with broad spectrum antibiotics if toxic or temperature >102°F

Initial Work-up: History and physical examination; Complete blood count with differential; Blood cultures; Blood urea nitrogen and serum creatinine levels

From Bia, M.J. and Flye, M.W. (1989). Infectious complications in renal transplant recipients. In M.W. Flye (Ed.). *Principles of Organ Transplantation* (p. 300). Philadelphia: W.B. Saunders.

Assessment of Renal Function

In the intermediate postoperative period, assessment of renal function continues as described above. Daily laboratory values, including serum electrolyte, BUN, creatinine, and glucose levels, are monitored. A normally functioning transplanted kidney will maintain serum electrolyte levels within normal limits. Any electrolyte imbalances are treated as needed. Serum BUN and creatinine levels should return toward normal and then stabilize. Continued ATN often requires dialysis, and patient support is critical. It is important to explain to the patient why dialysis is necessary, and that it should be temporary. Increases in serum BUN and creatinine levels may be caused by cyclosporine toxicity, rejection, or a technical complication. If cyclosporine toxicity is suspected, dose adjustments are made.

Strict fluid intake and output recordings should be made every shift, and recipients should be weighed daily in a consistent manner. A decrease in urine output or a weight gain of greater than 1 kg per day should be reported and further assessed. Fluid restrictions are required for patients with ATN or symptoms of fluid overload. Fluid intake should be encouraged in patients with adequate diuresis.

Assessment of Other Laboratory Parameters

Daily white blood cell (WBC) counts should be monitored. A decreased WBC count (leukopenia) may indicate bone marrow depression secondary to immunosuppression, or it may be a sign of viremia. The presence of leukopenia necessitates a decrease in immunosuppression in order to minimize the chance of infection. A WBC count of less than 2000/μl may necessitate reverse isolation. An increased WBC count (leukocytosis) often occurs as a result of prednisone therapy while prednisone doses are high, but it may also indicate bacterial infection. Monitoring of the differential count may aid diagnosis. Hemoglobin concentration and hematocrit are obtained daily and may provide clues regarding fluid volume or blood loss. Daily platelet counts provide information regarding the effects of antilymphocyte globulin.

Liver function tests and calcium, phosphorus, total protein, albumin, and amylase levels are monitored at regular intervals. Abnormalities are assessed and treated appropriately. The nurse must carefully monitor for potential posttransplant complications. Prevention of complications is critical, but when they do occur, rapid diagnosis and appropriate treatment are essential. Nursing care for the transplant recipient is summarized in Table 6–5.

Discharge Teaching

Patient education is a critical part of posttransplant nursing care. Components of patient education include (a) knowledge of medication dosages, effects, and adverse reactions; (b) ability to recognize signs and symptoms of rejection and infection; (c) ability to perform blood pressure, pulse, and temperature monitoring; (d) knowledge of how to avoid complications; (e) dietary recommendations; and (f) general health care guidelines (see Chapter 15).

LONG-TERM CARE

The nursing interventions for patients in the distant postoperative period center around the medical problems listed in Table 6–6. Many of these problems are discussed in previous chapters or in more detail in other sources.

Laboratory evaluation of the patient assists in monitoring overall health parameters, but it is the regular clinic visit from which much information is garnered. The clinic visit is also a time in which reinforcement of patient teaching takes place.

Over the long term, patient visits to the transplant clinic decrease. Many centers refer patients back to their original care providers and act only as a consultation service.

In the long-term posttransplant period success rates remain quite high. Patient survival has been reported to be between 70 per cent and 85 per cent at 15 years after transplantation, with major causes of morbidity and mortality including vascular catastrophes, sepsis, liver failure, hypertension, and rejection (Rao & Andersen, 1988; Toussaint, Kinnaert & Vereerstraeten, 1988). Patients also report a significantly improved quality of life with a kidney transplant as compared with dialysis (Simmons, Anderson, Kamstra, & Ames, 1985; Simmons, Anderson, & Kamstra, 1984). Quality of life is perceived as of even greater significance with the use of cyclosporine as compared with conventional immunosuppression (Simmons, Abress, & Anderson, 1988). Such data speak highly for the benefits of kidney transplantation, both physical and psychological.

COMPLICATIONS

Urologic Complications

Urine Leaks

Urine leaks are uncommon, but can be troublesome occurrences after kidney transplant. Decreased urine output, lower abdominal tenderness,

TABLE 6–5. NURSING CARE PLAN FOR KIDNEY TRANSPLANT RECIPIENT

Nursing Diagnosis	Predisposing Factors	Signs and Symptoms	Nursing Interventions
Potential fluid overload	Acute tubular necrosis secondary to prolonged cold or warm ischemic time and/or drug-induced nephrotoxicity Intraoperative fluid administration Postoperative fluid administration	↑ CVP ↑ BP ↓ Hgb/Hct Pulmonary edema ↓ u/o	Monitor for signs and symptoms of hypervolemia. Administer diuretics as ordered. Monitor electrolytes. Auscultate lungs. Maintain fluid restrictions/replacement as ordered. Maintain strict intake/output. Obtain daily weights on same scale. Provide patient support and education if temporary dialysis is necessary.
Potential for dehydration	Osmotic diuresis with functioning kidney Diuretic administration	↓ u/o ↓ CVP ↓ BP ↑ Hgb/Hct	Monitor for signs and symptoms of hypovolemia. Monitor electrolytes. Maintain strict intake/output. Replace fluids as ordered. Obtain daily weights on same scale.

Nursing diagnosis	Related to	Signs and symptoms	Interventions
Altered immune system: potential for organ rejection	T and B cell activity Immunosuppressive therapy	↓ u/o Swelling and tenderness at graft site ↑ BUN, ↑ Cr Fever Weight gain Lower extremity edema Scrotal edema in males Anorexia, malaise	Monitor signs and symptoms of rejection. Administer immunosuppressive medications as ordered. Monitor lab values, assessing renal function and medication side effects.
Potential for infection	Immunosuppression Anesthesia Decreased mobility Intravenous and Foley catheters Preoperative status of patient (e.g., nutritional status, diabetes)	↑ Temp Tachycardia ↑ WBC (as seen with bacterial infections) ↓ WBC (may be seen with viral infections) Lesion eruption	Monitor for signs and symptoms of infection. Be aware that many signs and symptoms of infection are masked by high steroid doses. Pan culture when temperature reaches 100.5° F. Instruct and encourage use of incentive spirometer. Encourage coughing and deep breathing. Encourage ambulation. Assess type of sputum. Auscultate lungs. Assess mucous membranes for redness, drainage, pain, lesions. Maintain sterile technique with dressing and line changes. Maintain strict Foley care. Administer antimicrobials as ordered.

CVP, central venous pressure; BP, blood pressure; Hgb, hemoglobin; Hct, hematocrit; BUN, blood urea nitrogen; Cr, creatinine; u/o, urine output.

pain, distention, dysuria, elevated serum BUN and creatinine levels, and fever may signal a urine leak somewhere in the upper urinary tract. Such complications usually occur within 30 days postoperatively (Malkowicz & Perloff, 1985; Palmer & Chatterjee, 1978). Diagnosis of a urine leak is made by cystography or fluoroscopic percutaneous nephrostogram, assessing for urine extravasation along the urinary tract.

Bladder leaks are prevented by careful bladder anastomosis during implantation, as well as by decompression by means of a Foley catheter postoperatively. Bladder overdistention must be avoided. It is important to monitor for blood clots occluding the catheter, which may prevent adequate drainage and contribute to bladder distention. If a bladder leak does develop, treatment usually consists of long-term Foley catheter drainage. Occasionally surgical reanastomosis is required.

Ureteral leaks may be caused by ureteral devascularization during the donor nephrectomy and preservation. When ureteral leaks do occur, percutaneous nephrostogram fluoroscopy, with placement of an internal-external stent to promote drainage and healing, is performed (Ehrlichman, Bettman, Kirkman, & Tilney, 1986; Liberman, Glass, Crummy, Sollingers, & Belzer, 1982). The stent is generally left in place for several weeks as healing occurs; care must be taken to prevent infection. The insertion site of an external stent must be dressed and cared for using sterile technique. Routine urine cultures should be obtained to monitor for contamination. Occasionally surgical repair is necessary, but it is not without significant risk of graft loss.

Obstruction

Obstruction in the urinary tract can arise from a variety of sources. Ureteral stenosis can occur either early or late in the posttransplant course. The patient may present with decreased urine output (or anuria if the obstruction is complete) and a rise in serum BUN and creatinine levels. Ultrasonography demonstrates a dilated ureter above the stenosis, with marked narrowing at the point of obstruction and hydronephrosis.

TABLE 6–6. MEDICAL PROBLEMS IN KIDNEY TRANSPLANT RECIPIENTS

Infection
Liver disease; acute hepatitis and chronic liver disease
Hypertension
Cardiovascular disease; hyperlipidemia
Metabolic defects (bone disease, renal tubular defects, erythrocytosis, steroid-related complications)
Graft dysfunction (acute and chronic rejection, de novo and recurrent glomerulonephritis, obstruction, cyclosporine nephrotoxicity, renal artery stenosis)
Sexual dysfunction
Malignancy

If the obstruction is not complete, acute relief may be obtained by means of a percutaneous antegrade or cystoscopically placed retrograde stent. The stent is left in place for several weeks. Restenosis after stent removal is not uncommon. Surgical repair with reimplantation or native nephrectomy with ureteropyelostomy may be required (Malkowicz & Perloff, 1985).

Lymphocele

Because renal lymphatics and lymphatics in the iliac fossa are disrupted during surgery, and all may not be adequately ligated, postsurgical lymphoceles can form. Depending on the size and location of the lymphocele, varying degrees of obstruction may form along the urinary tract. The patient may present with genital or ipsilateral lower extremity edema or edema in both areas, as well as decreased urine output and a rise in serum BUN and creatinine levels. Diagnosis is made by ultrasonography, which demonstrates the lymphatic fluid collection and, depending on the location of the collection, a dilated ureter with or without hydronephrosis. Percutaneous drainage may relieve the collection and obstruction, but the relief is usually temporary. Surgical repair with a transabdominal peritoneal marsupialization is generally the definitive procedure for repair.

Vascular Complications

Vascular complications are relatively rare, but renal artery stenosis or venous thrombosis may occur. They are generally caused by complications in donor procurement, preservation, or implantation.

Renal Artery Stenosis

Renal artery stenosis may form early or late in the posttransplant course. It is evidenced by severe hypertension, renal dysfunction, and often an audible bruit. The effects of renal artery stenosis may be exacerbated by such angiotensin-converting enzyme inhibitors as captopril (Capoten) and enalapril (Vasotec). Diagnosis is made by angiography, and correction by balloon angioplasty or surgical resection of the stenosed artery.

Venous Thrombosis

Venous thrombosis, usually in the renal vein and occasionally in the iliac vein, is diagnosed by venography. Patients present with graft swelling, oliguria, significant proteinuria, and lower extremity edema. A thrombectomy may be performed and anticoagulant treatment initiated. Unfortunately, graft loss is most often the consequence.

Hypertension

Hypertension is commonly seen in the posttransplant recipient. Several factors may contribute to the development of high blood pressure, including cyclosporine administration, vascular expansion owing to the steroid-related salt and water retention, obesity, increased renin production by the patient's native kidneys or by the transplanted kidney during rejection, and renal artery stenosis. Because of the systemic short- and long-term effects of hypertension, control is critical.

Treatment of mild hypertension begins with a salt-restricted diet with or without diuretic therapy. Weight loss is encouraged in the overweight patient. Cyclosporine doses may be decreased. Antihypertensive medications are added in a stepwise manner, with attempts made to prescribe the most effective agents in the least complicated manner in order to aid patient compliance. Patient education regarding the rationale for dietary discretion and medication administration, as well as assessment of patient compliance, is essential. Patients should be encouraged to report any side effects experienced as a result of their prescribed antihypertensive medication, and drug substitutions may be made as appropriate. In cases of refractory hypertension assessment for renal renin levels and renal artery stenosis is performed. Rarely is a native nephrectomy required.

Rejection

Rejection is fully discussed in Chapter 3 and is reviewed only briefly here.

Hyperacute Rejection

The antibody–complement system is activated in the presence of preformed antibodies on the donor kidney. This occurs as soon as blood flow to the transplanted kidney is reestablished. Cellular destruction is rapid by way of intrarenal thrombosis. The newly transplanted organ quickly "dies," since there is no successful treatment for hyperacute rejection. Because of accurate pretransplant crossmatching, preformed antibodies are almost always discovered before transplantation, with transplant pursued only in cases of negative donor–recipient crossmatches.

Accelerated Acute Rejection

Accelerated acute rejection, although rare, has been described in kidney transplantation. It also results from the presence of preformed antibodies, but is generally caused by an anamnestic response. Treatment may be attempted with high-dose steroids or antilymphocyte globulin, but success is limited. Graft removal is most often required.

Acute Rejection

Acute rejection episodes, although seen in decreasing frequency, are not uncommon. The risk of occurrence is greatest in the first months post transplant, but it can be seen at any time in the posttransplant course. It is a cell-mediated response, with production of cytotoxic T cells against donor antigens.

Signs and symptoms of acute rejection in the transplanted kidney may include elevated serum BUN and creatinine levels, decreased urine output, weight gain, malaise, graft tenderness, and fever. The latter two symptoms, however, may not be pronounced in a patient treated with cyclosporine.

Various protocols are used to treat acute rejection episodes. Increased doses of steroids may be administered either orally or as one- to three-day intravenous boluses. Antilymphocyte preparations may be used. More recently OKT3, a monoclonal antibody, has been used to successfully reverse some acute rejection episodes.

Most episodes are reversible when diagnosed and treated early. The major risk of treating rejection episodes is increased risk of infection. Additionally, rejection therapy is generally contraindicated when concurrent infection exists. If rejection is persistent or repeated, or the recipient is particularly prone to infectious complications (e.g., elderly, concurrent viremia), the decision may be made to abandon rejection therapy, restore the patient's health, and consider retransplantation when possible.

Chronic Rejection

Chronic rejection usually occurs months to years after transplantation. In kidney transplantation chronic rejection is evidenced by a slowly progressive decline in organ function, over variable lengths of time. Currently there is no successful treatment to reverse this process.

It is important to consider the differential diagnoses when renal dysfunction exists. Because infection and cyclosporine nephrotoxicity can also present with one or several of the signs and symptoms above, a percutaneous renal biopsy is often performed to provide a differential diagnosis as well as to guide treatment. For the renal biopsy, the transplanted kidney is frequently located by ultrasound and the skin marked. After injection of a local anesthetic a percutaneous biopsy needle is inserted into the kidney, and a small core of renal tissue is extracted. The tissue is reviewed under a microscope to ascertain that a section of glomeruli and cortex have been obtained. Further evaluation by light and electron microscopy and immunofluorescence is undertaken to determine the presence of lymphocytes, vasculitis, fibrin deposits, complement, and interstitial nephritis. Diagnosis of acute versus chronic rejection can thus be made. It is often difficult to differentiate between cyclosporine nephrotoxicity and acute rejection. Biopsy information is used in combination with clinical manifestations and treatment decisions are then made based on the observed histologic changes.

The main risk of percutaneous renal biopsy is bleeding. Postbiopsy nursing care includes hand pressure on the site for 20 to 30 minutes followed by placement of a sandbag over the biopsy site for several hours. Bed rest is recommended for one to three hours. Vital signs are monitored frequently during the first two to four hours. Serial urine samples are collected for several hours to assess for the presence of blood.

SUMMARY

Transplant is a viable therapy for patients with end-stage renal failure. The nurse's role in assisting the patient through evaluation and transplantation is crucial to a successful outcome.

References

Anderson, C.B., Tyler, J.D., Sicard, G.A., Anderman, D.K., Rodey, G.E., & Etheredge, E.E. (1984). Pretreatment of renal allograft recipients with immunosuppression and donor-specific blood. *Transplantation, 38,* 664–668.

Belzer, F.O. (1984). Advances in renal transplantation. In R.L. Jamison (Ed.). *Transplantation in the 80's: Recent Advances* (pp. 23–35). New York: Praeger.

Briggs, J.D. (1988). The recipient of a renal transplant. In P.J. Morris (Ed.). *Kidney Transplantation: Principles and Practice* (3rd ed.) (pp. 71–92). Philadelphia: W.B. Saunders.

Cook, D.J. & Takiff, H. (1986). Original disease of the recipient. In P.I. Terasaki (Ed.). *Clinical Transplants 1986,* (pp. 311–319). Los Angeles: UCLA Tissue Typing Laboratory.

Cosimi, A.B. (1988). The donor and donor nephrectomy. In Morris, P.J. (Ed.). *Kidney Transplantation: Principles and Practice* (3rd ed.) (pp. 93–121), Philadelphia: W.B. Saunders.

Ehrlichman, R.J., Bettman, M., Kirkman, R.L., & Tilney, N.L. (1986, February). The use of percutaneous nephrostomy in patients with ureteric obstruction undergoing renal transplantation. *Surgery, Gynecology and Obstetrics, 162,* 121–126.

Glass, N.R., Miller, D.T., Sollinger, H.W., & Belzer, F.O. (1985, February). A four-year experience with donor blood transfusion protocols for living donor renal transplantation. *Transplantation Proceedings, 17,* 1023–1025.

Iwaki, Y. & P.I. Terasaki (1986). Donor-specific transfusion. In P.I. Terasaki (Ed.). *Clinical Transplants, 1986* (pp. 267–275). Los Angeles: UCLA Tissue Typing Laboratory.

Jordan, M.L., Novick, A.C., Steinmuller, D., Braun, W., Buszta, C., Mintz, D., Goormastic, M., & Streem, S. (1985, August). Renal transplantation in the older recipient. *The Journal of Urology, 134,* 243–246.

Klintman, G., Brynger, H., Flatmark, A., Frodin, L., Husberg, B., Thorsby, E., & Groth C.G. (1985, February). The blood transfusion, DR matching, and mixed lymphocyte culture effects are not seen in cyclosporine-treated renal transplant recipients. *Transplantation Proceedings, 17,* 1026–1031.

Lee, H.M. (1988). Surgical techniques of renal transplantation. In P.J. Morris (Ed.). *Kidney Transplantation: Principles and Practice* (3rd ed.) (pp. 215–234). Philadelphia: W.B. Saunders.

Lieberman, R.P., Glass, N.R., Crummy, A.B., Sollinger, H.W., & Belzer, F.O. (1982, November). Nonoperative percutaneous management of urinary fistulas and strictures in renal transplantation. *Surgery, Gynecology and Obstetrics, 155,* 667–672.

Light, J.A., Metz, S.J., & Oddenino, K. (1983). Donor-specific transfusion with minimal sensitization. *Transplantation Proceedings, 15,* 917–923.

Malkowicz, S.B. & Perloff, L.J. (1985, June). Urologic considerations in renal transplantation. *Surgery, Gynecology and Obstetrics, 160,* 579–588.

Monaco, A.P. (1985, February). Clinical kidney transplantation in 1984. *Transplantation Proceedings, 17,* 5–12.

Opelz, G. Sengar, D.P.S., Mickey, M.R., & Terasaki, P.I. (1973, March). Effects of blood transfusions on subsequent kidney transplants. *Transplantation Proceedings, 17,* 1015–1022.

Opelz, G. (1985, February). Current relevance of the transfusion effect in renal transplantation. *Transplantation Proceedings, 17,* 1015–1022.

Palmer, J.M. & Chatterjee, S.N. (1978, April). Urologic complications in renal transplantation. *Surgical Clinics of North America, 58,* 305–319.

Rao, K.V. & Andersen, R.C. (1988). Long-term results and complications in renal transplant recipients: Observations in the second decade. *Transplantation, 45,* 45–52.

Simmons, R.G., Abress, L., & Anderson, C.R. (1988). Quality of life after kidney transplantation: A prospective, randomized comparison of cyclosporine and conventional immunosuppressive therapy. *Transplantation, 45,* 415–421.

Simmons, R.G., Anderson, C.R., Kamstra, L.K., & Ames, N.G. (1985). Quality of life and alternate end-stage renal disease therapies. *Transplant Proceedings, 17,* 1577–1588.

Simmons, R.G., Anderson, C.R., & Kamstra, L.K. (1984). Comparison of quality of life of patients on continuous ambulatory peritoneal dialysis, hemodialysis, and after transplantation. *American Journal of Kidney Diseases, 4,* 253–255.

Sollinger, H.W., Kalayoglu, M., & Belzer, F.O. (1986, September). Use of the donor specific protocol in living unrelated donor-recipient combination. *Annals of Surgery, 204,* 315–321.

Staff. (1989, May). UNOS releases 1988 transplantation statistics. *UNOS Update, 5*(5), 1.

Starzl, T.E. (1964). Role of excision of lymphoid masses in attenuating the rejection process. In T.E. Starzl (Ed.), *Experiences in Renal Transplantation* (pp. 126–129). Philadelphia: W.B. Saunders.

Starzl, T.E. (1985, April). Will live organ donations no longer be justified? *Hastings Center Report, 15*(2), 5.

Sterioff, S., Engen, D.E., & Zincke, H. (1986). Current status of renal transplantation—1986. *Mayo Clinic Proceedings, 61,* 573–578.

Stuart, F.P., Reckard, C.R., Ketel, B.L., & Schulak, J.A. (1980). Effects of splenectomy on first cadaver kidney transplants. *Annals of Surgery, 192,* 553–561.

Toussaint, C., Kinnaert, P., & Vereerstraeten, P. (1988). Late mortality and morbidity five to eighteen years after kidney transplantation. *Transplantation, 45,* 554–558.

Vincenti, F., Amend, W.J.C., Kaysen, G., Feduska, N., Birnbaum, J., Duca, R., & Salvatierra, O. (1983). *Transplantation Proceedings, 36,* 626–629.

Weiland, D., Sutherland, D.E.R., Chavers, B., Simmons, R.L., Ascher, N.L., & Najarian, J.S. (1984). Information on 628 living-related kidney donors at a single institution with long-term followup in 472 cases. *Transplantation Proceedings, 16,* 5.

7

Liver Transplantation: Nursing Diagnoses and Management

Sandra Staschak and Karen Zamberlan

This chapter reviews the nursing care of the liver transplant patient. The nursing management for each phase of the transplant process is addressed. Using a nursing diagnoses framework developed by Carpenito (1987), the indications, referral, evaluation, and preoperative, postoperative, and rehabilitative needs of the patient undergoing liver transplantation are thoroughly detailed.

First, however, in order to better comprehend the complex nursing needs of the patient with end-stage liver disease who undergoes liver transplantation, a review of the anatomy and physiology of the liver is presented.

ANATOMY AND PHYSIOLOGY OF THE LIVER

The numerous functions performed by the liver have been categorized by Guyton (1981) into vascular, secretory, and metabolic. The vascular functions are for storage and filtration of blood. The secretory function is secretion of bile into the gastrointestinal tract. The metabolic functions provide for the utilization of nutrients and their conversion to fuel for energy, and the detoxification of drugs.

The liver is the largest organ in the body, weighing about 1.5 kg in the adult. Located in the upper right quadrant of the abdomen, it lies directly below the diaphragm. The falciform ligament secures the liver to the diaphragm and the abdominal wall. There is a large right lobe and a small left lobe; in addition, the caudate and quadrate lobes, the gallbladder, and the portal triad (passage site composed of portal vein,

140

hepatic artery, and bile duct) are located on the visceral surface of the liver. The inferior vena cava passes through the posterior surface of the liver, which is protected by the rib cage. In healthy people the liver cannot be palpated (Fig. 7–1).

The dual blood supply to the liver is provided by the hepatic artery and the portal vein. Oxygenated blood from the aorta flows by way of the celiac axis into the common hepatic artery, accounting for 30 per cent of the blood supply to the liver. The portal vein supplies the remaining 70 per cent of the blood, which is rich in absorbed nutrients from the stomach, intestines, spleen, and pancreas (Fig. 7–2). The portal

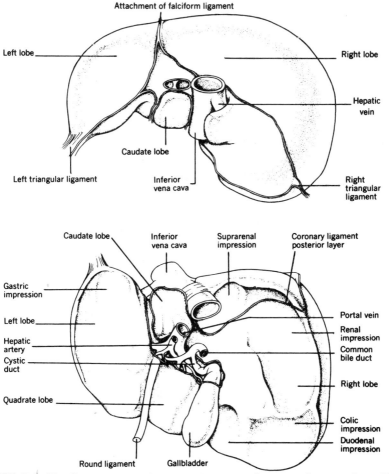

FIGURE 7–1. The liver, top, superior, posterior aspect; bottom, inferior surface. (From Chaffee, E.E. & Lytle, I.M. (1980). Basic Physiology and Anatomy (4th ed.). Philadelphia: J.B. Lippincott Company.)

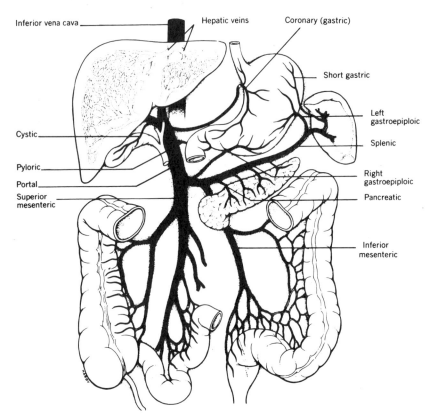

FIGURE 7–2. The portal and hepatic venous system. (From Chaffee, E.E. & Lytle, I.M. (1980). Basic Physiology and Anatomy (4th ed.). Philadelphia: J.B. Lippincott Company.)

system plus the arterial blood to the liver constitute part of the splanchnic circulation. The hepatic artery and portal vein enter the liver at the porta hepatis and divide into interlobular branches as they follow the septa formed by connective tissue throughout the liver. Blood is removed from the liver lobules by central veins that empty into sublobular veins and, finally, the hepatic veins. The hepatic veins drain into the vena cava, entering just below the diaphragm. About 50 per cent of the population have typical vasculature; the remainder have aberrant or anomalous vessels.

The liver produces approximately 600 to 1000 ml of yellow-green bile each day. Bile is produced in the liver lobules and contains water, bile salts, bilirubin, cholesterol, and various inorganic acids. As the bile is produced, it drains into the canaliculi (spaces between the rows of hepatic cells), interlobular bile ducts, right and left common bile ducts, and, finally, into the common hepatic duct, and is stored in the gallbladder. The bile flow follows the branches of the hepatic artery and portal vein within the liver; however, this bile flow is in the opposite direction of the hepatic blood flow (Guyton, 1981).

Bile salts are formed from cholesterol, which is either supplied by the diet or synthesized by the liver. Bile salts aid digestion by emulsifying dietary fats and are necessary for the formation of the micelles that transport fatty acids and fat-soluble vitamins to the surface of the intestinal mucosa for absorption. About 90 per cent of the bile salts excreted into the gastrointestinal tract are reabsorbed into the portal circulation in the distal ileum. They are reabsorbed by the liver and re-excreted in a process called the enterohepatic circulation. Bile salts can be recycled approximately 18 times before they are lost in the feces (Orr, Shinert, & Gross, 1981).

Bilirubin, a component of bile, gives bile its yellow color. It is derived from the heme portion of hemoglobin released from the break-down of red blood cells. Unconjugated, or indirect, bilirubin, which is insoluble in plasma, is transported, bound to albumin, and removed from the blood by the liver. Once inside the hepatocytes, bilirubin is conjugated with glucuronic acid so that it becomes bile- and also water-soluble. This conjugated, or direct, bilirubin is excreted in bile directly into the intestinal tract. In the intestines, normal bacterial flora aid in the breakdown of bilirubin into urobilinogen. Urobilinogen is excreted in feces and oxidized to stercobilin, which produces the brown color of stool. Bilirubin excreted from the blood by way of the kidneys provides the yellow color of urine. In liver disease, inability to secrete bilirubin results in its deposition in body tissues, producing the yellow discoloration of skin known as jaundice.

Bile is continually secreted by hepatocytes, and stored in the gall-bladder until fat in the duodenum stimulates its release. The primary stimulus for the secretion of bile from the gallbladder is release of the hormone cholecystokinin from the intestinal mucosa. This hormone promotes contraction of the gallbladder, forcing bile toward the duo-denum. Vagal stimulation associated with gastric secretion aids gallblad-der contraction. This contraction of the gallbladder and relaxation of the sphincter of Oddi permits the concentrated bile to enter the duodenum.

The liver is composed of 50,000 to 100,000 functional cylindrical units called lobules. Each lobule is several millimeters in length and 0.8 to 2.0 mm in diameter. The liver lobules are each constructed around a central vein that empties into the hepatic veins and, eventually, into the vena cava (Fig. 7–3). The lobule is composed of hepatic plates that radiate centrally like the spokes of a wagon wheel. Between each hepatic plate are small bile canaliculi that empty into terminal bile ducts originating in the septa between adjacent liver lobules. Blood from portal venules and arterioles empties into channels called sinusoids, which run

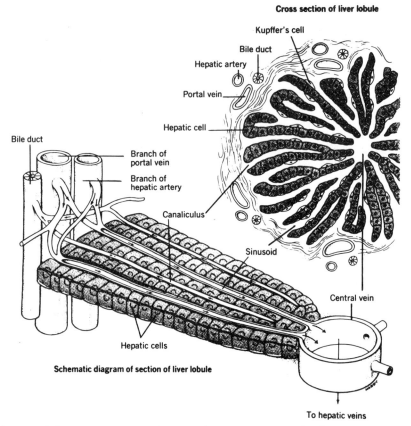

FIGURE 7–3. Schematic diagram of section of liver lobule. (From Chaffee, E.E. & Lytle, I.M. (1980). Basic Physiology and Anatomy (4th ed.). Philadelphia: J.B. Lippincott Company.)

along the sides of the hepatic plates and empty into the central veins (Guyton, 1981).

Lining the walls of the venous sinusoids are endothelial cells and phagocytic Kupffer's cells, which are part of the reticuloendothelial system. Bacteria and other foreign matter in the blood are filtered and removed here so that virtually no bacteria reach the general systemic circulation. Between the endothelial cells and the hepatocytes is a narrow space called the space of Disse, which collects plasma proteins and connects freely with the lymphatics to remove excess fluid (Guyton, 1981).

The liver is important in carbohydrate metabolism, particularly the maintenance of a normal blood glucose concentration. Glycogenesis is the process of glycogen formation. Glucose that is not used for energy is converted into glycogen by the hepatocytes. All cells of the body are capable of storing at least some glycogen, but hepatocytes can store up to 8 per cent of their weight as glycogen. When the blood glucose level increases to above normal (80–120 mg/dl), glucose is quickly stored as glycogen. When the blood glucose level decreases to below normal, then glycogen stored in the liver is rapidly converted back to glucose for energy. Insulin also causes uptake of glucose by hepatocytes to form glycogen. This permits the liver to act as a glucose buffer system (Orr et al., 1981).

Glycogenolysis is the process whereby glycogen is converted to glucose. The breakdown of glycogen to form glucose is catalyzed by the enzyme phosphorylase, which splits glucose molecules off the glycogen chain one at a time. This conversion occurs when the blood glucose level markedly falls, resulting in the release of the hormone glucagon by the pancreas. Within minutes, glucagon causes a series of reactions in the hepatocytes that lead to a rapid production of glucose. Certain stimuli to the sympathetic nervous system cause the adrenal medulla to secrete epinephrine, which has an effect similar to that of glucagon. The result is conversion of glycogen stored in muscle cells to glucose for quick energy. The liver functions as the glycogen-storage organ for the body because all of the enzymes necessary for the conversion of monosaccharides and fructose into glucose are present in the liver. If glycogen stores are depleted, the liver can make glucose from deaminated amino acids and the glycerol part of fats. This process, known as gluconeogenesis, occurs in response to a decrease in the blood glucose concentration.

The most important functions of the liver in protein metabolism are deamination of amino acids, formation of urea for the removal of ammonia from the blood, formation of plasma proteins, and interconversions among the different amino acids. Amino acids must be deaminated before they can be used for energy or converted into carbohydrates or fats. Ammonia is released during deamination. The remaining keto acid is then oxidized in the citric acid cycle for energy. Ammonia is removed from the blood by conversion to urea in the liver. The urea diffuses out of the hepatocytes into the blood and is excreted by the kidneys. Moderate amounts of ammonia are also continually formed in the intestines by bacteria and are then absorbed into the blood. Therefore, without this function of the liver, the plasma ammonia concentration rapidly rises, which may lead to hepatic coma and death.

Except for the gamma globulins, which are produced in lymph tissue, hepatocytes produce most of the proteins in the blood. Plasma protein depletion causes mitosis of the hepatocytes and growth of the liver, to increase plasma protein output. The three types of plasma proteins are albumins, globulins, and fibrinogen. Albumin maintains the blood oncotic pressure to prevent plasma loss from the capillaries. Globulins are present in large quantities in both the plasma and the cells.

Fibrinogen helps to form blood clots by polymerizing into long threads (Guyton, 1981).

Although fat metabolism can take place in almost all cells of the body, certain aspects of fat metabolism occur much more rapidly in the liver. The liver is involved in three functions of fat metabolism: (1) oxidation of fatty acids and formation of acetoacetic acid; (2) formation of lipoproteins, cholesterol, and phospholipids; and (3) conversion of carbohydrates and proteins to fat.

Lipoproteins, phospholipids, and cholesterol are formed in the liver. The lipoproteins function to carry lipid substances to other cells from the liver. Phospholipids are thought to aid in the transport of fatty acids through the intestinal mucosa and serve various structural purposes in intracellular organelles and cell membranes. Cholesterol is supplied in the diet and produced by hepatocytes. Of the cholesterol produced in the liver, 80 per cent is converted to cholic acid and secreted in bile salts to aid in intestinal absorption of fat-soluble substances. The remainder enters the blood, transported in the lipoproteins.

Miscellaneous metabolic functions of the liver include (1) storage of vitamins; (2) formation of blood coagulation factors; and (3) detoxification of drugs, hormones, and toxic substances. The liver has a propensity for storage of vitamin A, vitamin D, and vitamin B_{12} for as long as four months (Orr et al., 1981). Hepatocytes also contain 15 per cent to 30 per cent of the total iron supply of the body, stored in the liver as alpha ferritin. The liver is the site of synthesis of fibrinogen, prothrombin (factor II), accelerator globulin (factor V), and factors VII, VIII, IX, and X. Factors II, VII, IX, and X require vitamin K for synthesis. Vitamin K is fat-soluble, and can be absorbed from the intestinal tract only in the presence of bile salts. The liver also removes active clotting factors from the circulation, thereby preventing intravascular clotting.

Blood that enters the liver through the portal circulation is filtered by the phagocytic action of the Kupffer cells that line the sinusoids. These cells engulf foreign particles. This filtration removes intestinal or foreign bacteria present in the blood as well as endotoxins. Drugs, hormones, poisons, and other toxic substances are metabolized in the liver and converted into inactive forms for excretion. The liver accomplishes this through conversion of these fat and soluble compounds, which can readily be excreted in bile and urine.

PATHOPHYSIOLOGY OF HEPATIC FAILURE

Table 7–1, which reviews the major functions of the liver, serves as a framework to explain the symptoms of liver disease. Cholestatic liver disease is usually manifested by impairment of excretory function with

TABLE 7–1. FUNCTIONS OF THE LIVER AND MANIFESTATIONS OF ALTERED FUNCTION

FUNCTION	MANIFESTATIONS OF ALTERED FUNCTION
Production of bile salts	Malabsorption of fat and fat-soluble vitamins
Elimination of bilirubin	Failure to eliminate bilirubin elevates serum bilirubin level and causes jaundice
Metabolism of steroid hormones	
Estrogen and progesterone	Disturbances in gonadal function, including gynecomastia in the male
Testosterone	Signs of Cushing's syndrome
Glucocorticoids	Sodium retention and edema; hypokalemia
Aldosterone	
Metabolism of drugs	Decreased plasma binding of drugs due to decreased albumin production
	Decreased removal of drugs that are metabolized by the liver
Carbohydrate metabolism	Hypoglycemia may develop when glycogenolysis and
Stores glycogen	gluconeogenesis are impaired
Synthesizes glucose from amino acids, lactic acid, glycerol	Abnormal glucose tolerance curve may occur because of impaired uptake and release of glucose by the liver
Fat metabolism	
Formation of lipoproteins	Impaired synthesis of lipoproteins
Conversion of carbohydrates and proteins to fat	
Synthesis of cholesterol	
Formation of ketones from fatty acids	
Protein metabolism	
Deamination of proteins	
Formation of urea from ammonia	Elevated blood ammonia level
Synthesis of plasma proteins	Decreased levels of plasma proteins, particularly albumin, which contribute to edema formation
Synthesis of clotting factors	Bleeding tendency
Fibrinogen	
Prothrombin	
Factors V, VII, IX, X	
Storage of minerals and vitamins	Signs of deficiency of fat-soluble and other vitamins that are stored in the liver
Filtration of blood and removal of bacteria and particulate matter by Kupffer cells	Increased exposure of the body to colon bacilli and other foreign matter

(Reprinted with permission from Porth, C. M. (1986). Pathophysiology: Concepts of Altered Health States. Philadelphia: J.B. Lippincott) preservation of synthetic and metabolic functions. In contrast, hepato-cellular disease is manifested by synthetic, metabolic, and filtration dysfunctions. Therefore, patients with cholestatic disease appear health-ier than comparable patients with hepatocellular disease (Table 7–2). A third category includes diseases of the biliary tree, tumors, and hepatic receptor defects (Van Thiel, Tarter, & Stone, 1986).

The hepatocytes constantly produce and secrete bile. In hepatic failure adequate amounts of bile salts cannot be manufactured. Obstruc-tion of bile flow into the ducts (cholestasis) or a paucity of intrahepatic bile ducts leads to cirrhosis of the hepatic lobule and subsequent blockage of the bile canaliculi by scar tissue. Insufficient quantities of bile salts are available for fat emulsification in the small intestine.

Bile salts increase fat solubility, and form micelles with fatty acids to enhance absorption of lipids through gastrointestinal mucosa (Orr et al., 1981). Fat malabsorption occurs because limited bile is available to aid in this process. The patient has fatty stools, known as steatorrhea, which are greasy, large, and foul-smelling. Furthermore, reduced absorp-tion of the fat-soluble vitamins (A, D, E, and K) occurs.

Bile salts are conserved by reabsorption in the intestines, and returned to the liver by way of the enterohepatic circulation. In the liver the bile salts containing cholesterol are then extracted from the portal circulation and recycled by the action of an enzyme, glucuronyl trans-ferase. The cause of cholestatic pruritus is unclear but may be due to retained bile salts or unusual physiochemical forms of bile acids pro-duced in hepatic disease (Novak & Balistreri, 1985). Rising plasma levels of bile salts lead to deposition in the skin, presumably causing pruritus. Serum cholesterol levels five times the normal limit are associated with cutaneous xanthomas, fatty, tumor-like deposits in the skin (Keith, 1985).

TABLE 7–2. ADULT DISEASE-SPECIFIC INDICATIONS FOR LIVER TRANSPLANTATION

CHOLESTATIC DISEASES
Primary biliary cirrhosis
Sclerosing cholangitis

HEPATOCELLULAR DISEASES
Postnecrotic cirrhosis
Fulminant hepatic failure
Wilson's disease
Tyrosinemia
Alpha$_1$-antitrypsin deficiency
Hemochromatosis

OTHER DISEASES
Caroli's disease
Intrahepatic cholelithiasis
Hepatoma
Secondary biliary cirrhosis

Cutaneous xanthomas usually accompany pruritus and can occur anywhere on the body. They are more noticeable on the face (eyes and lips), arms, legs, and back.

Elevated Bilirubin Level

The destruction of senescent red blood cells in the reticuloendothelial system releases free, unconjugated bilirubin, which is bound to albumin in the plasma (Keith, 1985). The iron released from the red cell destruction is routinely stored in hepatocytes as ferritin (Orr et al., 1981). Hepatic disease reduces the liver's ability to conjugate bilirubin or store iron liberated from the degradation of hemoglobin. Jaundice is caused by elevated unconjugated bilirubin levels in the serum. This form of bilirubin (fat-soluble) has a special affinity for elastin tissue, such as the sclera and the oral membranes. The diseased liver attempts to conjugate bilirubin so that it can be excreted. Because the conjugated bilirubin is water-soluble, it is excreted by the kidneys, producing dark, tea-colored urine. Chronically jaundiced patients possess a long-lived bilirubin molecule linked to their plasma proteins, which presumably explains the slow resolution of prolonged jaundice after liver transplantation (Van Thiel et al., 1986).

Decreased Albumin Synthesis

Albumin is responsible for maintaining plasma colloid pressure. The normal liver synthesizes 12 g of albumin per day. The diseased liver is unable to synthesize adequate amounts. Fluid is then free to pass into the peritoneal cavity, causing ascites. Ascites is also enhanced by increased portal pressure and sodium retention owing to the secretion of aldosterone. Increased intrasinusoidal pressure within the liver because of cirrhosis can increase the ascitic fluid production and protein loss. Ascites causes abdominal swelling characterized by increasing abdominal girth. Increased fluid accumulation may cause pressure on the diaphragm, leading to respiratory and nutritional difficulties. The associated hypoproteinemia from albumin loss may lead to anasarca, or generalized edema due to fluid movement into all interstitial compartments (Bullock & Rosendahl, 1984).

Altered Clotting Ability

The liver synthesizes many of the clotting factors, such as fibrinogen, prothrombin, and factors V, VII, IX, and X. Various somatomedins essential for growth of tissues and organs are also synthesized. Liver disease interferes with the hepatocytes' ability to make glucose available for energy; thus low blood glucose levels are common. Patients with hepatocellular disease have more profound synthetic dysfunction than patients with cholestatic disease. The former have diminished plasma albumin levels and greater abnormalities of their prothrombin times. Vitamin K administration will not correct clotting defects in patients with hepatocellular disease. In addition, the diseased liver is unable to adequately remove clotting factors from the blood. Prolonged bleeding time, abnormal prothrombin time and partial thromboplastin time, and even disseminated intravascular clotting can result. The platelet count may also be low because of hypersplenism, which frequently accompanies liver failure.

Diminished Phagocytic Activity

The cleansing action of the Kupffer cells and the reticuloendothelial system is responsible for the liver's vascular filtration function. Patients with impaired vascular filtration are more prone to bacterial infections, especially spontaneous bacterial peritonitis, or cholangitis because of the diminished capacity of functioning cells.

Portal Hypertension

Obstruction of the blood flow in the liver increases the portal venous pressure. Portal hypertension leads to formation of a collateral venous system, which returns blood to the heart, bypassing the liver. The vessels most often affected are the esophageal, splenic, small bowel, and hemorrhoidal veins. Varices form, and bleeding may occur spontaneously or be precipitated by vomiting or coughing. Severe clotting defects may contribute to significant hemorrhage as well as make it difficult to arrest the bleeding.

As collaterals develop because of the high portal pressure, blood is shunted directly into the inferior vena cava, bypassing the liver. The shunted blood contains large amounts of ammonia and other products that cannot be metabolized in the liver, and this may lead to hepatic encephalopathy and in end stage disease, to coma.

Malnutrition

Nutrients are absorbed from the portal circulation, and they are processed and stored or distributed for use by other tissues. Impairment in the ability to produce glucose by the liver causes the blood glucose level to fall. Interference with the production of glucose (glycogenolysis or gluconeogenesis) or the utilization of glucose (glycogenesis) is reflected in hyperglycemia or hypoglycemia.

Other substances such as vitamins and drugs are metabolized and stored in the liver. Hepatocellular disease limits the liver's storage ability, and biliary obstruction reduces the uptake of fat-soluble vitamins, leading to various vitamin-deficiency syndromes. Administration and absorption of drugs that are metabolized in the liver can lead to toxic drug levels. The use of even small amounts of certain sedatives or antiemetics can lead to profound coma.

Failure to Absorb Vitamin D

The liver plays a critical role in the activation of vitamin D, without which there is decreased serum calcium. The body attempts to compensate by stimulating the parathyroid hormone, which increases resorption of calcium from the bones. If this process is longstanding, severe osteoporosis can result.

INDICATIONS FOR LIVER TRANSPLANTATION

The indications for orthotopic liver transplantation have become less restrictive as the success of this procedure has increased. A number of technical refinements have contributed to the improved results. These include the introduction of the veno-venous bypass, improvements in biliary tract reconstruction, and the development of techniques for multiple-organ procurement.

Liver transplantation should, ideally, be considered for any premoribund patient with progressive liver disease for whom the standard therapy for that particular condition is no longer successful. In practice, the two major disease categories are severe parenchymatous liver disease and primary malignancy of the liver. Despite these broad indications, practically every type of advanced and irreversible liver disease has been included in the indications for orthotopic liver transplantation (Table 7–3).

During the early period of liver transplantation many patients were already in a terminal stage of disease by the time a decision for referral had been made. This in part contributed to the poor survival statistics after transplantation (Starzl, Iwatsuki, Van Thiel, Gartner, Zitelli et al., 1982).

The problem of choosing the optimum time for transplantation is

TABLE 7–3. INDICATIONS FOR ORTHOTOPIC LIVER TRANSPLANTATION

Elevated serum bilirubin level
Decreased serum albumin level
Prolonged prothrombin time
Incapacitating hepatic encephalopathy
Portosystemic shunt procedures—if shunt procedures are contemplated, then the patient
  should be referred for transplant (unless it is a lifesaving procedure)
Primary hepatocellular carcinoma with absence of other indications
Spontaneous bacterial peritonitis
Incapacitating bone pain or spontaneous fractures
Intractable ascites with maximum medical therapy
Severe pruritus that causes the patient to entertain suicidal ideations

particularly difficult in cirrhosis, in which the clinical course and life expectancy are so variable. Only too often death follows a sudden and unpredictable clinical deterioration (e.g., variceal hemorrhage).

Patients with cirrhosis from any cause who, at the time of consideration for transplantation, already have a major bleeding tendency, evidence of sepsis, severe renal failure, or other disease, including malnutrition, are not the most ideal candidates for transplantation. Conversely, it is for patients in whom clinical deterioration is more gradual, with progressive worsening of liver function tests, ascites requiring increasing doses of diuretics, or chronic hepatic encephalopathy necessitating repeated hospital admissions, that liver transplantation should be considered (Calne & Williams, 1988).

Clinical expertise reflects that certain factors may adversely affect survival beyond six months. A pragmatic guide for identifying those patients who are at greatest risk and may require elective liver transplantation may be summarized as follows:

(1) inability to conduct a normal life-style;

(2) incapacitating encephalopathy;

(3) disabling lethargy;

(4) bone pain and spontaneous fractures;

(5) small liver volume with poor synthetic function;

(6) refractory ascites;

(7) variceal bleeding not controlled by sclerotherapy; and

(8) spontaneous bacterial peritonitis.

REFERRAL, RISK FACTORS, AND EVALUATION

Patients who present with end-stage liver disease are usually referred for evaluation when symptoms appear or acute decompensation is experienced. Referral is made by the primary care physician to the transplant center. A brief history and assessment of the patient's status from the referring physician determine how soon the patient will be seen at the transplant center.

The generally accepted risk factors that may exclude or decrease the chance of successful liver transplantation are listed in Table 7–4. With further refinements in the surgical technique and improvements in the postoperative management, fewer patients will be excluded as candidates for liver transplantation.

Orthotopic liver transplantation may be associated with significant morbidity and mortality. Patients with severely compromised and uncorrectable cardiac and respiratory function may not be able to tolerate such a major procedure, and thus are not accepted for liver transplantation.

Active infection outside the liver is a relative exclusion factor for liver transplantation, since the immunosuppressive therapy used in the posttransplant period could lead to rapidly progressive, overwhelming sepsis and death. However, these patients may be transplanted as soon as the sepsis is controlled.

Patients with alcoholic liver disease present an interesting dilemma. Although patients with this diagnosis have not been categorically eliminated from consideration for liver transplantation, some rules do apply. It is important to distinguish between "active alcoholism" (those patients actively drinking) and alcoholic liver disease (those patients sustaining severe liver damage from prior abuse), and to evaluate each candidate individually. The patient with alcoholic liver disease should ideally have a verifiable period of sobriety and successfully complete the preoperative evaluation. However, experience has demonstrated that pretransplant sobriety is not a good indicator of posttransplant compliance (Starzl, Van Thiel, Tzakis, Iwatsuka, Todo et al., 1988). Alcoholic liver disease can be cured by liver transplantation, but alcoholism must be treated before and after transplantation.

Without family support and strong self-motivation, and without

TABLE 7–4. RISK FACTORS IN LIVER TRANSPLANTATION

EXCLUDE	MAY EXCLUDE
General	**General**
Advanced cardiac disease	Portal vein thrombosis
Advanced vascular disease	Age >65 years*
Advanced respiratory disease	Hepatobiliary sepsis
Advanced neurological disease	Stage IV, hepatic coma
Active extrahepatobiliary sepsis and infection	Psychological factors
Specific	Financial factors
Extrahepatic malignancy	Previous abdominal surgery
Metastatic liver disease	**Specific**
AIDS/ARC	Active HBV replication

AIDS, acquired immunodeficiency syndrome; ARC, AIDS-related complex; HBV, hepatitis B virus.
*The chronological age may be older if physiologically fit.

continued therapy, these patients are likely to return to their prior habits. Additionally, alcohol abuse has frequently injured not only the liver, but also the lungs, heart, and kidneys to the extent that the patient's ability to undergo transplantation is adversely affected. Consultations for these patients may include a cardiology evaluation, a pulmonary evaluation, and a psychiatric assessment.

Metastatic liver disease is usually an exclusion for liver transplantation. Exceptions may be slow growing tumors such as neuro-endocrine tumors of the pancreas. The immunosuppressive therapy used after the transplant may lead to either recurrence of the original tumor or rapid progression of the existing disease.

An adequate portal and arterial blood supply is essential for a successful outcome. Patients with thrombosis of the portal vein have historically been unsuitable candidates for liver transplantation, since the necessary portal venous vascular input and all of its contained nutrients, hormones, and hepatotrophic factors will be absent. However, successful liver transplantation has recently been performed in these patients by either thrombectomy of the occluded portal vein or resection of the thrombosed portion of the vein and reconstruction with a vein graft.

Historically, patients over age 55 have also been excluded as candidates. However, the patient's state of health, rather than chronological age, appears to be clearly more important, and a number of patients over age 65 have been successfully transplanted (Starzl, Todo, Gordon, Makowka, Tzakis et al., 1987).

Previous abdominal surgery in the area of the hepatic hilum is a relative contraindication to liver transplantation. The adhesions from previous surgery in the presence of portal hypertension add to the complexity of the procedure and often lead to excessive blood loss (Starzl, Iwatsuki, Van Thiel, Gartner, Zitelli, et al., 1982).

Patients with active hepatitis B virus infection are at increased risk because the virus universally reinfects the transplanted liver, with recurrence of the disease (Starzl, Iwatsuki, Shaw, Gordon & Esquivel, 1985). Alpha-interferon has been used experimentally without obvious success in an attempt to prevent recurrence of the hepatitis B virus by augmenting immunity. Experimental therapy with antihepatitis B monoclonal antibody is currently under investigation (T.E. Starzl, personal communication, February 20, 1988). Fortunately, despite the high rate of recurrence, the disease is not as fulminant, and long-term survival may be possible (Van Thiel, 1985).

Patients who are in a hepatic coma are considered high-risk candidates. Once stage IV coma is reached, irreversible brain injury, brain stem herniation, or intracerebral hemorrhage may occur, making recovery impossible.

Financial consideration, relating both to the transplant and hospitalization as well as to the cost of medication after the transplant, may be prohibitive. If the patient is unable to accept these responsibilities, this may be a risk factor, excluding them as a transplant candidate.

A psychological assessment should be done. A history of a major psychiatric illness or apparent poor motivation for the procedure may also be considered a risk factor. Although these patients can be managed in the hospital, noncompliance after discharge can jeopardize the patient's life.

Consideration of the psychological, family, and social situation is of importance during assessment. Liver transplantation inevitably imposes great stress on the whole family, and it is essential that families receive necessary counseling and support. Because the operation is available in only a few centers, most families have to travel long distances and spend long periods away from home with an extremely ill family member. Families are often separated, particularly if a healthy spouse must return to children, job, or other family responsibilities. There may be prolonged interruption of careers, with resulting job loss. Problems with transportation and accommodations may add to the difficulties. For families from abroad there may also be language problems, which may cause further isolation (see Chapter 19). All of these factors contribute to the emotional and financial stress on the family unit. After transplantation, continued support is essential to help the family cope with any complications that may occur and with frequent hospital visits. Many families find it difficult to adjust after such disruption to family life (Calne, 1987).

PREOPERATIVE EVALUATION

The purpose of the preoperative evaluation is threefold: (1) to confirm the diagnosis, (2) to evaluate the patient's quality of life, and (3) to assess the progression of the disease. Evaluation includes medical and surgical assessment, psychosocial assessment, diagnostic testing, and nutrition screening.

The following mandatory factors in selecting candidates have been reported by Van Thiel and associates (1984):

1. Irreversible, chronic progressive liver disease
2. Progression of disease to a stage where all other forms of therapy are exhausted
3. No contraindications for orthotopic liver transplantation
4. Ability to accept the procedure and understand its nature and costs

A reasonable guide for the preoperative evaluation of potential liver recipients has been reported by Iwatsuki, Shaw, & Starzl (1983), with appropriate care being given to the state of hydration, renal status, and presence or absence of encephalopathy. The evaluation may be carried out on an inpatient or outpatient basis, depending on the severity of the patient's illness. The tests outlined in Table 7–5 should provide sufficient data to determine whether or not the patient is a transplant candidate.

Colonoscopy is indicated in sclerosing cholangitis and in all cases complicated by lower gastrointestinal bleeding. Angiography is reserved for cases in which patency of the portal or hepatic veins cannot be determined with less invasive techniques such as sonography, dynamic computed tomography (CT) scanning, or magnetic resonance imaging. Van Thiel (1985) suggests that cholangiography be performed only if insufficient data are available about the anatomy of the biliary tree, or if a concern about the presence of cholangiolar carcinoma exists.

Although not included as an evaluation requirement for liver trans-

TABLE 7–5. PREOPERATIVE EVALUATION OF LIVER TRANSPLANT RECIPIENTS

Complete history and physical examination to include:
  Review of past medical/surgical records
  Determination of body weight and height, measurement of chest circumference
  Nutritional evaluation
Basic laboratory data to include:
  Complete blood count with platelet count
  Electrolytes, BUN, creatinine, glucose, magnesium, calcium, phosphorus, and uric acid
    levels
  Protein electrophoresis; bilirubin, gamma glutamyl transpeptidase, amylase, and fasting
    blood ammonia levels; prothrombin time; partial thromboplastin time; coagulation
    profile; arterial blood gas determination; and indocyanine green clearance
  Hepatitis A and B serologic screens
  RPR and HIV status
Cultures as indicated: blood, urine, sputum, ascitic fluid, etc.
Blood typing, HLA typing, and cytotoxic antibody screen
Special studies for liver disease as indicated:
  Ceruloplasmin
  Alpha$_1$-antitrypsin level and phenotype
  Antimitochondrial, antithyroid, and antinuclear antibodies
  Iron, iron binding capacity and saturation, ferritin
  Quantitative immunoglobulins
Radiologic procedures
  Posteroanterior and lateral chest
  Abdominal ultrasound
  Abdominal CT
  Cholangiography (not all cases)
  Angiography (not all cases)
Consultant procedures and evaluations as indicated
  UGI panendoscopy
  Colonoscopy
  ERCP
  Ophthalmologic examination
  Neuropsychiatric evaluation
  EEG
  Social service

plantation, the importance of candidates meeting previous recipients during the candidates' evaluation cannot be stressed enough. Fears and anxieties are either heightened temporarily or relieved immediately.

CRITERIA FOR CANDIDACY AND THE WAITING PERIOD

After the evaluation, each patient's case may be discussed by the multidisciplinary transplant team, composed of physicians, social workers, clergy, nurses, and representatives of other relevant disciplines. The purpose of this transplant conference is to communicate, plan, evaluate, and educate. Throughout the case presentations, the necessary data are collected. This includes portal vein patency, laboratory assessment, liver volume, chest circumference, historical data (e.g., surgery and gastrointestinal bleeding), and other significant clinical data, such as recurrent bleeding, cholangitis, ascites, hepatitis screen, human immunodeficiency virus status, current clinical information, and medical urgency status.

If a patient is accepted, her name is activated on the computerized waiting list at the center where the transplant will occur. This information is entered into the UNOS (United Network for Organ Sharing) computer system, in which candidates can be identified and possibly matched if and when suitable donor organs become available.

Sometimes the more urgent candidates must remain in the hospital during the waiting period, and are managed by the transplant team. If a candidate's condition is relatively stable but urgent, she may remain in the local area and be followed as an outpatient in the clinic or private office of the transplant service. Even when the candidate returns home, the transplant service, usually through the coordinator, will continue to monitor the candidate in conjunction with the primary care physician. Information relevant to the candidate's condition is reviewed by the transplant team, and her medical urgency status is either confirmed or changed accordingly.

It is important to define the candidate's current status on the transplant list. An active candidate is ready for transplantation; a candidate who is in some way physically or emotionally unable to go through the procedure is considered inactive. Some candidates are considered inactive simply because they are too healthy or because they have not exhausted all options of traditional medical therapy. If a patient has been referred early for transplant, she may be listed as low priority, and is periodically reevaluated through contact with the primary care physician. These patients may also be reexamined as outpatients, depending on their condition, at various intervals.

Because of the shortage of acceptable donor organs and the ever-increasing size of waiting lists, many weeks or months may go by before the candidate is called for transplantation. This is a tense and emotional period for the candidate and for the family, who suffer equally as the wait continues. An important aspect of the transplant coordinator's and transplant social worker's roles is to monitor candidates' emotional and social stability during the waiting period, providing constant reassurance that they have not been forgotten in a large and complex system. Some facilities use the skills and expertise of a psychiatric liaison nurse or clinical nurse specialist who will interface with the candidates and their families.

The event that the candidate has long been awaiting, the proper donor match, triggers a series of responsibilities in which complicated arrangements must be intricately set into motion. Because of limited notification time, candidates must be available to travel the moment they are alerted by the transplant center. The initial selection of the recipient is based on a computerized point system, combining logistics, medical urgency, waiting time, the size of the recipient and donor, and ABO compatibility (Starzl, Gordon, Tzakis, Staschak, Fioravanti et al., 1988). The final decision, however, rests with the transplant surgeon and team. Their judgment and experience add the crucial human element vital to the selection process.

PREOPERATIVE PREPARATION

When a liver becomes available the patient is notified and returns to the transplant center. From this moment there is little time to further evaluate the patient. Preoperative preparation is brief and usually consists of obtaining blood samples, taking a chest x-ray, having an anesthesia consultation, and inserting intravenous lines. Once the patient is in the operating room, the anesthesia team assumes responsibility for her care.

ANESTHESIA

The characteristic multiple-organ involvement of end-stage liver failure requires a thorough preoperative assessment of the transplant recipient. Ideally, patients should be assessed when they are seen for their initial screening as transplant candidates. A thorough examination of all organs and systems is routine at this time because the urgency of surgery may preclude a lengthy assessment immediately before surgery. This examination is aimed at both revealing risk factors and noting the progress of secondary effects of the liver disease. If the patient has correctable disease, attempts can be made to optimize the patient's condition.

A second preoperative assessment is made before surgery, when a donor organ has been found for the patient. At this time the previous evaluation information is compared with the current physical status. Generally, a light preoperative medication is recommended because of the patient's overall poor physical condition and encephalopathy. An antacid may be included, particularly if the patient has eaten recently, since gastric emptying is usually prolonged in patients with liver disease.

The usual preoperative anesthesia procedure is followed; however, because of the extremely wide range of parameters that must be constantly evaluated, additional invasive monitoring devices are necessary. The specific monitoring is categorized into cardiovascular, ventilatory, temperature, neuromuscular, biochemical, hematologic, and fluid balance. Maintaining a close-to-normal physiologic state is a major determinant of successful outcome. The primary difficulties encountered during anesthesia for liver transplantation are cardiovascular instability, hypotension, arrhythmias, massive fluid shift, electrolyte imbalance, and coagulopathy.

According to Kang and Gelman (1987), the operation can be divided into three distinct stages, based on the characteristic physiologic changes. Stage one, the preanhepatic phase, extends from induction of anesthesia to complete dissection of the hepatic vasculature. Stage two, the anhepatic phase, begins when hepatic circulation is interrupted or when the native liver is removed and ends when the donor liver is reperfused. Stage three, the postanhepatic phase, is the period between reperfusion of the graft liver and the end of the surgery.

Unless unusual surgical or medical complications occur, the patient's clinical condition stabilizes, most of the physiologic variables are normalized, and the new liver begins to produce bile within several hours of reperfusion. At the conclusion of surgery, patients are transported to the intensive care unit (ICU) with several monitoring devices in place. Mechanical ventilation is provided until the patient recovers from hypothermia and the influence of drugs and anesthetic agents (Kang & Gelman, 1987).

INTRAOPERATIVE NURSING MANAGEMENT

The goals of nursing management during the operative phase of liver transplantation are support of the surgical team, emotional support and preparation of the patient, and prevention of complications. The provisions for the surgery are begun well in advance to prepare the room and instruments for the procedure. Once the room is set up, the patient is moved into the suite and preliminary preparation is initiated. Careful positioning of the patient becomes the operating room nurse's primary responsibility. The use of padding, pillows, and foam protectors prevents potential pressure areas or nerve injury secondary to prolonged immobility. The operating room nurse may also assist with the insertion of access lines, urinary catheters, and monitoring devices.

Hypothermia blankets are applied to maintain neutral body temperature during the operative procedure. Esophageal and rectal temperatures are recorded hourly. The large abdominal incision and lengthy surgery not only predispose the patient to hypothermia, but may also increase the risk of wound infection.

Hepatitis and acquired immunodeficiency syndrome precautions must be maintained throughout the long operative procedure to protect the patient and all staff members. Whether scrubbed or circulating, all operating room personnel should avoid direct contact with the patient's blood and secretions. The administration of recombinant hepatitis B vaccine (Heptavax-B), which promotes active immunity to hepatitis B, is recommended for health care providers who routinely care for transplant patients.

SURGERY

Rapidly developing surgical technology and major immunologic advances have improved survival statistics dramatically from 34 per cent one-year survival in 1978 to more than 70 per cent one-year survival in 1987. Each potential donor is carefully screened by history and laboratory parameters as to suitability of various organs for transplant (see Chapter 2). After certification of brain death, cardiopulmonary support of the donor must be adequately maintained up to and including the time of recovery.

Donor Hepatectomy

Careful hemodynamic support of the donor is essential during the entire recovery sequence to ensure optimal organ preservation and function after reimplantation. Operative exposure is obtained through a continuous midline sternotomy and laparotomy incision. This allows wide exposure for adequate organ assessment and more precise skeletonization of the blood supply to the various organs. After laparotomy and careful inspection of the liver, the recipient hospital is notified that the organs are suitable for transplantation. This information allows the recipient team to begin the recipient hepatectomy.

Two basic techniques of liver procurement have been described: the standard, or traditional, technique and the rapid technique. The first step in removing the donor liver using the standard technique is meticulous dissection of the hepatic artery down to and including the celiac axis and aorta. Extreme care is taken to identify all arterial anomalies and to maintain uninterrupted blood flow to all organs that will be used as grafts. The common bile duct is divided as far distally as possible and a small hole is made in the gallbladder to allow drainage and flushing of bile from the biliary tree. Any retained bile could potentially cause autolysis of the bile duct epithelium during transport. The pancreas can then be divided over the portal vein to allow visualization of the splenic and superior mesenteric veins. A blunt-tip intravenous tube is inserted into the ligated splenic vein for eventual cooling of the liver. This line is kept open with a slow drip of chilled lactated Ringer's solution until the final phases of the recovery. The ligamentous attachments of the liver to the diaphragm are divided, and the posterior portion of the liver and vena cava are mobilized. If it is in accordance with the local renal procurement practice, the kidneys may now be mobilized along with the ureters from their retroperitoneal positions. This also allows exposure of the aorta and vena cava down to their bifurcations in the pelvis.

The donor is systemically heparinized with 300 U/kg of intravenous heparin, and cannulae are placed in the aorta (Fig. 7–4). Cooling of the organs may now begin as the final phase of the procedure. After ligation of the superior mesenteric vein 2 to 4 liters of an iced lactated Ringer's solution at 4° C is rapidly infused by way of the splenic vein cannula to initiate cooling of the liver and to reduce the core body temperature to 30° to 31° C. Next, the aorta is clamped proximal to the celiac axis to stop arterial inflow to the abdominal organs and to allow perfusion and cooling of the liver and kidneys through the distal aortic cannula. The infusate used for this purpose is a cold modified Collins solution, which is high in potassium and resembles the intracellular electrolyte composition. Fluid distention of the organs is prevented by venting the venous return through the vena cava. Placement of a second clamp above the renal arteries but below the celiac axis allows continued slow flushing of the kidneys while the liver is being removed with its remaining vascular attachments. After removal of the liver, Viaspan solution is usually infused through the retained splenic vein cannula while the donor nephrectomy is carried out. The liver is double-bagged in Viaspan solution and placed in an ice chest for transport.

When the rapid technique is used no preliminary dissection is undertaken. The inferior mesenteric vein and distal aorta are cannulated and the proximal aorta encircled. When the cardiac team is ready to arrest the heart the proximal aorta is clamped and rapid cold infusion through both cannulas is begun. While the heart is being removed the

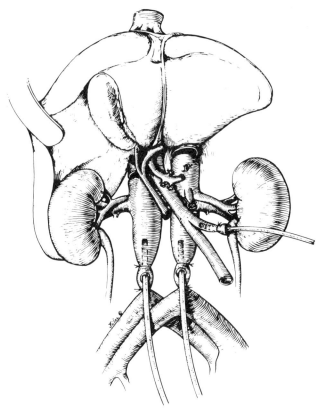

FIGURE 7–4. Sites of cannula placement for en bloc cadaveric organ profusion. (By permission of Surgery, Gynecology & Obstetrics from Shaw, B.W., Jr., Hakala, T., Rosenthal, J.T., Iwatsuki, S., et al. (September, 1982). *Surgery, Gynecology & Obstetrics, 155*, 321.)

liver and kidneys become completely flushed and cold. After the heart is removed the hepatic hilar dissection can be performed safely and rapidly in a bloodless field. The liver is then removed as already described for the standard technique. Depending on the type of preservation solution used, the liver may be preserved for up to 24 hours, although, ideally, the liver should be transplanted as soon as possible.

The iliac vessels are removed as potential vascular graft material, while the spleen and lymph nodes are removed for immunologic purposes. The recipient hospital is notified during crucial phases of the donor hepatectomy so that they may better plan the sequencing of the recipient operation.

Recipient Hepatectomy and Graft Insertion

Concurrent with the performance of the donor hepatectomy, a separate team begins the recipient hepatectomy. Severe portal hypertension

and coagulation disturbances present in the recipient as a direct consequence of end-stage liver disease make this part of the operation extremely hazardous and time-consuming. These problems are compounded in patients with previous upper abdominal surgeries by the
dense variceal collaterals that have developed in surgical adhesions.
Large-bore intravenous lines and blood infusion pumps are essential
components in the anesthetic support of the patient during this phase of
the operation.

The surgical exposure is performed as a bilateral subcostal incision
with midline extension and removal of the xiphoid process. Skeletonization of the hepatic artery, portal vein, and common bile duct high in
the hilum is the first step in preparing for removal of the liver. These
structures are not divided until the donor liver has actually arrived in
the operating room suite and has been satisfactorily reinspected. Careful
ligation and division of the extremely vascular ligamentous attachments
of the liver allow exposure of the vena cava above and below the liver.

Coincident with the arrival of the donor liver the recipient organ is
removed. Vascular clamps are placed in sequence on the hepatic artery,
portal vein, and suprahepatic and infrahepatic vena cava, and the liver
is removed. Crossclamping of the portal vein and infrahepatic vena cava
may lead to further venous hypertension, circulatory instability, and
excessive bleeding. In adults these complications have been ameliorated
by the veno-venous bypass system. Heparin-bonded Gott shunts inserted
into the left common femoral vein and the left axillary vein allow pump-
assisted venous return of systemic blood from the lower part of the body
back to the heart during the anhepatic phase of the procedure. An
additional Gott shunt placed in the portal vein allows effective decompression of the portal system. This bypass system is assisted by an
in-line Biomedicus pump head and does not require systemic heparini-
zation (Griffith, Shaw, Hardesty, Iwatsuki, Bahnson & Starzl, 1985) (Fig.
7–5).

The donor organ is removed from the transport cooler, checked for
defects, and readied for implantation. In sequence, the suprahepatic vena
caval anastomosis is performed, followed by the infrahepatic vena caval
anastomosis. An important step before completion of this latter anastomosis is flushing of the donor organ through the retained splenic vein
cannula to remove trapped air bubbles and potassium from the preservation solution. Failure to do so may lead to cardiac arrest from air
embolization or hyperkalemia. After this is done the portal venous
anastomosis is completed, portal venous blood flow is reestablished to
the graft, and veno-venous bypass is discontinued. The organ can be
observed to change color at this time, although patchy islands of poorly
perfused parenchyma may persist until hepatic arterial inflow is reestablished. The hepatic artery anastomosis, particularly in pediatric recipi-

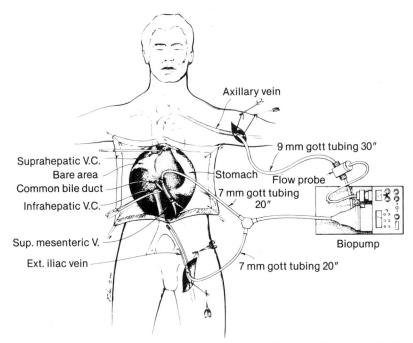

FIGURE 7–5. Veno-venous bypass system. (By permission of Surgery, Gynecology & Obstetrics from Griffith, B.P., Shaw, B.W., Jr., Hardesty, R.L., Iwatsuki, S., et al. (March 1985). *Surgery, Gynecology & Obstetrics*, *160*, 270–272.)

ents, must be performed with great care. Before bile duct reconstruction is started careful attention is paid to hemostasis. "Drying up" is an extremely time-consuming, although important, part of the operation. A properly preserved and functioning implanted liver will improve coagulation abnormalities within a short time and assist in this phase of the operation.

Biliary Reconstruction

Typically, biliary reconstruction is performed with an end-to-end anastomosis of the donor and recipient common bile ducts (choledochocholedochostomy), stented with a T tube (Fig. 7–6A). This reconstruction cannot be used if the recipient bile ducts are diseased (sclerosing cholantitis) or absent (biliary atresia) or if a great size discrepancy exists between the two ducts. In such situations the donor common bile duct is anastomosed to a Roux-en-Y limb of jejunum (choledochojejunostomy) (Fig. 7–6B). With few exceptions, donor cholecystectomy and operative cholangiography are performed before completion of this phase of the surgery. If a T tube is placed in the biliary tract, it is brought to the

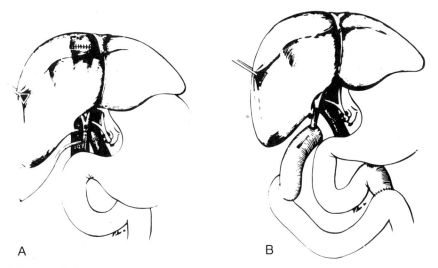

FIGURE 7–6. Anastomosis. A, Bile duct reconstruction with choledochocholedochostomy. B, Bile duct reconstruction with Roux-en-Y with choledochojejunostomy. (From Starzl, T.E., Iwatsuki, S., Shaw, B.W., Jr., Gordon, R.D., et al. (1982). *Hepatology*, 2, 614.)

outside and empties into a bile bag. Three Jackson-Pratt drains are placed: one under the right diaphragm, one under the left diaphragm, and one infrahepatically near the bile duct reconstruction.

The difficulty of the surgery and the blood replacement depend on the disease process, previous surgery, and the donor organ function (Marsh, Gordon, Stieber, Esquivel & Starzl, 1988). The donor and recipient operations require meticulous and time-consuming attention to detail. With operating time ranging from 6 to 24 hours, orthotopic liver transplantation is one of the most exhausting feats in surgery (Maletic-Staschak, 1984).

NURSING DIAGNOSES AND POSTOPERATIVE MANAGEMENT

Acute Phase

Immediately after surgery the liver transplant recipient is admitted to the ICU for monitoring and stabilization. The length of stay in the ICU is individualized but may average from two to five days. The critical care nurse must be knowledgeable of the operative procedure and prepared to utilize the nursing process that is outlined, to provide for the extensive nursing management of the liver transplant recipient (Table 7–6). This

TABLE 7–6. NURSING CARE PLAN FOR LIVER TRANSPLANT RECIPIENT

NURSING DIAGNOSIS	PREDISPOSING FACTORS	SIGNS AND SYMPTOMS	NURSING INTERVENTION
Potential for injury	Poor nutritional status Prolonged operative procedure Hypothermia Prolonged immobility	Redness or sores at bony prominences	Position patient properly on operative table. Use padding, pillows, and foam protectors during periods of prolonged immobility. Assess for signs and symptoms of injury. Reposition patient. Monitor vital signs every hour.
Potential for alterations in oxygenation	Prolonged immobility Mechanical ventilation Hypoventilation secondary to right phrenic nerve damage	Abnormal arterial blood gases Cyanosis Abnormal breath sounds	Monitor arterial blood gases every 2 h and as needed. Monitor respiratory settings and change as ordered. Auscultate lungs.
	Pain Abdominal distention Anesthesia Pretransplant nutritional status	Abnormal respiratory rate and rhythm Asymmetrical chest expansion	Monitor respiratory status. Monitor for pain; evaluate analgesic requirements. Reposition patient every 2 h. Suction patient as needed. Perform chest physiotherapy every 2–4 h and as needed. Monitor chest tube patency and drainage if tube inserted. Measure abdominal girth at same location every 12 h. Auscultate bowel sounds every 4 h.
Potential for alterations in cardiovascular status	Arrhythmia Hypertension Hypotension	Abnormal EKG ↑ Blood pressure ↓ Blood pressure	Monitor EKG. Monitor mean arterial pressure, central venous pressure. Administer antihypertensive agents, vasopressors, or volume expanders as ordered.
	Hemorrhage	Oozing from suture sites Sanguineous drainage from drains ↓ Hemoglobin/hematocrit	Monitor drainage characteristics every hour. Replace drainage as ordered. Monitor hemoglobin, hematocrit, platelets, and coagulation times.
	Thrombus	Unexplained fever ↑ Transaminase ↓ or ↑ Central venous pressure ↓ or ↑ Blood pressure ↓ Urine output	
Potential for fluid and electrolyte imbalance	Intraoperative fluid loss/ administration Hepatorenal syndrome Acute renal failure		Monitor for signs and symptoms of hypervolemia or hypovolemia. Monitor electrolyte levels. Maintain strict intake/output.

Nursing diagnosis	Related factors	Defining characteristics	Interventions
	Antibiotic/cyclosporine nephrotoxicity		Check weight daily. Monitor drug levels. Provide emotional support if dialysis is necessary.
Alterations in nutrition	Abdominal complications Preexisting malnutrition Stress of surgery	Increasing abdominal girth Fever Chills Right upper quadrant pain ↑ Serum bilirubin level Bilious drainage from abdominal drains ↓ Serum albumin, total protein levels	Monitor gastric pH every 2 hr. Administer antacids as ordered. Monitor abdominal girth. Monitor drainage characteristics. Monitor for signs and symptoms of biliary leaks or strictures. Monitor laboratory values. Administer parenteral or oral nutrition as ordered. Maintain calorie counts.
Potential for perceptual alterations	Graft failure Seizures Encephalopathy Brachial plexus injuries	Abnormal level of consciousness	Perform neurologic assessments every 2–4 h. Monitor serum ammonia level. Monitor liver function tests. Monitor cyclosporine levels. Adjust cyclosporine dose as ordered when anticonvulsants are administered concomitantly.
Alterations in immunity	Immunosuppressive therapy Anesthesia ↓ Mobility Intravenous, Foley, and drainage catheters	↑ Temperature Tachycardia ↑ or ↓ White blood cell count Redness and purulence at catheter sites	Monitor for signs and symptoms of infection. Maintain good handwashing technique. Maintain sterile technique with dressing and line changes. Change intravenous line tubing every 24 h. Monitor oral cavity for herpetic and fungal lesions. Pan culture with temperature of >100.5° F. Monitor culture results. Encourage pulmonary hygiene. Encourage ambulation. Administer antimicrobial agents as ordered.
	Preexisting nutritional status	Odorous drainage Lesions	
Altered immunity potential for rejection	T and B cell activity	Fever Abdominal pain ↑ Transaminase level ↑ Bilirubin level ↑ Alkaline phosphatase level Histologic findings on biopsy	Monitor for signs and symptoms of rejection. Administer immunosuppressive medications as ordered. Monitor laboratory values. Monitor for adverse effects of medications. Provide emotional support. Encourage active participation in self-care.
Knowledge deficit related to self-care maintenance after liver transplantation			Provide teaching as outlined in Chapter 15.

nursing management is directed toward meticulous observation for early recognition of potentially life-threatening complications.

A nasogastric tube is connected to suction, and a urinary catheter is attached to a urinometer for hourly urine output readings. An endotracheal tube attached to a ventilator provides respiratory support and airway protection. Cardiac rhythm and rate are monitored by electrocardiography. Jackson-Pratt drains are used to evacuate blood and ascites from the abdominal cavity. A T tube may be present to allow egress of bile from the biliary system. Intra-arterial and intravenous lines are placed for monitoring central venous pressure and arterial pressure and for fluid replacement. A pulmonary artery catheter is used for pulmonary artery and pulmonary artery occlusion pressures and cardiac output measurement.

Potential for Alterations in Oxygenation

The goals of nursing management of the respiratory system are to maintain adequate oxygenation and accurately measure for signs of hypoxemia and hypoventilation during weaning from mechanical ventilation. After transplantation, the patient is admitted to the ICU with an endotracheal tube and placed on mechanical ventilation. Prolonged anesthesia, in conjunction with impaired hepatic drug metabolism, necessitates ventilatory support. Endotracheal tube cuff pressure is monitored every two hours to prevent aspiration and tracheal ischemia. Most adults and more than 50 per cent of the children can be weaned from mechanical ventilation and extubated by the end of the second postoperative day (Shapiro, Wood, Shaw & Grenvik, 1986; Thompson, 1987). Arterial blood gas (ABG) values are monitored on admission and every four to six hours, or as needed, to maintain adequate oxygen levels.

Nursing management facilitates adequate oxygen delivery to the patient. Baseline assessment of the respiratory status, the chest x-ray interpretations, and the determination of the ABG values are ascertained. Continued consequences of operative hypothermia may include metabolic alkalosis, decreased anesthetic metabolism, and altered oxygen consumption. The nurse carefully evaluates the need for analgesics. Respiratory assessment includes auscultation of the chest for abnormal breath sounds, rate and rhythm of respirations, and symmetrical expansion of the chest. Careful attention should be given to an aggressive pulmonary toilet regimen. Endotracheal suctioning should be performed every two hours and as needed. The lungs should be hyperinflated with oxygen prior to endotracheal suctioning. The patient should be repositioned every two hours and aggressive chest physical therapy is given to loosen and mobilize secretions. Occasionally severe metabolic alkalosis with compensatory respiratory acidosis occurs in primary graft failure (Marsh, Gordon, Steiber, Esquivel, & Starzl, 1988).

Atelectasis and pleural effusions are the most commonly seen early postoperative respiratory complications. Pleural effusions almost invariably develop on the right side but may be seen on the left as well. They are probably caused by ascitic fluid passing across the raw surface of the diaphragm in the bed of the liver. Paralysis of the right diaphragm is evidenced by an elevated right diaphragm on chest x-ray and decreased expansion of the right lower lobe with spontaneous respirations.

Pleural effusions frequently require drainage but may resolve with diuresis. Small-bore pigtail catheters are used to provide continuous pleural drainage when large effusions compromise respiratory function and delay extubation. The catheters are attached to a closed gravity drainage system and require little additional care aside from ensuring patency and integrity of the system.

Chest tubes are occasionally placed during the transplant procedure to treat pneumothorax or severe pleural effusions that compromise oxygenation or ventilation during anesthesia. Routine chest tube care is required.

Persistent hypoventilation may be experienced from right phrenic nerve damage, incisional pain, or abdominal distention due to persistent ascites, bleeding, an ileus, a large donor liver, or intra-abdominal sepsis (Thompson, 1987). Patients who are severely malnourished and debilitated may have generalized muscle weakness, necessitating prolonged mechanical ventilation. Accurate recording of abdominal girth every 12 hours, auscultation of bowel sounds every four hours, and daily weights will assist in the evaluation of these complications. After extubation, patients are carefully monitored, and if difficulties are encountered with oxygenation, prompt reintubation or subsequent tracheostomy may be required.

Most important, persistent postoperative hepatic encephalopathy may result in lethargy, hypoventilation, and poor pulmonary toilet. In severe cases aspiration may result from diminished airway reflexes (cough and gag). The ensuing pneumonia may lead to the patient's demise. Any degree of persistent encephalopathy should result in prompt evaluation of the patient for reintubation.

Potential for Alterations in Cardiovascular Status Secondary to Arrhythmia, Hypertension/Hypotension, Hemorrhage, or Thrombus

The goals of nursing management of the cardiovascular system are to maintain adequate cardiac functioning and tissue perfusion while monitoring for complications. Liver transplant recipients may have normal sinus rhythm postoperatively, but bradycardia, tachycardia, and premature ventricular contractions have occurred. Traiger and Bohachick (1983) noted that most patients manifest sinus tachycardia for the first 48 hours because of sympathetic stimulation due to the stress of surgery.

Cardiovascular monitoring includes measurement of heart rate by electrocardiography, mean arterial pressure and blood gas analysis by way of an intra-arterial catheter, and central venous pressures and waveforms by way of a central venous line. A pulmonary artery catheter is routinely used. Analysis of the cardiopulmonary laboratory values aids in the judicious administration of vasoactive agents. All lines are sutured in place and povidone-iodine (Betadine) ointment is applied to each site.

Hypertension is a common development in patients undergoing a successful liver transplantation. It is severest in the first postoperative week, with mean systolic pressures greater than 150 mm Hg and arterial pressures greater than 95 mm Hg. The cause of hypertension is unclear but appears to be cyclosporine-related. Other factors such as pain, hypothermia, and fluid overload must also be evaluated. Preliminary studies have negated renin, angiotension, or catecholamines as factors (Thompson, 1987). Often the hypertension persists for many months, gradually becoming less severe, but requiring medication and blood pressure monitoring for adequate control.

Hypertension must be prevented in the acute phase, as these patients are at risk for intracerebral hemorrhage and major neurologic complications, such as seizures and coma (Marsh et al., 1988; Thompson, 1987). It is common for patients to require up to three antihypertensive medications and a diuretic for adequate blood pressure control (Wood, Shaw & Starzl, 1985). The drugs of choice will depend on the patient's degree of hypertension, response to medication, and physical condition.

Hypotension may also occur in the acute postoperative period, most often caused by intra-abdominal bleeding. Hypotension is managed with volume expanders, packed red blood cells, and fresh-frozen plasma to correct any existing coagulopathy. Vasopressor support may increase cardiac output, raising the blood pressure, but it should not be used in lieu of intravascular volume replacement. Reexploration and repair of the bleeding site will be necessary in the face of persistent hemorrhage.

Nursing management should be directed at strict monitoring for signs of hemorrhage. Increasing abdominal girth, blood oozing from suture or intravenous lines, or the presence of large amounts of sanguineous drainage in the Jackson-Pratt drains is indicative of hemorrhage. The abdominal drainage is measured hourly, and a hematocrit obtained from the drains is compared with that of serum. Variceal hemorrhage is uncommon after liver transplant. Gastrointestinal hemorrhage may result from gastritis, stress ulceration, or peptic ulcer. Occasionally bleeding from a Roux-en-Y anastomosis may also result in brisk gastrointestinal hemorrhage. Investigation is warranted with a nuclear medicine gastrointestinal bleed study, endoscopy, or both.

Portal vein thrombosis is a rare but dramatic complication. Sudden severe hypotension, rapid accumulation of ascites, and, possibly, variceal hemorrhage suggest thrombosis of the portal vein. Urgent retransplantation is required if the patient is to survive this catastrophe.

Hepatic artery thrombosis complicates 7 per cent of the liver transplants in adults but is common in children (Marsh et al., 1988). Unexplained fever, a rise in the transaminase level, and the absence of hepatic artery pulsations on a Doppler ultrasound are suggestive of hepatic artery thrombosis. Angiography is required to confirm the diagnosis. Retransplantation is usually required.

Potential for Fluid and Electrolyte Imbalances Related to Operative Factors

The goal of nursing management is to retain homeostatic fluid and electrolyte balance. Extensive volume loss can occur intraoperatively in patients with massive ascites or significant blood loss from coagulopathy or adhesions. Another complicating factor is third-spacing of fluids into the interstitial compartment after the portal vein and inferior vena cava clamps are removed intraoperatively (Starzl et al., 1982).

Metabolic and electrolyte disturbances are frequent consequences in the early postoperative period. Hyperglycemia is common in the early postoperative period and is monitored by blood glucose levels as well as Dextrostix reagent strips every two hours. Glucose homeostasis is easily sustained by maintenance infusions of glucose (Thompson, 1987). Profound hypoglycemia is an ominous finding, and may indicate massive hepatic necrosis or sepsis. Hypokalemia is the most frequently observed electrolyte disturbance in the acute postoperative period and may be related to chronic diuretic therapy or intraoperative volume replacement, or both. Hypocalcemia may be apparent if the patient has received large volumes of blood containing citrate preservatives, which decrease ionized calcium levels. Vitamin D deficiencies and respiratory or metabolic alkalosis may also cause hypocalcemia. Magnesium deficiency is common and may potentiate the tendency of cyclosporine to induce seizures. Normal serum magnesium levels should be maintained.

Nursing management includes strict hourly intake and output measurements. A urinary catheter facilitates monitoring for oliguria, and pale yellow urine is suggestive of a functioning graft. Fluid collected in the abdominal drains is measured every one to two hours, and in the event of excessive drainage may be replaced with plasma protein fraction at 0.5 ml per milliliter of drainage every four hours. The drains are stripped to prevent clots, and the color should change from sanguineous to serous in several days.

Alteration in Kidney Function Related to Hepatorenal Syndrome, Acute Renal Failure, and Antibiotic or Cyclosporine Nephrotoxicities

Nursing management of the patient with renal impairment is directed toward monitoring hourly urinary output and the serum creatinine level. Acute renal failure after liver transplantation is less common since the institution of veno-venous bypass. However, the patient with preexisting renal disease, hepatorenal syndrome, and antibiotic and cyclosporine toxicities may be at higher risk. Usually patients with adequate liver graft function have resolution of hepatorenal syndrome. Antibiotic or cyclosporine toxicity may exacerbate acute tubular necrosis, which may have resulted from intraoperative hypotension. Acute tubular necrosis is more likely to resolve if the cyclosporine dose is reduced, and if nephrotoxic antibiotic drugs are eliminated or given in renal doses (Marsh et al., 1988).

Comparative intake and output measurements are recorded until normal kidney function is established. Nursing assessment includes checking urine specific gravity, daily weights, and evaluation of central venous pressure and pulmonary artery occlusion pressure for evidence of fluid overload. Fluids or diuretics are administered as necessary, and the patient is carefully observed for hypokalemia. As the cyclosporine dose is adjusted, the nurse should monitor the serum creatinine for improvements in renal function. Renal failure that is unresponsive to treatment may require temporary dialysis.

Alterations in Nutrition Secondary to Abdominal Complications and Preexistent Malnutrition

Nursing management is directed toward providing adequate nutrition to promote wound healing and recognition of abdominal complications. Gastric pH is checked every two hours, and antacids are given to reduce gastric acidity. The most common gastrointestinal tract complications are bleeding and biliary leaks or strictures (Wood et al., 1985). Bleeding may necessitate reexploration in the early postoperative period. Candida or enteric organisms cultured from abdominal drainage are strongly suggestive of a bowel perforation. An abdominal ultrasound or CT scan may assist in determining hepatic artery patency, infarction, or intra-abdominal abscess.

Biliary leaks or strictures can occur at the anastomosis site or from the T tube insertion site. The patient may present with fever, chills, right upper quadrant pain, sepsis, elevated serum bilirubin level, and bilious drainage from the abdominal drains. Surgical correction of the leak is required. A leak may be repaired by reinforcement of the T tube suture; however, it may require conversion to a Roux-en-Y choledochojejunostomy. Bile duct strictures are usually later complications owing to ischemic injury to the biliary tree or premature removal of the T tube. Percutaneous dilation with a biliary catheter, or surgical revision of the duct may be necessary (Marsh et al., 1988).

Parenteral nutritional support may be required while the gastrointestinal tract recovers and to provide adequate caloric intake for healing. The nurse should be aware of the patient's intake, and calorie counts may be indicated. High-calorie fluid supplements are usually encouraged (Guenter & Slocum, 1983). An aggressive pretransplant nutritional support program can be successful in controlling the malnutrition in end-stage liver disease; thus minimal nutritional support may be needed after transplantation (Shronts, Teasley & Cerra, 1987).

Potential for Perceptual Alterations Due to Graft Failure or Seizures

The aim of nursing management for the neurologic system is to assess for signs of adequate function. The most serious complications that patients experience are seizures, strokes, encephalopathy, peripheral neuropathy, and brachial plexus injuries (Marsh et al., 1988). Intracranial bleeding is a rare but devastating event. Seizures are more common in children than in adults, but they usually result in no permanent sequelae. Cyclosporine toxicity or a low serum magnesium level has been implicated. Usually the seizure responds to treatment. Such drugs as Valium, phenobarbitol, phenytoin, or magnesium replacement may be prescribed. Medication provided for seizure control requires blood level monitoring. Cyclosporine pharmacokinetics may also be altered with the use of phenobarbital or phenytoin.

Level of consciousness is an important indicator of graft function. Neurologic checks should be performed every two to four hours to assess for compromise. Depressed detoxification in the new liver prolongs the effects of anesthesia and may result in elevated serum ammonia levels. After the transplant most patients are awake within four to eight hours. Laboratory assessment of liver function provides critical information about the new graft's function.

Postoperative Recovery and Discharge Phases

When the patient has achieved stable hepatic and cardiopulmonary function, she is transferred from the ICU to the surgical floor. Complications at any time during the recovery period could necessitate a return to the ICU for stabilization. Many patients are hospitalized for four to six weeks on the postsurgical unit, depending on their unique needs. Sometimes rehabilitation may be necessary at a rehabilitation institute or on an outpatient basis for a complete recovery. This section discusses some of the prevalent nursing diagnoses specific to the postsurgical recovery period. Discharge teaching that is unique to the needs of the patient and family is addressed.

Alteration in Immunity

The goals of nursing management are to monitor for signs of infection and to administer prescribed immunosuppressive therapy. The patient usually completes a high-dose steroid cycle, tapered over several days to a maintenance dose. Additionally, cyclosporine or other immunosuppressive agents are given in divided doses. Opportunistic infections may arise from the wound, drains, or invasive catheters. The immunosuppressed host has an altered ability to combat infection, and therefore, infections must be diagnosed early. Typical infections in the postsurgical recovery period are due to bacterial, viral, and fungal organisms (see Chapter 5).

Liver transplant patients are usually not placed in isolation after transplantation. Aseptic handwashing technique should be enforced. All intravenous lines and drains are inspected daily, and Betadine ointment is applied to all intravenous sites. Central and peripheral intravenous line tubing is changed every 24 hours, and Betadine ointment is applied to all connections. The patient's mouth is assessed daily for any evidence of herpetic or fungal lesions, and a prophylactic oral antifungal agent is used.

Potential Loss of the Transplanted Organ Graft Due to Rejection, Infection, or Ischemic Injury

Rejection can occur at any time, but it is most likely to occur at 10 to 14 days postoperatively and up until the end of the third postoperative month (Esquivel, Jaffee, Gordon, Iwatsuki, Shaw & Starzl, 1985). The goals of nursing management are to monitor for potential signs of rejection or infection, and administer appropriate therapy. Early postoperative signs of rejection may include fever, ascites, abdominal pain, a decreased quantity or quality of bile, and elevations in transaminases, bilirubin, and alkaline phosphatase levels. Ischemic injury may mimic rejection, and the differential diagnosis is usually confirmed by biopsy.

Treatment of a rejection episode may consist of a steroid recycle, changing or increasing the immunosuppressive drugs, or the administration of monoclonal antibody. Treatment of rejection may substantially increase the patient's risk for development of opportunistic infections. If this occurs, decreased maintenance immunosuppression may be required (Esquivel et al., 1985).

Because the diagnosis of rejection or infection is devastating to the patient and family, additional emotional support by staff and support liaison services should be available. During the wait for laboratory tests to confirm the diagnosis the patient may become acutely ill, which increases anxiety and fear.

Knowledge Deficit Related to Self-Care Maintenance After Liver Transplantation

Before discharge the patient must be knowledgeable about all aspects of her care. As soon as possible after the surgery the patient is encouraged to actively participate in an intensive patient education program. Prevention, recognition, and early treatment of complications can be accomplished with a teaching/learning program that involves the transplant nurse, physician, patient, and family. The following sections discuss information that is essential for the patient to master before discharge.

Medications. A successful recovery with continued function of the new liver depends on strict adherence to the prescribed medication regimen. Foremost are the immunosuppressant drugs that the patient will take for the rest of her life. The patient should be instructed as to the dosage, purpose, timing, precautionary measures, and side effects (see Chapter 3).

T Tube Care. Any patient who has a duct-to-duct (choledochocholedochostomy) reconstruction will have a T tube placed at the time of surgery. This tube generally remains in place for several months. Before discharge the tube will be clamped and the patient will be taught how to care for the T tube.

It is important to observe the T tube insertion site every day for any signs of infection, such as redness or drainage. The site must be cleaned daily with antimicrobial solution. If T tube cholangiography is performed, antibiotics will be prescribed before the procedure to prevent infection.

Infection. Patients must be taught about the potential seriousness of infections because of their immunodeficient state. Teaching should include some parameters concerning temperature, exposure to communicable diseases, vaccinations, and contact with people who have episodic illness.

Particular attention should be paid to any prolonged low-grade fevers or sudden high fevers. Routine investigation of childhood illnesses should be conducted before the patient leaves the area. If the patient is exposed to mumps, measles, or chickenpox and lacks antibodies against them, she may require special immunizations for self-protection.

Activity and Exercise. Once patients are discharged, they are encouraged to return to normal activities, with some moderations. The following points are emphasized to patients (Staschak & Formella, 1988):

1. Long walks or walking up and down the stairs is permitted.

2. A regular exercise program that is geared to the patient's progress is recommended. Active physical exercise is emphasized if the patient's medical condition permits. An exercise program is necessary to maintain normal weight and to minimize the destructive effects of prednisone on muscles and bones.

3. Driving is permitted only after the abdominal incision is well healed and minimal side effects from the medications are experienced. Caution and restraint in the early postoperative period will help to assure personal safety and the safety of others.

Sex and Birth Control. After a successful transplant, patients are instructed to resume sexual activity when they feel comfortable. They should be reassured that sexual intercourse will not harm their new livers.

Women generally resume their menstrual cycle after liver transplantation. Birth control pills and intrauterine devices should be avoided because of their potential side effects. The suggested methods of birth control are foam with a condom, "the sponge" with a condom, and a diaphragm with spermicidal gel. Permanent methods of birth control should be discussed with the patient's gynecologist (Staschak & Formella, 1988).

The decision whether or not to have children is influenced by many factors. It is not known whether immunosuppressants increase the risk of premature delivery and low birth weight for the female recipient.

Rejection. Rejection is the most common complication in the posttransplant period, and nearly all patients will experience one or more episodes. The chances of rejection diminish with time, but rejection can occur at any time. Therefore, it is important to make the patient aware of the most common signs and symptoms, such as fatigue, lethargy, fever, abdominal tenderness, light-colored stools, dark-colored urine, jaundice, and abnormalities in liver function tests. The onset of rejection does not mean that the patient's graft will be lost; however, the diagnosis of rejection may precipitate an emotional crisis with both the patient and family. The nurse must learn to effectively assist the patient and family to cope.

Follow-up Medical Care. Health prevention and maintenance must be promoted in the outpatient setting. The following guidelines may be used:

1. Routine eye examinations, which include cataract and glaucoma screening, are encouraged because of long-term steroid therapy.

2. Maintaining good oral hygiene and follow-up dental care are particularly important. Gum hyperplasia postoperatively, in combination with poor dental hygiene related to liver disease in the preoperative period, may make frequent dental visits necessary. The patient should be advised to take prophylactic antibiotics before any dental treatment.

In conclusion, nurses have a major impact on the success of the transplant and the subsequent recovery of the transplant recipient. Postoperative teaching and participation in long-term follow-up care are vital to assure that the patient maintains optimal health.

Rehabilitation. Patients who are severely debilitated preoperatively or those patients who suffer major complications after transplantation may require a more intensive or prolonged recovery. After discharge from the hospital these patients may require transfer to a rehabilitation institute for a complete recovery. The rehabilitative medicine specialists, physical therapists, and social workers may assist the transplant team in obtaining placement in a specialized facility.

THE FUTURE OF LIVER TRANSPLANTATION

Increased experience indicates that fewer transplants will be performed for end-stage liver disease, while more will be performed for selected indications. It appears that the focus of treatment for liver disease will shift from crisis management to disease control. It has been speculated that artificial livers, each performing one or more hepatic functions, could be on the horizon. As a result, liver transplantation for fulminant hepatic failure will be used less often but applied more frequently for the problem of subacute hepatic failure.

With further research provided by opportunities unique to the transplant center, new insights into the specific pathogenesis of individual liver diseases and their complications may be realized. New and better methods of rejection control will be found. Experiments are currently being conducted with FK 506 (see Chapter 4), a Japanese-produced immunosuppressant that is 100 times more powerful than cyclosporine.

Xenografts may begin to find room in this ever-expanding clinical arena of transplantation. Human monoclonal antibodies for treatment and prevention of future cancers and hepatitis B may soon become a reality.

Liver transplantation, since its auspicious beginning in 1963, has reached successful heights that far exceed one's expectations. Today many patients enjoy restored health and a satisfactory quality of life despite the complexity of this procedure. As a member of the health care team, the transplant nurse has a unique opportunity to experience the continued success of liver transplantation.

Acknowledgments: We thank J. Wallis Marsh, M.D., Linda Sher, M.D., Olga C. Maletic, Ellen Lang, Shun Iwatsuki, M.D., Todd Howard, M.D., and Thomas E. Starzl, M.D., for their assistance in preparing this manuscript.

Dedication
To Jeffrey, Zachary, Ashleigh, and Garry for their patience.

References

Bullock, B. & Rosendahl, P.P. (1984). *Pathophysiology: Adaptations and Alterations in Function*. Boston: Little, Brown.

Calne, R. (1987). *Liver Transplantation* (2nd ed.). Orlando: Grune & Stratton.

Calne, R. & Williams, S. (1988). Liver transplantation. In L.H. Blumgart (Ed.). *Surgery of the Liver and Biliary Tract* (pp. 1509, 1510). New York: Churchill Livingstone.

Carpenito, L.J. (1987). *Handbook of Nursing Diagnosis*. Philadelphia: J.B. Lippincott.

Chaffee, E.E. & Lytle, I.M. (1980). *Basic Physiology and Anatomy* (4th ed.). Philadelphia: J.B. Lippincott.

Esquivel, C.O., Jaffee, R., Gordon, R.D., Iwatsuki, S., Shaw, B.W., & Starzl, T.E. (1985). Liver rejection and its differentiation from other causes of graft dysfunction. *Seminars in Liver Disease, 5*(4), 369–374.

Griffith, B.P., Shaw, B.W., Jr., Hardesty, R.L., Iwatsuki, S., Bahnson, H.T., & Starzl, T.E. (1985). Veno-venous bypass without systemic anticoagulation for human liver transplantation. *Surgery, Gynecology, & Obstetrics, 160,* 270–272.

Guenter, P. & Slocum, B. (1983). Hepatic disease: Nutritional implications. *Nursing Clinics of North America 18*(1), 71–81.

Guyton, A.C. (1986). *Textbook of Medical Physiology* (7th ed.). Philadelphia: W.B. Saunders.

Iwatsuki, S., Shaw, B., & Starzl, T. (1983). Current status of hepatic transplantation. *Seminars in Liver Disease, 3*(3), 173–180.

Kang, Y.G. & Gelman, S. (1987). Liver transplantation. In S. Gelman (Ed.). *Anesthesia and Organ Transplantation* (pp. 139–186). Philadelphia: W.B. Saunders.

Keith, J.S. (1985). Hepatic failure: Etiologies, manifestations and management. *Critical Care Nurse, 5*(1), 60–86.

Kusne, S., Dummer, J.S., Singh, N., Iwatsuki, S., Makowka, L., Esquivel, C., Tzakis, A.G., Starzl, T.E., & Ho, M. (1988). Infections after liver transplantation. *Journal of Medicine, 67,* 132–143.

Maletic-Staschak, S. (1984). Orthotopic liver transplantation. *Journal of the Association of Operating Room Nurses, 39,* 35–39.

Marsh, J.W., Gordon, R.D., Stieber, A., Esquivel, C.O., & Starzl, T.E. (1988). Critical care of the liver transplant patient. In W. Shomaker, S. Ayres, A. Grenvik, P. Holbrook, & L. Thompson (Eds.). *The Society of Critical Care Medicine* (2nd ed.) (pp 1329–1333). Philadelphia: W.B. Saunders.

Novak, D.A., & Balistreri, W.F. (1985). Management of the child with mild cholestasis. *Pediatric Annals, 14*(7), 488–492.

Orr, M.E., Shinert, J., & Gross, J. (1981). *Acute Pancreatic and Hepatic Dysfunction.* Bethany, Conn.: Fleschner Publishing.

Porth, C.M. (1986). *Pathophysiology: Concepts of Altered Health States.* Philadelphia: J.B. Lippincott.

Shapiro, M.J., Wood, R.P., Shaw, B.W., Jr., & Grenvik, A. (1986). Postoperative care of liver transplantation patients. In P.M. Winter, Y.G. Kang (Eds.). *Hepatic Transplantation: Anesthetic and Perioperative Management* (pp. 177–201). New York: Praeger.

Shaw, B.W., Jr., Hakala, T., Rosenthal, J.T., Iwatsuki, S., Broznick, B., & Starzl, T.E. (1982). Combination donor hepatectomy and nephrectomy and early functional results of allografts. *Surgery Gynecology & Obstetrics, 155,* 321–325.

Shronts, E.P., Teasley, K.M., & Cerra, F.B. (1987). Nutrition support of the adult liver transplant candidate. *Journal of the American Dietetic Association, 87*(4), 441–451.

Starzl, T.E., Gordon, R.D., Tzakis, A., Staschak, S., Fioravanti, V., Broznick, B., Makowka, L., & Bahnson, H.T. (1988). Equitable allocation of extrarenal organs: With special reference to the liver. *Transplantation Proceedings, 20*(1), 131–138.

Starzl, T.E., Iwatsuki, S., Shaw, B.W., Gordon, R.D., & Esquivel, C.O. (1985). Immunosuppression and other nonsurgical factors in the improved results of liver transplantation. *Seminars in Liver Disease, 5*(4), 334–343.

Starzl, T.E., Iwatsuki, S., Van Thiel, D.H., Gartner, J.C., Zitelli, B.J., Malatack, J.J., Schade, R.R., Shaw, B.W. Jr, Hakala, T.R., Rosenthal, J.T., & Porter, K.A. (1982). Evolution of liver transplantation. *Hepatology, 2*(5), 614–636.

Starzl, T., Todo, S., Gordon, R., Makowka, L., Tzakis, A., Iwatsuki, S., Marsh, W., Esquivel, C., & Van Thiel, D. (1987). Liver transplantation in older patients. (Letter to Editor) *New England Journal of Medicine, 315,* 481–482.

Starzl, T.E., Van Thiel, D.H., Tzakis, A., Iwatsuki, S., Todo, S., Marsh, J.W., Konero, B., Staschak, S., Steiber, A., & Gordon, R. (1988). Orthotopic liver transplantation for alcoholic cirrhosis. *Journal of the American Medical Association, 260,* 2542–2544.

Staschak, S. & Formella, L. (1988). Liver transplantation: Patient education manual. Pittsburgh: Department of Surgery, University of Pittsburgh.

Thompson, A. (1987). Aspects of pediatric intensive care after liver transplantation. *Transplantation Proceedings, 19,*(4, Suppl 3), 34–39.

Traiger, G.L., & Bohachick, P. (1983). Liver transplantation: Care of the patient in the acute postoperative period. *Critical Care Nurse, 3*(5), 96–103.

Van Thiel, D.H. (1985). Liver transplantation. *Pediatric Annals, 14*(7), 474–478, 480.

Van Thiel, D.H., Schade, R.R., Gavaler, J.S., Shaw, B.W. Jr., Iwatsuki, S., & Starzl, T.E. (1984). Medical aspects of liver transplantation. *Hepatology, 4*(1), 79s–83s.

Van Thiel, D.H., Tarter, R., & Stone, B.G. (1986). Pathophysiology of liver disease. In P.M Winter, Y.G. Kang (Eds.). *Hepatic Transplantation: Anesthetic and Perioperative Management* (pp. 19–32). New York: Praeger.

Wood, R.P., Shaw, B.W., & Starzl, T.E. (1985). Extrahepatic complications of liver transplantation. *Seminars in Liver Disease, 5*(4), 377–384.

8

Heart Transplant

Patricia Gamberg and Kimberly Walton

The 1980s have placed heart transplantation in the forefront of surgical intervention for advanced cardiac failure. Improved surgical techniques and immunosuppressive regimens have enabled heart transplant recipients to return to a normal productive life-style. The recipient currently experiences shorter hospital stays and reduced morbidity and mortality.

Survival in heart transplantation has demonstrated a steady improvement since 1967. The International Society for Heart Transplantation Registry reports five years' actuarial survival of 72 per cent for all patients undergoing orthotopic or heterotopic heart transplantation from 1967 through 1986. For the year 1987 the International Heart Transplant Registry reported 1436 procedures performed in 109 centers throughout the world. One year's actuarial survival for the calendar year 1986 was 82 per cent.

The earliest experiments in heart transplantation were carried out by Carrel and Guthrie (1905). The heart of a donor dog was placed in the neck of the recipient animal. This non-anatomical, or heterotopic, placement set the stage for future heart transplants and proved that the denervated heart could indeed beat again after removal from the body.

As described in Table 8–1, three decades of inactivity passed before Mann and associates (1933) reported up to eight days of survival following canine heterotopic heart transplantation. These authors also provided the first description of heart rejection as observed in the canine model.

Attempts at canine orthotopic transplantation were reported by Goldberg and associates (1958). However, the heart was unable to support the animal hemodynamically. The first successful canine orthotopic heart transplants were described by Lower and Shumway (1960). They also demonstrated histologic changes now known to be characteristic of rejection. The use of immunosuppressive therapy was first reported by Reemtsma and colleagues (1962).

180

TABLE 8–1. EARLY EXPERIENCE IN HEART TRANSPLANTATION

INVESTIGATOR	DATE	CONTRIBUTION
Carrel	1905	Canine heterotopic transplant
Mann	1933	Canine heterotopic transplants Modification
Goldberg	1958	Orthotopic transplant using pump oxygenation
Lower & Shumway	1960	Successful orthotopic transplant in canine
Reemtsma	1962	Use of immunosuppression in canine
Barnard	1967	First human cardiac allograft

The first human heart transplant was performed in Mississippi in 1964. This was a xenograft procedure using a chimpanzee heart in a 68-year-old recipient who lived only a matter of hours.

The first successful human heart allograft procedure was performed by Christiaan Barnard at Capetown, South Africa, in 1967. Intensive worldwide activity followed this initial effort. The next year, 101 heart transplants were performed by 64 teams in 22 countries. Following this initial enthusiasm, the extremely poor survival rates made it evident that the procedure was not a panacea for end-stage heart patients. By 1970 heart transplantation was deemed by some a dismal failure. Few institutions maintained programs after these initial two years. Over the next decade heart transplantation continued to develop in only a handful of centers worldwide. Baumgartner and associates (1979) reported five active centers in January 1978 with one-year patient survival of 50 per cent to 60 per cent (Baumgartner, Reitz, Oyer, Stinson & Shumway, 1979).

In 1980, clinical trials using cyclosporine-based immunosuppression began. A marked improvement in mortality and morbidity was reported, resulting in a dramatic increase in activity in the field of heart transplantation. One-year survival rates were now 80 per cent (Gamberg, 1983). At the last report of the International Heart Transplant Registry in 1988 there were 109 centers performing heart transplantation in the United States and 79 centers in other countries. Twenty-two hundred procedures were performed in 1987 (Kaye, 1987).

In the discussion to follow, the current status of heart transplantation is described in detail. Patient evaluation of pediatric and adult recipients is included along with the preoperative care that is needed to manage a heart transplant patient. Heterotopic and orthotopic surgical procedures are presented with illustrations to provide clear understanding of the anatomy involved. Immediate and long-term postoperative care is also discussed. Finally, potential complications of a heart transplantation, survival statistics, and future direction in this field are presented.

PRETRANSPLANT EVALUATION

The evaluation process is usually initiated when a patient is referred to a heart transplant center. A careful history of the underlying cardiac problem is obtained, and the patient's physical status and current medication regimen, as well as her compliance with that regimen, are evaluated. Previous diagnostic tests and cardiac procedures are reviewed for evidence of systemic diseases, active infections, pulmonary hypertension, and marked obesity, which may preclude transplantation.

Patients are evaluated on an individual basis according to established criteria that address medical, psychosocial, and financial issues. The medical criteria for transplant recipients are similar in most transplant centers and have been developed based on early experience in the field. These criteria are summarized in Table 8–2.

After medical selection criteria have been considered, further assessment is needed to determine the patient's suitability for transplantation. Patients with ischemic cardiac disease and cardiomyopathy constitute the majority of the adult recipients. The children considered are those with cardiomyopathy or endomyocardial fibrosis and relatively normal lungs. The children with congenital heart disease with associated pulmonary vascular disease should be considered for heart-lung transplantation. The acceptable age range for recipient selection is in a state of flux, and criteria vary at different centers. The older patient had previously been thought to be at higher risk for postoperative complications, and patients over age 50 were excluded from consideration. In the cyclosporine era, carefully selected older patients have enjoyed survival rates equal to those of young patients and most centers have relaxed the criteria to include those in the 50- to 60-year range. A limited number of centers have active heart transplant programs for infants and neonates. The issues of compliance and drug effects on growth and development, and the special problems associated with pediatric care make this a challenging group of patients for select centers. Because corticosteroids have been the mainstay of immunosuppression, insulin-dependent diabetes has usually been considered a contraindication to heart transplantation. Those patients who do not demonstrate severe complications of diabetes are now considered candidates for heart transplantation at some centers.

TABLE 8–2. RECIPIENT SELECTION CRITERIA

1. End-stage cardiac disease with limited life expectancy
2. Cardiac disease not amenable to more conventional therapy
3. Absence of significant systemic disease
4. Absence of active infection
5. Pulmonary vascular resistance <4 Wood units
6. Absence of unresolved pulmonary infarcts

Psychosocial evaluation is an integral part of the evaluation procedure. This may be done by a psychiatrist, psychologist, social worker, transplant nurse, or physician. Issues that should be addressed in the psychosocial evaluation are those that would impact on postoperative morbidity or mortality. Preoperative compliance with the current medical regimen is a good indicator of future compliance essential for survival in heart transplant patients. The emotional stability of the recipient and her understanding of the prognosis and risks of the transplant procedure need to be assured. Patients with a history of depression or other disabling psychiatric disorders are not often accepted because of the risk of recurrence or intensification of symptoms with subsequent steroid therapy and the stresses of the postoperative period. Some programs may refuse to consider candidates with a history of alcohol or drug abuse. Substance abuse is often difficult to assess, and individual decisions may be made on a case-by-case basis.

Family support is also paramount during the entire transplant process. Although patients need not be part of a traditional family unit, an acceptable network of support and caring is essential for a successful outcome.

The issue of ability to pay is an extremely troublesome one. The health care system in the United States is complex and perplexing, and does not necessarily ensure equitable medical care for all. Medicare's and other insurance carriers' acceptance of the procedure as therapeutic is just beginning to resolve this issue. Currently Medicare funding is limited to centers that fulfill the requirements established by the National Organ Transplant Act. Many patients must resort to public appeal, fund raising, or other private sources.

An explanation of predicted survival rates should be given. The patient who is being evaluated needs adequate information in order to give informed consent either for or against heart transplantation. Immediate postoperative care should be explained; a tour of the postoperative unit may be helpful to give patients and their families an idea of what to expect. Potential late postoperative complications such as infection, malignancy, and hypertension need to be explained in detail.

The time spent waiting for a donor heart can be stressful. In addition to making sure optimal medical care is maintained, attention must be given to the psychological state of the waiting recipient. Gallows humor during this time is common, especially among those with a prolonged waiting period. Such comments as "It is raining; that should bring a donor" may be expressed by a patient. Some patients can more easily verbalize these thoughts to the transplant team. It is important to treat such comments as acceptable behavior and offer the candidate assurance and support. Questions about the approximate length of the waiting period need to be answered. One needs to make sure patients know who will contact them and where to report when called.

OPERATIVE PROCEDURE

There are two operative procedures for heart transplantation: orthotopic and heterotopic (Fig. 8–1A and B). Orthotopic transplantation refers to the placement of the heart in the correct anatomical position. Heterotopic transplantation refers to placement of the donor heart in a nonanatomical location in the body. Successful heart transplantation can be obtained by using either procedure.

Orthotopic heart transplantation has remained the standard procedure for many years. Originally described in a canine model in 1960, the recipient's own heart is replaced with a donor heart (Lower & Shumway, 1960). Using the orthotopic procedure, the superior and inferior vena cava and aorta are clamped and the patient is placed on cardiopulmonary bypass. The heart is then excised at the midatrial level, leaving the posterior right and left atrial walls and their venous connections intact.

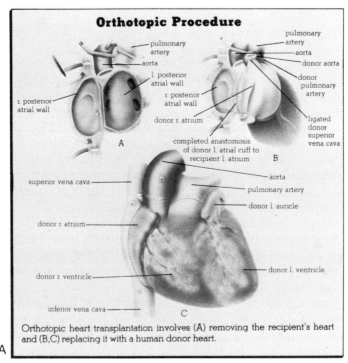

FIGURE 8–1. Heart transplant. A, Orthotopic procedure. B, Parallel procedure. (Reprinted from American Journal of Nursing, October 1980, by permission of Masako Herman, artist.)

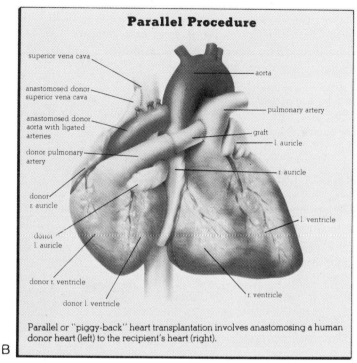

Parallel Procedure

superior vena cava

aorta

anastomosed donor superior vena cava

pulmonary artery

anastomosed donor aorta with ligated arteries

graft

l. auricle

donor pulmonary artery

r. auricle

donor r. auricle

l. ventricle

donor l. auricle

donor r. ventricle

r. ventricle

donor l. ventricle

Parallel or "piggy-back" heart transplantation involves anastomosing a human donor heart (left) to the recipient's heart (right).

B

FIGURE 8–1 *Continued*

A similar transection and excision of the donor heart leaves the sinus node and the blood supply intact. After the heart is excised it is immersed in a cooling solution and the atrial remnants are trimmed to fit those of the recipient. In the event of distant heart procurement the donor heart is transported in a cooling solution. Cold ischemic times of up to seven hours have resulted in excellent graft function, although ischemic times of less than three hours are generally preferred. With implantation of the donor heart, anastomosis of the left atrium, right atrium, and the great vessels is performed sequentially. Defibrillation may be required if spontaneous defibrillation does not occur. Isoproterenol is generally started at this time and titrated as necessary to maintain heart rate initially.

As a precautionary measure, epicardial pacing wires are implanted on the donor right atrium and brought to the external chest wall to be used in the event of bradycardia in the postoperative period. Chest tubes are inserted, and the chest is closed.

The heterotopic, or parallel, procedure may be indicated for patients with an extremely small donor or, occasionally, in patients with a high pulmonary vascular resistance. This procedure involves placing the donor heart in the right chest cavity and performing end-to-side anastomosis of the donor heart's superior vena cava and aorta with recipient vessels. The pulmonary artery is also anastomosed end-to-side but may require a small Dacron graft for lengthening purposes.

This heterotopic procedure results in the donor heart effectively being used to assist the failing ventricle of the recipient. The potential for clot formation in the failing recipient ventricle remains high, and patients require systemic anticoagulation.

IMMEDIATE POSTOPERATIVE CARE

Immediate postoperative nursing care of a heart transplant recipient is similar to that of a patient who has undergone routine cardiac surgery. Care of a heart transplant recipient, however, does involve several differences and considerations. These include differences in physiologic and pharmacologic responses of the transplanted heart because of its denervated status and the increased susceptibility to infectious complications seen in all patients after institution of immunosuppressive therapy.

Because the technique of heart transplantation does not involve anastomosis of neural structures, the heart is denervated and thus lacks the normal physiologic responses to sympathetic and parasympathetic nerve stimulation. Nerve receptors in the transplanted heart do remain intact, and the heart is normally responsive to endogenously or exogenously administered catecholamines. Isoproterenol is routinely used to maintain heart rate in this early postoperative period until the donor sinoatrial (SA) node assumes a normal rate.

The parasympathetic nervous system normally slows the heart, and in its absence the transplanted heart beats at a rate higher than normal (90–110 beats per minute). Neither the Valsalva maneuver nor carotid massage will slow heart rate, since both act through reflexes that depend on the parasympathetic nervous system. Atropine does not increase the heart rate in the transplanted heart, since it acts by blocking parasympathetic impulses.

The effects of denervation also include the absence of reflex tachycardia in response to orthostatic changes in blood pressure. This may cause orthostatic hypotension, especially in the early postoperative phase when the patient is deconditioned. Venous pooling in the extremities may also occur, leaving the heart with a diminished preload. For these reasons, careful observation must be directed to the patient who needs assistance for her first time out of bed. As the patient achieves better cardiovascular conditioning this phenomenon will become less pronounced.

Unusual electrocardiographic activity is often noticed postoperatively in heart transplant recipients. Two sets of P waves at independent rates are often seen because of the presence of the remnant recipient atria and the donor atria, both of which maintain their electrical activity. The recipient's sinoatrial node is retained during the surgical procedure. It responds normally to autonomic stimulation and produces P waves, but the stimulation of these P waves does not cross the suture line, and thus they are not followed by QRS complexes. The donor P wave is followed by a QRS complex, and thus does stimulate ventricular contraction (Fig. 8–2). This phenomenon is mainly an electrocardiographic curiosity and does not seem to lead to any significant problems with beat-by-beat changes in output.

In the early postoperative phase such problems as hidden mediastinal bleeding and right heart failure may arise. The pericardial sac is often enlarged during illness to accommodate an enlarging heart, enabling it to conceal mediastinal bleeding that occurs postoperatively with placement of a normal-sized heart. Nursing intervention, therefore, would be to raise the head of the bed 30 degrees and turn the patient from side to side every hour to promote mediastinal drainage.

Another problem in the immediate postoperative phase may be right heart failure due to the inability of the normal donor right heart to increase its work load activity to cope with an increased peripheral vascular resistance in the recipient. By closely monitoring the patient's right atrial pressures and cardiac output this potentially fatal condition can be diagnosed early and appropriate measures taken. Trends or deviations in cardiac output and its relation to right atrial pressure may show a pattern that emerges clinically and necessitates a need to modify the volume status or intravenous inotropic support.

Inotropic support, such as isoproterenol or dobutamine, may be needed in the management of right heart failure. The recipient may be

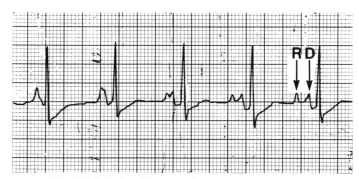

FIGURE 8–2. Atrial activity after heart transplantation.

placed on an infusion of prostaglandin E (PGE), a potent pulmonary vasodilator that reduces systemic blood pressure as well as pulmonary hypertension. Epicardial pacing may also be required by way of the surgically implanted wires for chronotropic support. Rarely, a patient requires permanent pacemaker placement for persistent bradycardia.

Protective Isolation

Protective isolation may be observed during the immediate postoperative phase. Increased susceptibility to infection because of the use of immunosuppressive medication renders a transplant patient vulnerable to opportunistic infections. Some centers require noncirculating room ventilation and the use of surgical gowns, gloves, masks, shoe covers, and cap to reduce the possible transmission of infection. Other centers institute more flexible procedures and restrict only staff and family members with an infection. Some centers may require their staff to wear a mask and gloves during dressing changes. Strict isolation may be required when the patient is being treated for an acute rejection.

Psychological Effects

Heart transplantation is not associated with serious psychological morbidity. The initial higher doses of steroids in the early postoperative period may play a part in an increased emotional response. Moods exhibited by the recipient, euphoria and depression, are most often an intensified form of their existing or appropriate mood. Relaxation of strict isolation procedures and shorter hospital stays have minimized these problems. Before transplantation, the recipient often wonders how she will react when a stranger's heart replaces hers. After transplant, however, the recipient quickly considers the new heart her own. The recipient often expresses gratitude to the donor family but rarely feels that the organ is not hers. An anonymous note of gratitude to the donor family can be forwarded by the donor coordinator, to help facilitate the expression of this gratitude.

Table 8–3 outlines potential problems that may arise during the postoperative phase. Nursing assessment and intervention highlight several areas that require attention. Optimal clinical management relies on clinical judgment as well as on measurements of the heart's function.

Immunosuppression

A major challenge in successful management of the heart transplant patient is balancing the immunosuppressive therapy. The purpose of immunosuppression is to prevent rejection of the graft. In the past, immunosuppressive therapy included high-dose steroids as well as azathioprine. The introduction of cyclosporine has resulted in markedly improved clinical results, and cyclosporine-based immunosuppression is used by most major transplant centers.

Most centers currently use a triple-drug regimen consisting of cyclosporine, azathioprine, and steroids. The specific regimen in each program is determined by the transplant physician. A few centers have been successful in eliminating steroids from their basic regimens (Renlund, O'Connell, Gilbert, Watson, & Bristow, 1987).

Rejection

Rejection describes the immunologic process that ensues when the recipient's immune system recognizes dissimilar graft tissue. Clinical and laboratory experience have confirmed three types of rejection in the heart transplant recipient: hyperacute, acute, and chronic. Hyperacute and acute rejection are discussed here, and chronic rejection is discussed in the next section.

Hyperacute rejection, the most serious and life-threatening type, occurs early and is usually the result of preformed antibodies; fortunately it is rare. It usually necessitates immediate retransplantation. To prevent a hyperacute rejection, patients with preformed antibodies are cross-matched with each possible donor before retrieval of the heart.

Acute rejection can occur at any time post transplant but is most common during the first three months. At Stanford University, for example, in the recent era of cyclosporine-treated patients, a linearized rejection rate of 2.4 events per 100 patient days is seen at one month postoperatively and declines thereafter. Patients may manifest signs of acute rejection with increased central venous pressure, decreased cardiac output, decreased myocardial compliance (ventricular gallop rhythm), and/or atrial arrhythmias. Cyclosporine-treated patients most often show no overt signs of rejection, except at the histologic level, that is, on cardiac biopsy surveillance. Clinical evidence is often not apparent unless the process is histologically severe.

A technique that is noninvasive and highly sensitive for diagnosing rejection is being sought in various transplant centers. One such technique that involves the monitoring of the urine polyamine levels has been evaluated. Changes in the cell growth–cell death ratio cause fluctuations in acetylated derivative components of urinary polyamines. Because rejection is expected to result in greater cell death, this would change the ratio (Womble, Copeland, & Fuller, 1984).

Cytoimmunologic monitoring represents a method for evaluation of

Text continued on page 196

TABLE 8–3. NURSING CARE PLAN FOR HEART TRANSPLANT RECIPIENT

Need, Problem, or Potential Problem	Assessment	Nursing Intervention

Potential low cardiac output related to:
 a. Hypovolemia due to increased intravascular space as patient warms, third-spacing, or bleeding
 b. Fluid overload
 c. Perioperative MI or ventricular dysfunction due to global ischemia related to organ storage preservation and anesthesia
 d. Tamponade
 e. Denervation of heart: cardiac response dependent on circulating catecholamines
	1. Vital signs as necessary, including the need for pacing and cuff BP, compare with preoperative level
	 2. Circulatory status (check strength of pulses, sensation, warmth, color, etc.)
	 3. Presence of arrhythmias
	 4. Decrease in hourly urine output
	 5. Changes in ABGs
	 6. Presence of S_3 or murmur
	 7. Signs and symptoms of MI
	 8. Signs and symptoms of CHF
	 9. Signs and symptoms of tamponade
		1. Notify charge nurse and physician of signs and symptoms of low cardiac output.
		 2. Optimize preload with fluids as ordered.
		 3. Optimize afterload as ordered.
		 4. Correct ABGs per order. Consult with physician about the need to change PEEP, as this may alter CO.
		 5. Obtain order for chest x-ray to rule out tamponade.
		 6. Administer inotropic agents within ordered guidelines; consult with physician concerning the need for digitalization, Ca^{++} administration, etc.
		 7. Consult with physician for measures to optimize heart rate, e.g., Isuprel, pacemaker.
		   a. Isuprel infusion 1–4 days for positive inotropic, chronotropic support
		   b. Atrial pacing wires
		   c. Vagal maneuvers or drugs for stimulating the vagus ineffective on denervated heart

Arrhythmia related to edematous suture lines in atria, electrolyte imbalance, sensitivity to ischemia	1. Effect on cardiac output 2. Possible causes 3. Effect of antiarrhythmic drugs and pacemakers	1. Notify charge nurse and physician of presence of arrhythmia. 2. Increase frequency of vital sign assessment and note perfusion. 3. Obtain rhythm strip q shift. Label with name, date, time, activity. 4. Maintain potassium scale as ordered or consult with physician for change. 5. Administer antiarrhythmic drugs as ordered or obtain order if necessary. 6. Obtain pacemaker; attach, set, and turn on as ordered.

Hypertension increasing myocardial work and oxygen consumption related to:
a. Vasoconstriction from hypothermia and drugs
b. Pain, anxiety, shivering
c. Essential hypertension related to cyclosporine
	1. MAP, pulse, and cuff BP
	2. Signs and symptoms of CHF and MI
	3. Temperature and warmth of extremities
	4. Signs of pain and anxiety
	5. Complaints of headache
	6. Complaints of nausea or vomiting
		1. Keep MAP within parameters with antihypertensive drugs as ordered.
		  a. Nipride, Arfonad—acute
		  b. Minipress, Captopril—later
		2. Record cuff BP q4h.
		3. Consult with physician for:
		  a. MAP, pulse pressure, and large discrepancy between MAP and cuff BP
		  b. MAP uncontrolled with current drugs or only with excessive drugs (e.g., 5 μg/kg/min of Nipride)
		  c. Signs and symptoms of CHF and MI
		  d. Increasing bleeding from chest tubes and/or line insertion site
		4. Use warm blankets to control shivering; consult with physician for need for hyperthermia unit, sedation.
		5. Use ordered sedation as needed to reduce pain, anxiety, or agitation.

Potential CT bleeding related to:
a. Heparin effect
b. Possible preoperative hepatic dysfunction
c. Abnormal coagulation studies
d. Insufficient cauterization during surgery
	1. PCV, PLT, and coagulation profile
	2. Need for Ca^{++} after multiple transfusions
		1. Notify charge nurse and physician for:
		  a. CT output 150 ml/h
		  b. Signs and symptoms of hypovolemia or tamponade
		  c. Bleeding from other sites
		2. Transfuse with whole blood or packed cells to maintain PCV, MAP, central venous pressure, as ordered.
		3. Use cytomegalovirus-negative blood only.

Table continued on following page

191

TABLE 8–3. NURSING CARE PLAN FOR HEART TRANSPLANT RECIPIENT *Continued*

Need, Problem, or Potential Problem	Assessment	Nursing Intervention
Atelectasis related to: a. Anesthesia b. Pneumonia c. Inadequate ventilation from: 1. Improper endotracheal tube placement 2. Splinting 3. Abdominal distention 4. Bronchospasm 5. Pneumothorax or hemothorax 6. Agitation 7. Decreased mobility 8. Pleural effusion associated with rejection	1. Breath sounds every 2 h, after respiratory treatment and as needed. 2. Rate, character, quality of chest expansion, presence of nasal flaring or crepitus, use of accessory muscles, etc. 3. Position of trachea 4. ABGs 5. Signs and symptoms of hypoxia, hypercarbia 6. Color, consistency, amount of sputum 7. Need for sedation 8. Lab, e.g. hemoglobin with oxygen-carrying capacity, Po_2 resulting in muscle weakness	1. Notify charge nurse and physician of changes in breath sounds, ABGs, and quantity or quality of sputum. 2. Consult with physician for: a. Culture and sensitivity results b. Need for respiratory therapy or modification thereof c. Need for culture and sensitivity of sputum d. Need for correction of abnormal ABGs e. Need for CT 3. For a patient on a ventilator: a. Bag, sigh, instill saline, and suction every 1–2 h and as needed. b. Position patient with affected side up as much as possible to improve V/Q relationship. 4. For extubated patient: Assist respiratory therapist with treatment as ordered (up in chair when possible).
Renal failure a. Prerenal failure related to prolonged hypovolemia or hypotension, or impeded blood supply to kidneys b. Renal failure related to nephrotoxic effect of cyclosporine	1. Fluid balance a. Signs and symptoms of hypovolemia b. Signs and symptoms of low perfusion state c. Signs and symptoms of hypervolemia 2. Blood and urine chemistry results	1. Administer or restrict fluids as ordered; obtain needed orders. 2. Report signs and symptoms of decreased perfusion state. 3. Record accurate I & O, weight, lab results, and specific gravity. 4. Creatinine clearance over 12 hours every day as ordered. 5. Adjust cyclosporine dose per order to minimize nephrotoxic effects without compromising immunosuppression.

Nursing diagnosis	Assessment	Intervention

Infection related to:
 a. Invasive lines and procedures
 b. Cellular susceptibility due to nutritional state
 c. Immunosuppression
	1. Temperature
	 2. Circulatory status
	 3. Pulmonary status
	 4. Amount, color, odor, and consistency of pulmonary/wound exudate
	 5. Appearance of wound incision sites
	 6. Appearance and odor of urine
	 7. Skin integrity
	 8. White blood cell count and cultures and sensitivity results, and related drug therapy
		1. Notify physician and charge nurse of signs and symptoms of infection.
		 2. Culture blood, sputum, urine, and wound as ordered.
		 3. Maintain sterile technique for all dressing and line changes.
		 4. Consult with physician for required changes in drug therapy.
		 5. Change bottles and tubing every 24 h.
		 6. Isolate patient as indicated:
		   a. All entering room should gown and glove
		   b. Reverse isolation, including masks, boots, caps, gowns, until first negative biopsy; then masks and boots.
		   c. Recipient wears above apparel if leaving room.
		   d. Routine room cleaning by RN.
		 7. All equipment entering room wiped with detergent germicide.
		 8. Oral care: antifungal agents administered orally three times a day.
		 9. Skin care: inspect integrity overall and mucous membranes.
		 10. Wound care: incisions cleansed daily with half-strength hydrogen peroxide and Betadine.

Rejection as evidenced by histologic changes per biopsy; later vital signs	Monitor and record results of weekly biopsies, daily lab studies.	1. Prepare patient for endomyocardial biopsy as ordered (routinely every 5–7 days in first 2 mo). 2. Follow changes in immunosuppressive regimen as ordered.

Table continued on following page

TABLE 8–3. NURSING CARE PLAN FOR HEART TRANSPLANT RECIPIENT *Continued*

Need, Problem, or Potential Problem	Assessment	Nursing Intervention
GI bleeding related to steroid therapy, preexisting medical problems	Signs and symptoms a. Change in bowel sounds b. Increasing abdominal girth c. Tympanic percussion of abdomen d. Rebound tenderness e. Positive guaiac of stool and/or NG drainage; ↓ pH of NG drainage f. Location and intensity of pain	1. Notify charge nurse and physician of signs and symptoms of GI bleeding. 2. Reposition, irrigate, and retape NG tube to secure patency. 3. Lavage NG as ordered until it is clear. Considerations: iced NS may be inappropriate because vascular reactivity is increased by heat, decreased by cold.
Anxiety related to: a. Depersonalization b. Dependent state c. Isolation d. Fear of graft rejection e. Body image changes	1. Orientation to time place, person, and situation 2. Psychosocial needs from patient, history, family, friends, etc. 3. Need for assistance from other resources, e.g., clergy, social worker, etc. 4. Effect of environment on patient	1. Reorient as needed. 2. Reduce unnecessary environmental stimuli. 3. Assure consistency in patient care routine and allow for scheduled periods of rest. 4. Encourage family and staff to communicate with patient through verbal and tactile stimuli. 5. Explain procedures. 6. Allow choices in care if possible. 7. Individualize environment. 8. Facilitate interaction between physician and patient and family. 9. Contact other resources as needed. 10. Monitor readiness for out of room as soon as possible. 11. Reassure patient that rejection is expected in first months post transplant. 12. Explain procedures using unit resources. 13. Provide primary nursing care. 14. Prepare patient for changes in nursing care post ICU.

Altered life-style requiring acquisition of new information and skills	1. Age, level of education
	2. Readiness for learning
	3. Family involvement
	4. Understanding of content presented by physical therapy
		1. Set priorities and goals with patient and family.
		2. Establish specific plan of teaching using unit resources.
		3. Record and communicate patient progress.
		4. Reinforce teaching throughout hospital stay:
		  a. Medications
		  b. Activities—exercise
		  c. Diet
		  d. When to notify physician
		  e. Signs and symptoms of infection
		  f. Late signs and symptoms of rejection

Neurologic dysfunction related to:
a. Low perfusion state
b. Cerebral thrombi
c. Air embolism
d. Drugs
	Assess the following every hour and as needed:
	1. LOC
	2. Pupils
	3. Movement, strength of extremities
	4. Signs and symptoms of increasing intracranial pressure
	  a. Bradycardia
	  b. MAP, pulse pressure
	  c. Decerebrate posturing (occurs with upper brain stem damage); extremities rigidly extended and arms hyperpronated
	  d. Decorticate posturing (accompanies damage above the brain stem to the corticospinal motor tract); legs stiffly extended and arms sharply flexed on chest
	  e. Abnormal reflex response
	5. History of preexisting neurologic problem
		1. Notify charge nurse and physician of abnormal changes in neurologic status.
		2. If possible, avoid sedation until patient reacts.
		3. Assure patient safety, e.g., seizure precautions.

Negative nitrogen balance from insufficient calories to meet the body's daily requirements	1. Daily weights, blood and urine chemistry results
	2. Wound healing
	3. Diet, in relation to caloric, mineral, and vitamin needs
		If patient is taking food by mouth:
		  a. Consult with dietitian to provide optimal diet; no added salt.
		  b. Provide nutritional snacks.
		  c. Organize nursing care to facilitate maximal intake at mealtime.

MI, myocardial infarction; BP, blood pressure; ABGs, arterial blood gases; CHF, congestive heart failure; PEEP, positive end-expiratory pressure; MAP, mean arterial pressure; CT, chest tubes; PCV, packed cell volume; PLT, platelets; NG, nasogastric lymphocyte activation. Determinations of the absolute concentration of circulating lymphoblasts and prelymphoblasts with the use of a mononuclear concentrate of the recipient's blood are made (Hammer, Reichenspurner, & Ertel, 1984).

Magnetic resonance imaging produces cross-sectional images without using ionized radiation or contrast material. The patient is placed in a magnetic field, and the response of protons to pulsed radiofrequency stimulations is used to generate an image. In addition, proton relaxation times may be determined for a given tissue and these changes may permit the detection of tissue necrosis (Eugene, Lechat, Hadjiisky, Teillac, Grosgogeat, & Cabrol, 1986).

The effectiveness of changes in diastolic function is also being evaluated as a noninvasive marker. A decrease in the isovolumic relaxation (IVR) time is used as a criteria for diagnosis of acute rejection. The IVR is defined as the time interval between aortic valve closure detected on the phonocardiogram and mitral valve opening identified on the echocardiogram. The IVR is thought to decrease with rejection because of change in the torque of the left ventricle (Dawkins, Olershaw, Billingham, Hunt, Oyer et al., 1984).

Further testing is needed to affirm if any of these procedures are sensitive or specific enough to reliably detect rejection and replace the cardiac biopsy in diagnosis of rejection.

Endomyocardial biopsy provides the most definitive evidence of acute rejection. Microscopic examination of myocardial tissue reveals interstitial and perivascular mononuclear cell infiltration and myocyte necrosis. It is also used to monitor the efficacy of rejection treatment. The biopsy procedure itself is invasive and involves percutaneous insertion of a biopsy forceps into the internal jugular vein (Fig. 8–3). The forceps is advanced across the tricuspid valve to the apex of the right ventricle, and samples of the endocardium are excised for microscopic examination. The biopsy can also be done from the femoral approach. The femoral approach is routinely used in young children and in adults whenever vascular access in the neck is difficult (Fig. 8–4).

The patient should be observed for possible complications of cardiac biopsy. These include pneumothorax, bleeding, atrial arrhythmias, and, most important, cardiac tamponade due to perforation of the heart. All of these complications are rare and are generally evident before the patient leaves the operating room or catheterization laboratory.

After diagnosing rejection by invasive and noninvasive methods, treatment in the early postoperative period may involve an increase in steroid therapy. A bolus of methylprednisolone for a period of three days is a common way of treating acute rejection in the early postoperative period. Later episodes may be treated with an increase in oral steroids

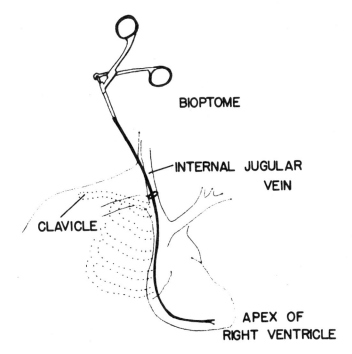

BIOPTOME

INTERNAL JUGULAR VEIN

CLAVICLE

APEX OF RIGHT VENTRICLE

FIGURE 8–3. Jugular biopsy procedure.

with a gradual taper. Orthoclone OKT3 or antithymocyte globulin may also be used.

POSTTRANSPLANT CARE

Physical therapy should be started soon after the patient is extubated. Bedside physical therapy can be instituted with progression from supine exercise to bicycle ergometry. An individualized program should be tailored to the patient's physical and medical status and age. Warm-up, peak-activity, and cool-down techniques and exercises are taught. Onset of leg pain and difficulty breathing are used as guides for progression and intensity of exercise. Patients are told they should not become so short of breath that they cannot converse. Written guidelines regarding activity progression should be given to the patient at discharge so that she can continue exercise routines at home.

Patients are taught to monitor their pulse rates and are made aware that there is a delay of five to ten minutes for the heart rate to increase, since the heart is denervated. They may also have a resting heart rate somewhat above normal.

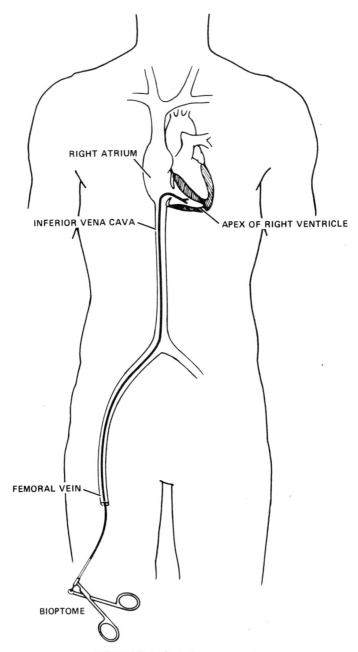

FIGURE 8–4. Groin biopsy procedure.

Education of the transplant patient and family is begun before transplantation, with orientation to the procedure and the nursing unit. A patient-teaching manual is given to the patient after she is extubated. Self-medication, along with teaching about the action and side effects of the drugs, is begun. The teaching involves patient participation with progression to independent care.

Temperature, pulse, and blood pressure monitoring is taught. Dietary teaching is begun, including diet restrictions, modification of fat intake, and maintenance of ideal weight.

The transition from hospital to home environment is made smoother when teaching is begun early. The medication routine must be adapted to the patient's life-style. Dosage times can be spaced to fit the work or school schedule, which helps to ensure compliance. The importance of early reporting of any symptoms needs to be stressed.

After discharge, patients are initially seen in the outpatient setting twice weekly. With clinical stability, frequency of visits is gradually reduced by three months postoperatively to a monthly schedule. After the first year, patients are generally seen every six weeks.

Blood work is drawn and evaluated for evidence of drug toxicity; renal, hepatic, or bone marrow dysfunction, electrolyte imbalance; and glucose intolerance. The electrocardiogram is examined for changes in rhythm as well as for ischemia. The chest x-ray detects pulmonary infection or malignant complications at an early and asymptomatic stage. The clinical examination, in addition to routine cardiovascular assessment, should place an emphasis on infection screening and attention to signs of malignancy and side effects of drugs. It is vital that patients play an active role in their health care. They need to be aware of their medical regimen and of potential complications. Additional functions of the clinical visit are to assess the patient's understanding and to expand on teaching begun in the hospital setting.

LONG-TERM COMPLICATIONS

As the patient returns to work or school, other complications may arise. Long-term complications of a heart transplant include steroid-related adverse effects (see Chapter 4), malignancy (see Chapter 4), graft atherosclerosis, infection, and hypertension. Three of these long-term complications are described with suggested treatment and measures to minimize their presence.

Graft Atherosclerosis

Graft atherosclerosis is a major cause of heart transplant morbidity and mortality. This accelerated form of coronary artery disease was described in the heart transplant literature as early as 1969 (Griepp, Stinson, Bieber, Reitz, Copeland, & Oyer, 1977).

Several measures undertaken early in 1970 attempted to slow the progress. Attention to risk factors was intensified. Most programs strongly advised patients to limit dietary intake of fats and encouraged maintenance of ideal weight and regular exercise. Dipyridamole and warfarin were prescribed in an attempt to reduce the possible thrombotic component of the lesion. Routine use of warfarin has been discontinued. Aspirin and dipyridamole are currently being used in some centers in an attempt to reduce the incidence of graft atherosclerosis.

Because the transplanted heart is denervated, atherosclerosis can progress without warning symptoms of ischemia. Symptoms of heart failure or arrhythmia may be the presenting complaint. Electrocardiographic evidence of ischemia has been seen in patients whose presenting complaint is a flu-like syndrome with breathlessness. The atherosclerosis is usually diffuse and concentric, and affects the entire length of the vessel. Coronary bypass grafting or angioplasty, therefore, is not feasible, and retransplantation is often undertaken when the disease is felt to be life-threatening. Screening for evidence of this process in the posttransplant patient is done by treadmill studies and myocardial scan. Because noninvasive screening has a low level of sensitivity, effective screening is accomplished mainly through regular coronary arteriography. Graft atherosclerosis is being studied in many centers with respect to cause, prevention, and treatment. Some investigators believe that it represents a chronic rejection process.

Infection

Infection remains the major cause of morbidity and mortality in the heart transplant recipient. The lung is the most frequent site of infection, with bacterial pathogens being the most common. Routine chest x-rays are important for surveillance of early asymptomatic pulmonary infection. Most recipients are instructed to wear a mask any time they return to the hospital as protection from hospital organisms. Careful assessment of the patient with particular attention to potential infection sites is vital. Skin care should be encouraged and dressings changed using sterile technique. Wounds should be closely observed for erythema, and appropriate cultures obtained. A dry cough or slight breathlessness may be indicative of an early *Pneumocystis* infection. A headache may represent early symptoms of meningitis or abscess. The nurse needs to be aware, and the patient must be educated to report all symptoms and not ignore a minor change in status. Any fever should be aggressively evaluated for a source of infection. *Legionella* has recently emerged as a prominent pathogen in some centers (Kirby, Snyder, Meyer & Finegold, 1980). An environmental evaluation of the possible sources (i.e., water supply) and measures to modify any source should be undertaken. Nocardia infection can present as a nodular pulmonary infection or a subcutaneous lesion. Toxoplasmosis is an infection that can be transmitted by way of the donor heart. Preoperative donor and recipient sera can be screened for the presence of antibody. If the donor is seropositive, prophylactic treatment may be instituted. Diagnosis of disease may be made when the organism is seen on routine cardiac biopsy. Refer to Chapter 5 for further information regarding infectious complications.

Hypertension

The approach to treating the hypertension exhibited by the heart transplant patient has been the administration of an individualized regimen of antihypertensive medications. Adequate control is important to preserve renal function, avoid peripheral vascular disease, and impact on the development of graft atherosclerosis. Home monitoring of blood pressure is thought to be important in devising a regimen to afford maximum control in this group.

LONG-TERM MANAGEMENT

Long-term care is usually given at a local medical facility close to the recipient's home rather than at the transplant center. The recipient leaves a highly protected, specialized environment and returns to her primary care physician, whose practice may not include any similar patients.

The transplant team members now assume the role of consultant in the care of each patient. The coordinator, together with the transplant physicians, serves as a resource to the local physician, the recipient, and the recipient's family.

In most cases the transplant recipient is cardiac functional class I and should have only minor life-style restrictions. Generally, the recipient can look forward to leading a relatively normal life and returning to the occupation and activities of her choice. Obvious sources of infection should be avoided and a regular exercise regimen pursued. Maintenance of ideal body weight and modification of fat intake are of utmost importance. Avoidance of smoking is stressed, since the lungs are a frequent site of infectious complications.

Those caring for heart transplant patients need to be alert to subtle changes in the patient's clinical course. Aggressive investigation of symptoms and institution of prompt treatment are vital to long-term survival.

ANNUAL REVIEW

Generally, each patient is evaluated around the anniversary of her transplant. Evaluation at that time includes right and left heart catheterization, coronary arteriography, and endomyocardial biopsy. This evaluation also serves as a general screening for infectious and malignant complications and for side effects or interactions of drug therapy. Additionally, research studies are often implemented during this stay.

THE FUTURE OF HEART TRANSPLANTATION

Certain hurdles must be overcome if progress is to be made in the field of heart transplantation. Practical issues include donor availability and development of methods for preserving the heart for long-distance retrieval and short-term storage. Advances in immunology, mechanical circulatory support systems, and cardiac xenografting may redirect and change the current methods of heart replacement. Surpassing clinical problems and developing new ways to meet the challenge of rejection may improve patient and graft survival.

Donor availability has been suggested as the primary determinant of the future of heart transplantation. Evans and associates (1986) describe the current dilemma of the donor shortage and how future heart transplantation will be dictated by the number of available donor hearts. Refer to Chapter 18 for further discussion of this issue.

Effective long-term preservation of the excised heart for transplantation remains an unsolved problem. Biodegradation, an accumulation of waste products, and acidosis eventually cause the preserved heart to function poorly. Quality of the heart before it is transplanted is affected by preservation time and, thus, may be compromised with extended preservation. Many attempts have been made to develop a solution that will prolong organ viability and allow for long-distance procurement. Some of the current solutions are the Bretschneider histidine-buffered, the Papworth, and the St. Thomas. These and other solutions are usually kept at lower temperatures to ensure hypothermia, and contain potassium as a common ingredient.

The role of mechanical circulatory support systems may also affect the future of heart transplantation. The total artificial heart and the left ventricular and biventricular extracorporeal assist devices have been used as bridges to heart transplantation at a small number of centers. In patients who receive assist devices the prognosis for survival without transplantation is less than one year (Pae & Pierce, 1986). The temporary "bridge" concept underscores the need for a suitable donor heart within stricter time constraints. Even though this aggressive, temporary, therapeutic modality may benefit a small number of patients, it requires further study with established protocols.

The future of these bioengineering devices is difficult to predict. Frequent use of these successfully implantable devices would strain the already limited number of available donor hearts. An advanced, permanent total artificial heart may become practical in the future as technology advances. If this should occur, the need for available donor hearts would diminish.

Another factor that may play a part in the future of heart transplantation is xenografts. An alternative to heart replacement, xenografts remain a scientifically feasible approach.

In summary, the therapeutic efficacy of heart transplantation has become accepted worldwide and is reflected in the increasing number of centers with successful programs. Improved long-term survival and quality of life afforded heart transplant patients will ensure that the procedure can be offered to an increasing number of patients.

References

Baumgartner, W.A., Reitz, B.A., Oyer, P.E., Stinson, E.B., & Shumway, N.E. (1979). Cardiac homotransplantation. Current Problems in Surgery, 16, 1–61.

Carrel, A., & Guthrie, C.C. (1905). The transplantation of veins and organs. American Journal of Medicine, 10, 1101–1102.

Dawkins, K.D., Oldershaw, P.J., Billingham, M.E., Hunt S., Oyer, P., Jamieson, S., Popp, R., Stinson, E., & Shumway, N. (1984). Changes in diastolic function as non-invasive marker of cardiac allograft rejection. Journal of Heart Transplantation, 3(4), 286.

Eugene, M., Lechat, P., Hadjiisky, P., Teillac, A., Grosgogeat, Y., & Cabrol, C. (1986). Nuclear magnetic resonance and proton relaxation times in experimental heterotopic heart transplantation. Journal of Heart Transplantation, 5(1), 39–45.

Evans, R., Manninen, D., Garrison, L., & Maier, A. (1986). Donor availability as a primary determinant of the future of heart transplant. Journal of the American Medical Association, 255(4), 1892–1898.

Gamberg, P. (1983). Clinical results: Cardiac transplantation. Transplant Proceedings, 15, 41–47.

Goldberg, M., Bergman, E.F., & Akman, L.C. (1958). Homologous transplantation of the canine heart. Journal of International College of Surgeons, 30, 575–586.

Griepp, R.B., Stinson, E.B., Bieber, C.P., Reitz, B.A., Copeland, J.G., & Oyer, P.E. (1977). Control of graft arteriosclerosis in human heart transplant recipients. Surgery, 81(3), 262–269.

Hammer, C., Reichenspurner, H., & Ertel, W. (1984). Cytological and immunologic monitoring of cyclosporine-treated human heart recipients. Journal of Heart Transplantation, 3(3), 228.

Kaye, M.P. (1987). The registry of the International Society for Heart Transplantation: Fourth official report. Journal of Heart Transplantation, 6(2), 63–67.

Kirby, B.D., Snyder, K.M., Meyer, R.D., & Finegold, S.M. (1980). Legionnaire's disease: Report of sixty-five nosocomially acquired cases and review of the literature. Medicine, 59, 188–205.

Lower, R.R., & Shumway, N.E. (1960). Studies on orthotopic transplantation of the canine heart. *Surgical Forum, 11,* 18–19.

Mann, F.C., Priestley, J.R., Markowitz, J., & Yater, W.M. (1933). Transplantation of the intact mammalian heart. *Archives of Surgery, 26,* 219–224.

Pae, W., & Pierce, W. (1986). Combined registry for the clinical use of mechanical ventricular assist pumps and the total artificial heart. *Journal of Heart Transplantation 5*(1), 6–7.

Reemtsma, K., Williamson, W.E., Iglesias, F., et al. (1962). Studies in homologous canine transplantation prolongation of survival with folic acid antagonists. *Surgery, 52,* 127–133.

Renlund, D.G., O'Connell, J.B., Gilbert, E.M., Watson, F.S., & Bristow, M.R. (1987). Feasibility of discontinuation of corticosteroid maintenance therapy in heart transplantation. *Journal of Heart Transplantation, 6,* 71.

Womble, J.R., Copeland, J.G., & Fuller, J.K. (1984). Urine polyamine test predicts rejection in cyclosporine-treated heart transplant patients. *Circulation, 70,* 11–17.

9

Heart-Lung and Unilateral Lung Transplantation

Janice A. Copeland

Heart-lung and unilateral lung transplantation have been under investigation for more than 40 years. Canine heart-lung transplantation was first attempted in 1946 by the Russian surgeon Demikhov (Demikhov, 1960). The first attempt at human heart-lung transplant was in 1968 by Cooley, in a two-month-old infant. The child died after 14 hours because of hemorrhage (Cooley, Bloodwell, Hallman, Nora, Harrison, & Leachman, 1969). The second human heart-lung transplant was performed by Lillehei in 1970. The 43-year-old recipient, who had a history of emphysema and pulmonary hypertension, lived for eight days. His death was caused by progressive respiratory failure. The next year Barnard, in Cape Town, performed a combined heart-lung transplant in a 49-year-old with chronic obstructive lung disease. This patient survived for 23 days before succumbing to complications secondary to infection (Barnard & Cooper, 1981).

Unilateral lung transplantation was first attempted in dogs in 1951 (Juvenelle, Citret, Wiles, & Stewart, 1951). In 1954 Hardin and Kittle demonstrated a technique of single lung transplant that has changed little even today. The first human lung transplant was performed by Hardy in 1963. The patient died of respiratory failure after 18 days (Hardy, Webb, Dalton, & Walker, 1963). After this first attempt, approximately 40 clinical human lung transplants were done over the next 20 years with only two recipients ever being discharged from the hospital. The longest survivor was a 23-year-old man with silicosis who underwent a right lung transplant by Derom, in 1968. The patient was discharged from the hospital after eight months but died of chronic rejection and sepsis two months later (Derom, Versieck, Rolly, Berzsenyl, Visermeire, & Vrints, 1971).

None of the precyclosporine attempts at unilateral or combined

205

heart-lung transplants were successful. The reasons for the early deaths were several: (1) bleeding and technical problems, (2) adverse effects of high steroid doses on the healing of bronchial or tracheal anastomoses, and (3) secondary complications of pulmonary infections.

Both heart-lung and unilateral lung transplantations treat end-stage pulmonary disease. Patient selection, operative procedures, and basic follow-up differ for the two procedures in many respects; therefore, these are discussed separately. First to be reviewed is heart-lung transplantation, which has been the more commonly used procedure. Then unilateral lung transplantation and, finally, new and future procedures for treatment of fatal pulmonary diseases are discussed.

HEART-LUNG TRANSPLANTATION

The clinical use of heart-lung transplantation for the treatment of certain end-stage pulmonary disease became feasible with the advent of cyclosporine. The Stanford group performed the first successful heart-lung transplant in 1981. Their first recipient was a 45-year-old woman with primary pulmonary hypertension. She underwent the transplant on March 9, 1981, and survived for five and one-half years, thus proving that long-term survival could be obtained with the use of cyclosporine for immunosuppression (Reitz, Wallwork, Hunt, Pennock, Billingham, et al., 1982).

More than 147 heart-lung transplants have been performed throughout the world since 1981. The one-year actuarial survival is 55.4 per cent, with a two-year rate of 51.9 per cent as of March 1987 (Kaye, 1987) (Figs. 9–1 and 9–2).

Many heart transplant centers are now performing heart-lung transplants. Recipient and donor selection plays an important role in determining a successful program.

Indications and Recipient Selection

There is a wide variety of end-stage cardiopulmonary diseases that, theoretically, could be treated with heart-lung transplantation (Table 9–1). However, the best results are found in patients with either primary pulmonary hypertension or Eisenmenger's syndrome who have not undergone prior chest surgery.

Eisenmenger's syndrome indicates any large congenital heart defect that allows free communication between the pulmonary and systemic circuits at the aortic, ventricular, or atrial level with a balanced or predominant right-to-left shunt secondary to marked elevation of pul-

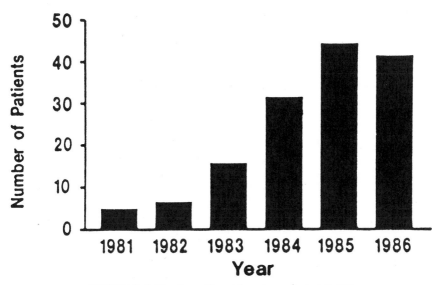

FIGURE 9–1. Number of heart-lung transplants per year.

monary resistance (Graham, 1979). These patients are good candidates because their cardiac function is usually impaired secondary to their pulmonary hypertension. They are generally young and can better tolerate the rigorous recovery period. The Stanford group found fatal hemorrhage

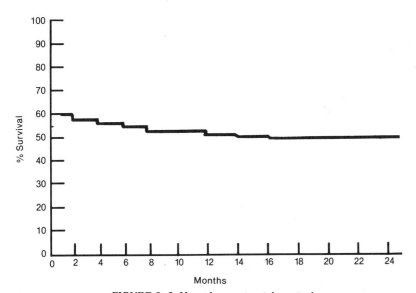

FIGURE 9–2. Heart-lung actuarial survival.

TABLE 9–1. INDICATIONS FOR HEART-LUNG TRANSPLANTATION

1. Primary pulmonary hypertension
2. Eisenmenger's syndrome
3. Chronic obstructive pulmonary disease
4. Pulmonary fibrosis
5. Cystic fibrosis

in those patients with Eisenmenger's syndrome who had previously undergone open-heart or thoracic surgery. This complication is due to adhesions, large collateral vessel development, and coagulation abnormalities resulting from hepatic dysfunction caused by previous surgical intervention (Jamieson, Baldwin, Stinson, Reitz, Oyer et al., 1984; Reitz et al., 1982). Others have been impressed with the incidence of this complication, which far exceeds that seen in conventional cardiac operations (Copeland, 1987).

Contraindications that are similar to those described in other organ transplantation are listed in Table 9–2. Patient selection is one of the most important considerations for long-term survival. Listed in Table 9–3 are the commonly accepted selection criteria.

Donor Selection and Retrieval

Specifically for heart-lung donors, the following criteria apply: (1) age less than 35 years; (2) a close size match in regard to the chest, the donor being slightly smaller than the recipient; (3) normal cardiac and pulmonary function as seen on the electrocardiogram; (4) clear chest x-ray; and (5) clinical examination. The lungs of the donor are the most critical and may be deemed unsuitable because of "neurogenic pulmonary edema," chest trauma, bacterial infection, atelectasis, or aspiration. Probably only 25 per cent of potential cadaver donors have lungs that are suitable for combined heart-lung transplantation (Reitz, 1982).

In the early years of heart-lung transplantation, because of inadequate lung preservation techniques, long-distance procurement was not feasible. Therefore, the donor was located at or transported to the transplant center. This factor eliminated possible donors because either the donor physician or donor family refused consent to transfer the donor, or if

TABLE 9–2. CONTRAINDICATIONS FOR HEART-LUNG TRANSPLANTATION

1. Systemic disease (i.e., sarcoidosis, alpha$_1$-antitrypsin deficiency)
2. Active infection
3. Psychological disorder
4. Alcohol or drug dependence
5. Life-limiting conditions (i.e., irreversible renal or hepatic failure, acquired immunodeficiency syndrome, malignancy)

TABLE 9–3. CRITERIA FOR ACCEPTANCE AS A HEART-LUNG RECIPIENT

1. End-stage cardiopulmonary disease
2. Age <50
3. No previous cardiac or thoracic surgery
4. Creatinine clearance >30 ml/min
5. Financial capability (insurance or personal)

consent was given, the donor lungs were unacceptable after the transfer because of aspiration, a positive Gram stain of the tracheal aspirate, or pulmonary edema occurring after the transport had started.

Today long-distance procurement is common. Several methods have been used. First, a method of autoperfusion of the heart-lung allograft has been reported. The heart and lungs were removed from the donor en bloc and placed in a normothermic crystalloid bath in which the donor blood was circulated through the heart and the lungs were ventilated with room air (Ladowski, Kopelanski, Tesdori, Stevenson, Hardesty, & Griffith, 1985). This technique is complex, however, and its clinical application is further complicated by the current need to share a rare resource, the organ donor. Furthermore, there is potential for mechanical failure, organ failure, and infection during transportation; therefore, it is no longer used (Adachi, Fraser, Kontos, Borkon, Hutchins et al., 1987).

The second technique is hypothermic cardiopulmonary preservation. In this procedure the donor is placed on cardiopulmonary bypass and cooled to 15° C. After a cold cardioplegic arrest of the heart the organs are further cooled by cardiopulmonary bypass and topical cooling. Then the heart and lungs are removed en bloc and placed in a cold (4° C.), sterile saline solution and transported to the transplant center in a small portable cooler. This technique is a simple and stable method and allows for multiple organ procurement (Adachi et al., 1987).

Even simpler and currently most popular are techniques that cool the lungs (Eurocollins solution) and the heart (cardioplegic solution) with separate fluids and then transport the heart-lung block in ice. Some programs do not perfuse and use only topical hypothermia.

The Waiting Period

During the evaluation phase the patient and his family are usually quite anxious. They are aware that the transplant procedure is the only option left to save the patient's life. Most are relieved when they find out they have been accepted as a candidate. However, as the waiting begins they are often discouraged by the length of time they may have to wait for a suitable donor. This is due to the lack of good pulmonary donors and to the length of each center's waiting list. Once a heart-lung transplant candidate has been accepted, the patient is immediately listed on the United Network for Organ Sharing national computer. The average waiting time is 12 to 18 months. The major limitation to heart-lung transplant is lack of suitable donors (Dawkins & Jamieson, 1984). Approximately 20 per cent to 25 per cent of potential recipients die while waiting.

In the early years patients and families were asked to live near the transplant center. This often required moving away from their homes and community support and added a financial strain to an already stressful situation. Currently, however, many centers will allow the patient to live at home and come only when a potential donor has been identified. Patients and their families are able to remain in familiar surroundings. The patient is usually unemployed because of medical disability, and this lessens the financial burden of paying for an apartment for an extended period of time in another city.

Many transplant centers have developed support groups for patients who are waiting or who have already had their transplants. Patients have found support groups to be beneficial (see Chapter 14). Those who live away from their transplant center may try to find another transplant support group near their home town.

One of the most difficult things to face as a caregiver is seeing a patient slowly deteriorate when a suitable donor cannot be found. The patient often becomes more cachectic, requires more oxygen, has increased shortness of breath, and may be hospitalized while waiting. This situation can invoke a feeling of helplessness, and caregivers often benefit from emotional support themselves.

Preoperative Preparation and Surgical Procedure

Recipient selection is determined by ABO compatibility, size match, severity of illness, and the length of time the patient has been waiting. A potential heart transplant recipient will also be notified in case the lungs are later deemed unacceptable. Thus there will be no waste of precious organs. The transplant will usually occur in the next six to ten hours. Preoperative orders are given, including blood, urine, and sputum cultures, prophylactic antibiotics, and immunosuppression, usually consisting of cyclosporine and azathioprine. Any coagulation deficit is corrected with fresh frozen plasma or vitamin K.

The heart and lungs are removed en bloc from the donor and placed into the recipient's chest. Care is taken not to injure the phrenic or vagus nerves. The anastomoses that join the donor organs to the recipient are at the trachea, left atrium, and aorta. The most common operative complication is excessive bleeding (Fig. 9–3).

Postoperative Management

Immediate postoperative care is similar to that of a heart transplant recipient. The isolation techniques in the intensive care unit vary from center to center but usually follow a protective protocol for 48 hours. The recipient is ventilated for 24 to 48 hours, depending on her arterial blood gas results. A sample immunosuppressive protocol is listed in Table 9–4. Corticosteroid administration is not initiated until approximately 14 days postoperatively to allow for adequate healing of the tracheal anastomosis.

Rejection episodes are one of the most difficult phenomena to diagnosis in heart-lung recipients. It has been shown that the heart and lungs can reject independent of each other (McGregor, Billingham, Yousem, Burke, Oyer et al., 1985). Heart biopsy is the primary means of diagnosing cardiac rejection. Diagnosis of lung rejection presents a more difficult problem. Usually the first sign is an increase in interstitial and perihilar edema. Daily chest x-rays are essential (Fig. 9–4).

Symptoms of rejection include shortness of breath, fatigue, and decreased exercise tolerance. Late symptoms show respiratory failure with need for ventilatory support along with hepatic failure and pulmonary edema.

Infection in a heart-lung recipient is potentially fatal if left undiagnosed. Any possible infection, particularly pulmonary infections, must be aggressively investigated so that treatment can be initiated as quickly as possible. Infection must be ruled out by weekly sputum cultures. Transtracheal aspiration, bronchial lavage, and needle aspiration of the lung are performed to assist in differentiating between infection and rejection. Open-lung biopsy is performed when no clear diagnosis can be made. Symptoms of infection of the lungs are the same as those of rejection except the patient may have a fever. If a nodule is seen on chest x-ray, then a pulmonary needle aspiration should be done to make a definitive diagnosis.

Patient and family education is essential for successful long-term rehabilitation and survival. Education includes learning about the immunosuppressive medications and other drugs, learning how to perform pulmonary toilet, knowing what to do if the patient becomes ill, and understanding the importance of avoiding infections. This and other nursing care are summarized in Table 9–5.

Discharge from the hospital usually occurs three to four weeks postoperatively in an uncomplicated transplant. The heart-lung recipient

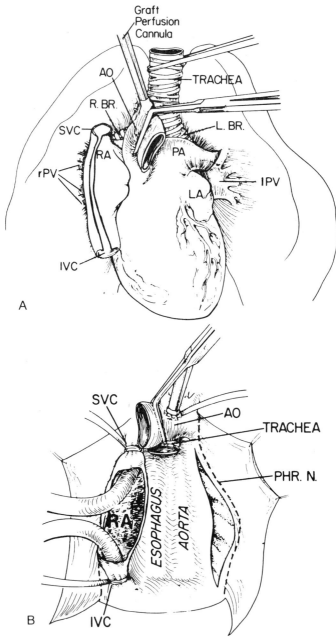

FIGURE 9–3. *A*, The heart-lung allograft. PA: pulmonary artery; Ao: aorta; LA: left atrium; RA: right atrium; SVC: superior vena cava; IVC: inferior vena cava; rPV and lPV: right and left pulmonary veins; R.BR and L.BR; right and left bronchi. *B*, The recipient's anterior mediastinum following excision of the recipient's heart and lungs. Ao: aorta; SVC: superior vena cava; RA: right atrium; IVC: inferior vena cava; PHR.N.: phrenic nerve. From Cabrol, C, et al (1984): Heart and heart-lung transplantation: Technique and safeguards. *Heart Transplantation, 3,* 110–114.

TABLE 9–4. IMMUNOSUPPRESSIVE REGIMEN

	FIRST 14 DAYS POSTOPERATIVE	AFTER FIRST TWO WEEKS
Cyclosporine	3–10 mg/kg/d PO	3–5 mg/kg/d—adjust to cyclosporine level PO
Azathioprine	1.5 mg/kg/d	1.5 kg/d PO (some centers discontinue)
Prednisone	—	60–100 mg/d—taper by 10 mg/d PO to 10–30 mg/d PO
Methyl prednisolone	250 mg every 8 h × 3 doses IV	
RATG (Rabbit anti-thymocyte globulin)	200 mg/d × 3 days IM	
Rejection episode	1 g Solu-Medrol × 3 days IV	1 g Solu-Medrol per day × 3 days IV

is then followed at the center's outpatient clinic. Assessment includes a weekly measurement of the cyclosporine level, which usually is maintained between 100 and 200 ng/ml, performed by fluorescent polarization, complete blood count, and electrolyte chemistries. The blood urea nitrogen (BUN) and creatinine levels are closely monitored because any elevation in either could signify cyclosporine toxicity. Chest x-rays are

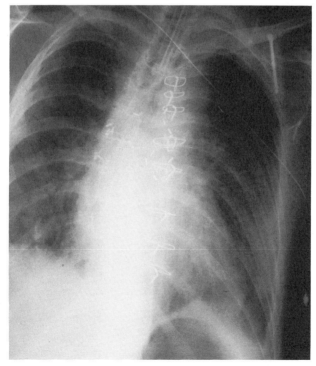

FIGURE 9–4. Chest x-ray showing pulmonary rejection.

TABLE 9–5. NURSING CARE OF HEART-LUNG RECIPIENT

Nursing Diagnoses	Predisposing Factors	Signs and Symptoms	Nursing Interventions
Altered hemodynamic status: cardiac output decreased	Cardiac tamponade	$\downarrow$ BP, $\uparrow$ CVP, $\uparrow$ HR, $\downarrow$ UO, sudden $\uparrow$ in chest drainage, pulsus alternans	Monitor vital signs closely. Monitor chest tube output. Monitor EKG.
	Excessive bleeding	$\downarrow$ BP, $\downarrow$ CVP, $\uparrow$ HR, $\downarrow$ UO, $\uparrow$ chest tube drainage	Monitor vital signs. Monitor EKG. Maintain hourly I & O. Monitor chest tube output.
	Cardiac arrhythmias, bradycardia	Irregular or slow heart rate	Monitor EKG rhythm. Monitor potassium levels. Maintain inotropic drips.
Altered respiratory status: breathing pattern ineffective	Denervated bilateral lungs	Slow respirations Fear of inability to breathe Pulmonary edema	Provide ventilatory support for 24–48 h postoperative. Turn, cough, and deep breathe frequently. Maintain PEEP on ventilator. Maintain low fluid intake volume. Provide incentive spirometry.
Airway clearance ineffective	Denervated carina	No deep cough reflex	Suction while on ventilator. Encourage coughing regularly post extubation; turn frequently, PP & D.
Gas exchange impaired	Ineffectual breathing	Low Po_2 $\uparrow$ CO_2	Monitor arterial blood gas measurements. Check for cyanosis in nail beds and lips.
Potential for infection	Immunosuppression Multiple IVs Catheters Intubation Surgical incision	Fever Redness and tenderness around IV sites and incision sites Excessive secretions from endotracheal tube $\uparrow$ Respiration rate Shortness of breath $\uparrow$ Fatigue	Monitor temperature with vital signs. Observe for local infections. Follow protective isolation procedures. Monitor WBC. Maintain skin integrity. Obtain ET cultures daily. Obtain chest x-ray daily. Observe strict pulmonary hygiene.

Potential for rejection	Cardiac dysfunction	Malignant arrhythmias	Monitor EKG.
			Monitor cardiac function.
	Immunosuppression	Shortness of breath	Supervise medication dosages.
	Infection	White-out on chest x-ray	Monitor CSA levels.
	Respiratory failure	Need for ventilatory support	Obtain daily chest x-ray.
		Fatigue, lethargy	Monitor exercise tolerance.
Alteration in fluid volume: excessive	Pulmonary edema	Frothing around endotracheal tube	Maintain PEEP while being ventilated.
	Impaired pulmonary lymphatic drainage	↑ Respiration rate	Monitor respiratory rate with vital signs.
	Reimplantation response	↑ Shortness of breath	Monitor I & O.
		Extremity edema	Obtain serial chest x-rays.
			Monitor extremities for pitting edema.
Self-concept: disturbance in body image, role performance, personal identity	Cushingoid appearance	Change in body fat secondary to steroids	Educate about medication side effects.
	Change in life-style	Change in body hair secondary to cyclosporine	Initiate physical rehabilitation program.
	Not chronically disabled	Able to return to normal activity, possibly return to work	Suggest support group for patient and family.
	Change in personality	Depression	Counsel on change in family dynamics.
Noncompliance: medication, hygiene, exercise, nutrition	Rejection	Respiratory failure	Monitor medication dosages, quiz patient.
	Infection	↑ Shortness of breath	Obtain routine chest x-rays.
	Obesity	Fever	Monitor vital signs at routine outpatient clinic visits.
	↓ Exercise tolerance	Need for rehospitalization post discharge	Monitor weight.
	Hypertension	Excessive, weight gain	Monitor physical rehabilitation schedule.
		↑ Fatigue, lethargy	Monitor nutrition; offer counseling.
		↑ BP	

BP, blood pressure; CVP, central venous pressure; HR, heart rate; UO, urinary output; PEEP, positive end-expiratory pressure.

important for weekly comparison of pulmonary, vascular, or cardiac changes. Patients are encouraged to join a cardiac rehabilitation program for exercise and to follow dietary guidelines.

If the patient is doing well, she is allowed to return home after three to four months. Follow-up care continues to be closely monitored by the original transplant center, which usually remains responsible for adjusting the immunosuppressive regimen. Pulmonary function tests are performed every three to six months to measure lung capacity. Some centers are even having patients perform and record the results of their pulmonary function tests on a daily basis to be able to follow their lung compliance more closely. Annual cardiac catheterization, chest x-ray, and laboratory tests are performed. These laboratory tests include the measurement of cyclosporine, electrolytes, BUN, and creatinine levels and a complete blood count. A 24-hour urine collection for creatinine clearance is also ordered along with chest x-rays. Pulmonary function tests for forced vital capacity and forced expiratory volume are obtained for comparison with earlier tests to note any changes in lung status. These tests assess signs of coronary atherosclerosis or airflow obstruction, which are often associated with chronic rejection.

These late complications are often fatal. Proliferative atherosclerosis is the major complication that affects the grafted heart. The long-term pulmonary sequelae of heart-lung transplantation include airflow obstruction secondary to obliterative bronchiolitis, recurrent respiratory infection, bronchiectasis, and pulmonary fibrosis (Dawkins, Jamieson, Hunt, Baldwin, Burke et al., 1985). The histologic similarity between the disease of the coronary and pulmonary vessels in these patients suggests that the causes may be similar, but the exact cause is a matter of speculation (Dawkins et al., 1985). If the airflow obstruction can be diagnosed early, aggressive medical management with steroids can often reverse the diseases. If the coronary artery disease or pulmonary airflow obstruction has become irreversible and the patient remains a good transplant candidate (i.e., has no active infection, reversible renal or hepatic failure, or both, or other life-debilitating complications), then retransplantation may be considered.

UNILATERAL LUNG TRANSPLANTATION

Indications and Recipient Selection

Unilateral lung transplantation is probably the best operation for those patients with end-stage pulmonary fibrosis. In other pulmonary diseases (e.g., emphysema, obstructive lung disease, and cystic fibrosis) the diseased lung that is not removed may compromise the donor lung, resulting in subsequent organ failure and death.

The major obstacle facing the success of single-lung transplantation is the proper selection of candidates. Listed in Table 9–6 are some recipient criteria and exclusions for unilateral lung transplants.

Donor Selection and Retrieval

Donor selection is similar to that described in heart-lung transplantation. Age restrictions are not as severe as for heart-lung donors, and donors up to 55 years of age would be acceptable. Size match is not as critical. A relatively oversized lung can be inserted, particularly on the left side.

The unilateral lung transplant procedure is quite different from a heart-lung transplant procedure. The lung is the only transplanted solid organ that does not have a systemic blood supply: the bronchial vessels are small and difficult to reconnect (Dark & Cooper, 1987). The chest is opened by means of a lateral thoracotomy. Coronary bypass is not needed, but femorofemoral bypass should be on standby in case anesthesia is not tolerated by the right ventricle. A pneumonectomy is performed on the recipient. The donor lung is anastomosed to the recipient heart at the left atrial cuff, and the bronchus and pulmonary artery are connected end to end. Finally, a pedicle of omentum is brought up from the abdomen and wrapped around the bronchial anastomosis. This technique, described by Cooper and associates in Toronto, restores bronchial artery circulation to the donor lung, improves bronchial healing, and affords protection against dehiscence, which may result from small bronchial vessels and steroid immunosuppression (Morgan, Lima, Goldberg, Ayabe, Ferdman, & Cooper, 1985).

TABLE 9–6. UNILATERAL LUNG CRITERIA

RECIPIENT CRITERIA	EXCLUSION CRITERIA
End-stage pulmonary fibrosis	Insulin-dependent diabetes
Age <55	History of alcohol or drug addiction
Not on steroids	Active infection
No other major organ dysfunction	History of malignancy
Psychological stability	Renal insufficiency with creatinine clearance <30 ml/min
	Myogenic respiratory disease (i.e., myasthenia gravis, muscular dystrophy)
	Cor pulmonale with gross cardiomegaly
	Chronic pulmonary emboli
	Lupus erythematosus
	Primary pulmonary hypertension
	Alpha$_1$-antitrypsin deficiency

It was further demonstrated that the immunosuppressant cyclosporine caused no adverse effects on bronchial healing (Goldberg, Morgan, Ayabe, Luk, Ferdman, & Peters, 1983). The left lung is usually chosen for transplant unless there has been a previous thoracotomy on that side (Fig. 9–5). It is possible to use the other donor lung for another recipient. If care is taken with the dissection, the heart can also be used, thus benefiting three patients (Dark & Cooper, 1987).

Postoperative Management

Isolation procedures for the lung recipient are the same as for the heart-lung recipient. Reverse isolation techniques are usually used for two to seven days as much to reduce casual traffic as to minimize the risk of infection.

Immunosuppression and the treatment of rejection are the same as for heart-lung transplantation. The unilateral lung recipient has several advantages when compared with a heart-lung recipient. First, the native lung provides a control for radiographic comparison with the donor lung in evaluating rejection. Second, clearance of secretions is not as significant a problem as with the heart-lung recipient because the carina remain innervated. The advantages of unilateral lung transplant are listed in Table 9–7 (Dawkins et al., 1985).

The patient's hospital stay would be much like that for any other

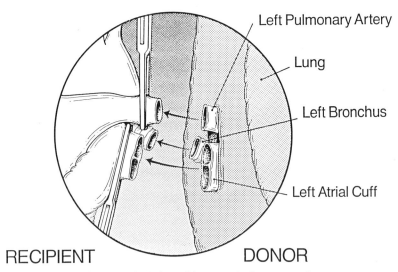

Left Pulmonary Artery

Lung

Left Bronchus

Left Atrial Cuff

RECIPIENT   DONOR

FIGURE 9–5. Unilateral lung surgical anastomosis.

TABLE 9–7. ADVANTAGES OF UNILATERAL-LUNG TRANSPLANTS

Innervated carina	Smoother postoperative course
Other lung retained	Some support available during severe rejection
	Provides control for radiographic comparison
Donor size not crucial	
Donor age up to 55 acceptable	
Heart available for another recipient	
Bypass not required	

transplant group. Prevention and treatment of infection, patient education, physical rehabilitation, and outpatient follow-up should be conducted in the same manner as for heart or heart-lung recipients. See Table 9–8 for a summary of recipient nursing care.

THE FUTURE

Heart-lung transplantation has been used in a limited manner for treatment of primary pulmonary hypertension. Unilateral lung transplantation is reserved for those patients with end-stage pulmonary fibrosis. Patients with terminal septic pulmonary diseases such as cystic fibrosis and alpha$_1$-antitrypsin deficiency, obstructive pulmonary disease, and emphysema usually have normal cardiac function and, therefore, do not need a heart-lung transplant. These patients are not candidates for single-lung transplantation either. For this group a double-lung transplant has been developed by Dark (Dark, Patterson, Al-Jilaihawi, Hsu, Egan, & Cooper, 1986).

A new surgical technique using heterotopic heart–single lung transplantation was described by Cooley and co-workers in 1987. This technique was used in a 34-year-old woman who had pulmonary hypertension but had undergone a patent ductus ligation at the age of five. The previous thoracotomy made her a high-risk heart-lung candidate, and this new procedure limits dissection in the vascular collateralized mediastinum and preserves the carina and left lung. Even though the patient died two hours postoperatively, secondary to diffuse hemorrhage and systemic acidosis, Cooley believes that this technique is a potential alternative for selected high-risk heart-lung transplant candidates (Cooley, Frazier, Macris, & Duncan, 1987).

It is likely that there will be a considerable expansion of transplantation for end-stage pulmonary disease in the near future. Because not all patients in need of lung transplants also require a simultaneous heart transplant, unilateral and bilateral lung transplants can be performed at centers without heart or heart-lung programs. In this way the greatest

TABLE 9-8. NURSING CARE OF THE UNILATERAL/BILATERAL LUNG RECIPIENT

Nursing Diagnosis	Predisposing Factors	Signs and Symptoms	Nursing Intervention
Altered hemodynamic status: decreased cardiac output	Excessive bleeding	Change in BP, ↑ HR, ↓ CVP, ↓ UO, ↑ in chest tube drainage	Monitor vital signs. Monitor EKG. Monitor chest tube drainage.
Altered respiratory status: ineffective breathing pattern	Denervated single lung	Pulmonary edema	Maintain PEEP on ventilator. Provide ventilatory support for 24–48 h. Maintain low fluid intake volume. Auscultate lung sounds. Turn, cough, and deep breathe. Provide incentive spirometry.
Impaired gas exchange	Ineffectual breathing	Low Po_2	Monitor ABGs. Check for cyanosis in nail beds and lips.
Alteration in fluid volume: excessive	Pulmonary edema Impaired pulmonary lymphatic drainage Reimplantation response	Frothing around endotracheal tube ↑ Respiration rate Shortness of breath Extremity edema	Maintain PEEP while being ventilated. Monitor respiratory rate with vital signs. Monitor I & O. Obtain serial chest x-rays. Monitor extremities for pitting edema.
Potential for infection	Immunosuppression Multiple IVs Catheters Intubation Surgical incision	Fever Redness and tenderness around IV sites and incision sites Excessive secretions from endotracheal tube ↑ Respiration rate Shortness of breath Fatigue	Monitor temperature with vital signs. Observe for local infections. Follow protective isolation procedures. Monitor WBC count. Maintain skin integrity. Obtain ET cultures daily. Obtain chest x-ray daily. Observe strict pulmonary hygiene.

Potential for rejection	Immunosuppression Infection Respiratory failure	Shortness of breath White-out on chest x-ray Need for ventilatory support Fatigue, lethargy	Supervise medication dosages. Monitor CSA levels. Obtain daily chest x-ray. Monitor exercise tolerance.
Altered self-concept: disturbance in body image, role performance, personal identity	Cushingoid appearance Change in life-style Not chronically disabled Change in personality	Change in body fat secondary to steroids Change in body hair secondary to cyclosporine Able to return to normal activity, possibly return to work Depression	Educate about medication side effects. Initiate physical rehabilitation program. Suggest support group for patient and family. Counsel on change in family dynamics.
Noncompliance: medication, hygiene, exercise, nutrition	Rejection Infection Obesity Exercise tolerance Hypertension	Respiratory failure Shortness of breath Fever Need for rehospitalization post discharge Excessive weight gain ↑ BP Fatigue, lethargy	Monitor medication dosages, quiz patient. Obtain routine chest x-ray. Monitor vital signs at routine outpatient clinic visits. Monitor weight. Monitor physical rehabilitation schedule. Monitor nutrition, offer counseling.

BP, blood pressure; HR, heart rate; CVP, central venous pressure; UO, urinary output; PEEP, positive end-expiratory pressure.

TABLE 9–9. POSSIBLE TRANSPLANTS FOR PATIENTS WITH END-STAGE PULMONARY DISEASE

TRANSPLANT	CRITERIA
Heart-lung	Primary pulmonary hypertension
	Eisenmenger's syndrome
	No prior thoracic surgery
Unilateral lung	Pulmonary fibrosis
Bilateral lung	Septic pulmonary disease
	Obstructive lung disease
	Emphysema
Heterotopic heart–unilateral lung	Pulmonary hypertension with history of prior thoracic surgery

number of recipients will benefit from the scarce donor organs. Table 9–9 summarizes the possible transplants for patients with end-stage pulmonary disease.

References

Adachi, H., Fraser, C.D., Kontos, G.J., Borkon, A.M., Hutchins, G.M., Galloway, E., Brown, J., Reitz, B.A., & Baumgartner, W.A. (1987). Auto perfused working heart-lung preparation versus hypothermic cardiopulmonary preservation for transplantation. *Journal of Heart Transplantation, 6,* 253–260.

Barnard, C.N. &, Cooper, D.K.C. (1981). Clinical transplantation of the heart: A review of 13 years' personal experience. *Journal of the Royal Society of Medicine, 74,* 670–674.

Cooley, D.A., Bloodwell, R.D., Hallman, G.L., Nora, J.J., Harrison, G.M., & Leachman, R.D. (1969). Organ transplantation for advanced cardiopulmonary disease. *Annals of Thoracic Surgery, 8,* 30–42.

Cooley, D.A., Frazier, O.H., Macris, M.P., & Duncan, J.M. (1987). Heterotopic heart–single lung transplantation: Report of a new technique. *Journal of Heart Transplant, 6,* 112–115.

Copeland, J.G. (1987). Heart-lung transplantation: Current status. *The American Journal of Heart Transplantation, 43,* 2–3.

Dark, J., & Cooper, J.D. (1987). Single-lung transplantation. *British Journal of Hospital Medicine, 5,* 443–445.

Dark, J.H., Patterson, G.A., Al-Jilaihawi, A.N., Hsu, H., Egan, T., & Cooper, J.D. (1986). Double lung transplantation. *The Annals of Thoracic Surgery, 42,* 395–398.

Dawkins, K.D., & Jamieson, S.W. (1984). The current status of heart-lung transplantation. *The International Journal of Cardiology, 5,* 406–410.

Dawkins, K.D., Jamieson, S.W., Hunt, S.A., Baldwin, J.C., Burke, C.M., Morris, A., Billingham, M.E., Theodore, J., Oyer, P.E., Stinson, E.B., & Shumway, N.E. (1985). Long term results, hemodynamics and complications after combined heart and lung transplantation. *Circulation, 71,* 919–926.

Demikhov, V.P. (1960). Some essential points of the techniques of transplantation of the heart, lungs, and other organs. In *Experimental Transplantation of Vital Organs.* Translated from Russian by Basil Haigh, Consultants Bureau, New York (1962) (pp 29–47). Moscow, Medgiz.

Derom, F., Versieck, J., Rolly, G., Berzsenyl, G., Visermeire, P., & Vrints, L. (1971). Ten month survival after lung homotransplantation in man. *Journal of Thoracic and Cardiovascular Surgery, 61,* 835–846.

Goldberg, M., Morgan, E., Ayabe, H.A., Luk, S., Ferdman, A., & Peters, W.J. (1983). A comparison between cyclosporine-A and methylprednisolone plus azathioprine on bronchial healing following canine lung auto-transplantation. *Journal of Thoracic and Cardiovascular Surgery, 85,* 821–826.

Graham, T.P., (1979). The Eisenmenger's reaction and its management. In W.C. Roberts, (Ed). *Congenital Heart Disease in Adults* (pp. 531–542). Philadelphia: F.A. Davis.

Hardin, C.A., & Kittle, C.F. (1954). Experiences with transplantation of the lung. *Science, 119*, 97–98.

Hardy, J.D., Webb, W.R., Dalton, M.L., & Walker, G.R. (1963). Lung homotransplantation in man. *Journal of the American Medical Association, 186*, 1065–1074.

Jamieson, S.W., Baldwin, J., Stinson, E.B., Reitz, B.A., Oyer, P.E., Hunt, S.A., Billingham, M.E., Theodore, J., Modry, D., Bieber, C.P., & Shumway, N.E. (1984). Clinical heart-lung transplantation. *Transplantation, 37*, 81–84.

Juvenelle, A.A., Citret, C., Wiles, C.E., & Stewart, J.D. (1951). Pneumonectomy with reimplantation of the lung in the dog for physiologic study. *Journal of Thoracic Surgery, 21*, 111–115.

Kaye, M.P. (1987). The registry of the international society for heart transplantation: Fourth official report—1987. *Journal of Heart Transplantation, 6*, 63–67.

Ladowski, J.S., Kapelanski, D.P., Tesdori, M.F., Stevenson, W.C., Hardesty, R.L., & Griffith, B.P. (1985). Use of auto perfusion for distant procurement of heart-lung allograft. *Journal of Heart Transplantation, 4*, 330–333.

Lillehei, C.W. (1970). Discussion of Wildevuur C.R.H., & Benfield, J.R. A review of 23 human lung transplantations by 20 surgeons. *The American Journal of Thoracic Surgery, 9*, 489–515.

McGregor, C.G.A., Billingham, M.E., Yousem, S.A., Burke, C.M., Oyer, P.E., Stinson, E.B., & Shumway, N. (1985). Isolated pulmonary rejection after combined heart and lung transplantation. *Journal of Thoracic and Cardiovascular Surgery, 90*, 623.

Morgan, W.E., Lima, O., Goldberg, M., Ayabe, H., Ferdman, A., & Cooper, J.D. (1985). Improved bronchial healing in canine left lung reimplantation using omental pedical wrap. *Journal of Thoracic and Cardiovascular Surgery, 89*, 734–742.

Reitz, B.A. (1982). Heart-lung transplantation: A review. *Journal of Heart Transplantation, 1*, 291–298.

Reitz, B.A., Wallwork, J.L., Hunt, S.A., Pennock, J.L., Billingham, M.E., Oyer, P.E., Stinson, E.B., & Shumway, N.E. (1982). Heart-lung transplantation. *New England Journal of Medicine, 306*, 557–564.

10

Pancreas Transplantation

Eileen DeMayo, Barbara Elick,
and Barbara Schanbacher

Diabetes mellitus is a major health problem and the third leading cause of death in the United States (American Diabetes Association, 1987). Because there is no known cure for type I diabetes, the only treatment is lifelong insulin injections given in an attempt to normalize the blood glucose and to reduce complications of the disease. Approximately 40 per cent of patients with insulin-dependent diabetes will develop devastating complications, such as renal failure, retinopathy, neuropathy, gastroenteropathy, and peripheral and cardiovascular disease. It is believed that the complications are secondary to disordered carbohydrate metabolism. Although the data are not conclusive, there is evidence that hyperglycemia and insulin deficiency are correlated with microangiopathic changes in diabetic patients and that meticulous control of the blood glucose has a favorable effect in delaying the development of complications (Davidson, 1978).

Nephropathy is a leading cause of morbidity in patients with insulin-dependent diabetes. It is estimated that 40 per cent to 50 per cent of such patients between the ages of 30 and 40 will develop nephropathy 15 to 25 years after the onset of the disease (Grenfell & Watkins, 1986). Twenty-five per cent to 30 per cent of patients with end-stage renal disease also have diabetes mellitus, and that number is increasing.

In the United States diabetic patients are twice as likely as nondiabetic patients to die of coronary artery disease (Christman & Bennett, 1987). Diabetic retinopathy is the number one cause of new blindness in people between the ages of 20 and 74 years, and approximately 5000 persons will lose their eyesight each year secondary to diabetes. Diabetic neuropathy is another common complication that affects either the autonomic or sensorimotor nervous system, or both, in end-stage diabetes. Pancreatic transplantation with restoration of normal glucose control offers select patients with diabetes the hope of prevention or delay of

224

the secondary complications of the disease. An important component is the selection of the appropriate candidate for this procedure (Corry, Nahiem, Schanbacher, & Gonwa, 1987).

HISTORICAL PERSPECTIVE

The first pancreas allograft transplant was performed by Kelly and associates at the University of Minnesota on December 17, 1966 (Kelly, Lillehei, Merkel, Idezuki, & Goetz, 1967). From December 1966 to June 1977 the American College of Surgeons and National Institutes of Health Organ Transplant Registry recorded 57 pancreas transplants in 55 diabetic patients (Sutherland, Kendall, Goetz, & Najarian, 1986). The early years of pancreas transplantation were discouraging because of low patient and graft survival rates.

Renewed interest in pancreas transplantation occurred in approximately 1982 after improvement in surgical techniques, the availability of new immunosuppressive drugs, and improved immune monitoring techniques. Approximately 1000 cases have been reported to date with more than 400 transplants carried out from 1983 through 1985 with a 44 per cent one-year graft survival rate (Sutherland, 1986). Over the past two years, with further improvements in surgical technique and diagnosis of rejection, 60 per cent to 70 per cent one-year graft survival rates have been reported (Sollinger, Stratta, Kalayoglu, Pirsch, & Belzer, 1987). At most major transplant centers, 90 to 95% one-year patient survival rates are being achieved (Sollinger, Stratta, Kalayoglu, & Belzer, 1987; Sutherland, Goetz, & Najarian, 1987). The longest functioning pancreatic allograft reported is ten and one-half years (D.E.R. Sutherland, personal communication, 1988).

Various surgical techniques for management of exocrine drainage have been used throughout the years, such as polymer injection into the pancreatic duct, anastomosis of the duct to recipient bowel or native ureter, and anastomosis of the donor duodenum encompassing the pancreatic duct to recipient urinary bladder. Each technique is described in detail later in this chapter. The worldwide experience has shown differences in graft survival rates between these three basic techniques, but many centers have currently reported excellent results with the urinary drainage technique (Sutherland, 1986; Sollinger, Stratta, Kalayoglu, & Belzer, 1987).

REVIEW OF ANATOMY AND PHYSIOLOGY

The pancreas is approximately six to eight inches in length, weighs between 100 and 150 g, and is divided into four parts: head, neck, body, and tail. The pancreas lies in back of the peritoneum behind the stomach and in front of the inferior vena cava, aorta, and left kidney. The head fills the loop formed by the duodenum and the tail reaches to the spleen (Fig. 10–1).

The pancreas is composed of two main ducts. The duct of Wirsung runs the full length of the gland, from the tail to the head. It empties digestive enzymes into the duodenum near or in conjunction with the common bile duct. These two ducts usually join at the ampulla of Vater. The second duct, the duct of Santorini, is an accessory duct and is not always present. This duct branches from the duct of Wirsung in the neck region and empties into the duodenum.

Blood is supplied to the duodenum and pancreas by way of branches of the celiac trunk and the superior mesenteric artery. The blood supply to the head of the pancreas comes from the branches of the gastroduodenal artery. The neck, body, and tail are supplied by the splenic artery and its branches, the superior and inferior pancreatic arteries.

The pancreas contains two types of tissue: (1) ducted or exocrine and (2) ductless or endocrine. The exocrine secretions empty into the duodenum and contain many of the digestive enzymes. The endocrine secretions empty into the venous system and are essential for the regulation of carbohydrate metabolism.

The exocrine cells of the pancreas, the acinar cells, function to produce enzymes that are needed for the digestion of carbohydrates

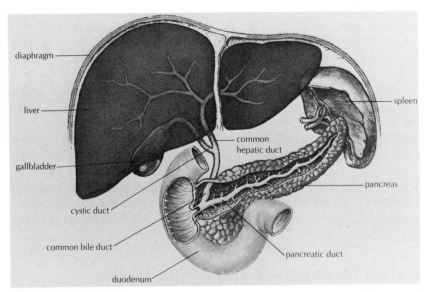

FIGURE 10–1. Anatomy of the pancreas. (Reprinted with permission from Memmler, R., Wood, D. (1987). *Structure and Function of the Human Body*. Philadelphia: J.B. Lippincott, p. 188.)

(amylase), proteins (trypsin), and fats (lipase). The protein-digesting enzymes are produced in inactive forms and are converted to active forms in the small intestine by the proper pH or presence of other enzymes (Memmler & Wood, 1987). When foods are eaten the pancreas secretes and releases digestive enzymes through the duct of Wirsung into the duodenum. These enzymes digest food into simpler substances that can then be absorbed into the bloodstream and transported throughout the body for direct use or storage.

The endocrine tissue of the pancreas has 1 to 2 million cluster cells, the islets of Langerhans, scattered throughout the pancreas. These islet cells constitute only 2 per cent of the pancreas tissue. The islets contain three types of cells: (1) alpha cells, which produce glucagon; (2) beta cells, which produce insulin; and (3) delta cells, which produce somatostatin (Fig. 10–2).

Glucagon increases the blood glucose level. This is in contrast to insulin, which decreases the blood glucose level. Glucagon is secreted in response to hypoglycemia by stimulating the rapid conversion of liver glycogen to glucose (glycogenolysis) and promptly raises the blood sugar level.

Insulin, released by the beta cells, regulates the amount of glucose in the bloodstream and aids in the utilization of glucose as an energy source by the cells. Insulin is active in the transport of glucose across the cell membrane. Once inside the cell, glucose can be used for energy metabolism or stored as glycogen. Insulin acts by (1) facilitating the conversion of glucose to glycogen in the liver and skeletal muscle (glycogenesis), (2) preventing breakdown of amino acids to glucose in the liver (gluconeogenesis), and (3) preventing breakdown of lipids into fatty acids.

When the pancreas does not provide adequate insulin, glucose is not released from extracellular fluid into the cells. Without glucose to

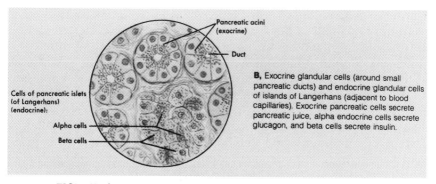

FIGURE 10–2. Anatomy and physiology of the islets of Langerhans.

metabolize, the cells become depleted of energy. To compensate for the lack of glucose, cells begin to oxidize fats and protein from adipose tissue and muscle.

Somatostatin inhibits either insulin or glucagon secretion according to the blood glucose levels. It also reduces the rate at which triglycerides are absorbed from the intestines after a fatty meal.

Diabetes is a condition in which either the pancreas does not produce enough insulin, or it produces sufficient insulin but the cells of the body are unable to use the insulin properly (Holleroroth, 1986). The glucose that cells are unable to use accumulates in the blood, a condition known as hyperglycemia. At this stage the strong osmotic pull of the glucose draws fluid from cells, causing cellular dehydration. When the blood sugar reaches approximately 160 to 180 mg/100 ml, the kidneys begin to excrete glucose, which carries water with it, resulting in symptoms of polyuria, glycosuria, polydipsia, and dehydration. Weight loss also occurs because of the utilization of stored fat and protein for energy. Polyphagia is experienced because glucose cannot be used by the cells and the use of body tissue results in a state of starvation.

CANDIDATE SELECTION

The majority of pancreas transplants performed have been in people who already have exhibited manifestations of the secondary complications of diabetes. Currently there are three groups of patients for which this procedure is considered: (1) simultaneous kidney and pancreas transplantation, (2) pancreas transplantation after successful kidney transplantation, and (3) pancreas transplantation before kidney transplantation for patients who are nonuremic and manifest other secondary complications of diabetes.

Most transplant programs in the United States and elsewhere are faced with an increasing number of patients with chronic end-stage renal failure as a result of longstanding type I diabetes mellitus. In some centers one-third to one-half of the kidney transplants are performed in patients with diabetes. Depending on the age of the patient and the duration of debilitating complications, some of these patients represent a substantial risk when subjected to an extensive operation and immunosuppressive therapy (Corry, Ngheim, Schulack, Beutel, & Gonwa, 1986). However, there are other patients with diabetes and renal failure who are relatively young and whose secondary complications have not progressed to total blindness, amputations, and debilitating neuropathy. This select group could benefit from simultaneous kidney and pancreas transplantation with its attendant advantages (Corry, 1987).

An additional advantage of the simultaneous kidney and pancreas transplant procedure is related to the influence of uremia on platelet function. Many patients with renal failure have disordered coagulation ability as a result of the physiologic effects of uremia; therefore, they may be at reduced risk for pancreas graft vascular thrombosis post transplant (Corry, Ngheim, Schanbacher, & Gonwa, 1987; Sutherland, Moudry, Elick, Goetz, & Najarian, 1988).

Caution must be exercised in the selection of candidates for the simultaneous transplant procedure, since not all patients are able to withstand the stress of a lengthy and extensive operation (Corry et al., 1986). Another important component in consideration for selection for the combined operation is the status of the candidate's renal insufficiency (Sutherland, 1986). The decision is clear if the patient is already maintained on dialysis. A dilemma, however, for the transplant clinician is the patient who shows evidence of early progression to renal failure. At which point is the simultaneous procedure justified? A serum creatinine level of 2 to 3 mg/dl or a creatinine clearance of less than 50 ml/min usually indicates impending renal failure and the need for kidney replacement therapy, generally within 12 to 24 months. Therefore, it is usually appropriate to offer the patient this therapeutic option.

Pancreas transplantation after successful kidney transplantation is the second most common approach to this procedure. Certainly any patient who is approaching renal failure should first be evaluated for living-donor kidney transplantation. The patient then may be a candidate for a subsequent cadaveric pancreas transplant or a living-donor transplant from the same kidney donor or another source. Until recently, most pancreas transplants have been performed in patients in the late stages of their disease, as described in the two groups discussed so far. In these cases the effects of diabetes are already manifest, and perhaps reversal or stabilization of the progression of end-stage diabetic disease is not possible. Ideally, pancreas transplantation should be offered before the secondary complications of diabetes are apparent. Although currently there are limited data supporting the efficacy of pancreas transplantation in delaying or reversing diabetic complications, prevention of recurrence of diabetic nephropathy in the kidney transplant by a pancreas transplant has been demonstrated (Mauer, Steffes, Sutherland, Najarian, Michael, & Brown, 1975). A continuing dilemma in the candidacy of the nonuremic diabetic is the uncertainty as to how to determine which segment of the diabetic population will develop complications. The smallest percentage of the total pancreas transplants performed is currently in this group of nonuremic diabetics. Another important consideration in offering pancreas transplantation to the nonuremic is the relative decreased successful grafting in this group. Immunosuppression is necessary to prevent graft rejection. Therefore, for nonuremic diabetic patients, pancreas transplant is appropriate only in those people whose complications are predictably more serious than the potential side effects of chronic immunosuppression (Sutherland, Moudry, Elick, Goetz, & Najarian, 1984).

DETERMINATION OF EXTENT OF DIABETIC DISEASE

The protocols for candidacy in most pancreas transplant centers require evidence of early nephropathy (elevated serum creatinine level, decreased creatinine clearance, proteinuria, and, usually, hypertension), preproliferative retinopathy, severe neuropathy, refractoriness to diabetic management, or a combination of any of these indications.

A thorough and meticulous pretransplant evaluation is essential for candidates considering this procedure. Not only does the evaluation determine the medical and psychological suitability for pancreatic transplantation, but the various tests provide a baseline by which the secondary complications can be monitored in the posttransplant period.

Generally, most of the evaluation can be completed on an outpatient basis; however, the evaluation protocol of many centers requires admission to the transplant hospital, frequently in a clinical research center unit. At this time accurate controlled testing can be accomplished. The typical pancreas transplant evaluation is outlined in Table 10–1, although variances may occur from center to center.

It is important to emphasize the cardiac evaluation component of the preparation for pancreas transplantation (Fig. 10–3). Although a patient may not exhibit any cardiac symptomatology before the transplant, there is evidence that it may exist. Weintrauch (1977) estimated that approximately 50 per cent of asymptomatic diabetics will have coronary artery disease at the time of onset of renal failure. In fact, many transplant programs require mandatory coronary angiography for diabetic kidney transplant candidates. An abnormal angiogram may indicate the need for pretransplant coronary artery bypass surgery or may disqualify a person from participating. At least two major pancreas transplant centers report higher patient mortality rates (after pancreas transplantation) from documented myocardial infarcts before the initiation of meticulous cardiac evaluation protocols (Conway & Davis, 1987; Smith, Wright, Schanbacher, & Corry, 1988).

EVALUATION PROCESS

A mandatory component of the pretransplant evaluation is a thorough psychosocial assessment of the patient and support systems. The social worker and psychologist or psychiatrist play an instrumental role

TABLE 10–1. PANCREAS TRANSPLANTATION EVALUATION

Endocrine/metabolic profile
    Glycosylated hemoglobin and islet cell antibodies
    Peptide measurement (urine and serum)
    Serum cholesterol and triglyceride levels
    Serum amylase and lipase levels
    Glucose tolernce test (oral, intravenous, or both)
Ophthalmologic
    Slit-lamp examination
    Intraocular pressure measurements
    Visual acuity determination
    Stereo color fundus photography
    Fluorescein angiography
Neurologic
    Clinical examination
    Nerve conduction velocities
    Autonomic testing
    Quantitation of sensory loss
Nephrologic
    Renal function testing
    Renal biopsy
Gastrointestinal
    Gastric emptying testing
    Upper and lower gastrointestinal contrast studies
Cardiovascular
    Electrocardiography
    Thallium stress testing
    Coronary angiography
    Clinical examination by cardiologists
Peripheral vascular
    Clinical examination
    Doppler studies
Psychosocial
    Social worker
    Psychologist/psychiatrist
Immunologic
    ABO testing
    Histocompatibility testing
    Cytotoxic screening
Gynecologic
Dental
Financial

in determining the patient's capacity for withstanding the potential emotional stresses attendant with the transplant process. Before the initiation of the evaluation process it is also necessary to conduct a financial investigation to determine payment for the procedure. Unlike the kidney transplant patient, who qualifies for coverage under a special Medicare program, there is no automatic funding mechanism for pancreas transplantation. This topic is addressed later in the chapter.

After completion of the evaluation and accumulation of data and records, the case is discussed by the transplant team, at which time a disposition is decided. Throughout the entire pretransplant phase the

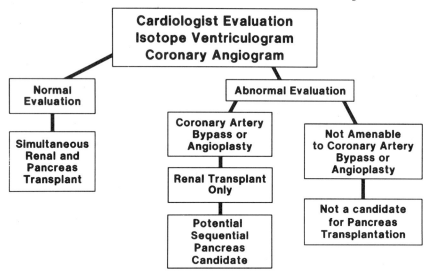

UNIVERSITY OF IOWA
Cardiac Evaluation and Policy

FIGURE 10–3. Cardiac evaluation policy.

referring physician must be kept abreast of the progression of the evaluation and the final disposition.

DONOR SELECTION

The first human pancreas transplant, performed by Kelly and associates, used a segmental cadaver graft, although 12 subsequent grafts involved whole cadaver grafts, including the duodenum (Kelly et al., 1967). The segmental graft can restore euglycemia to a diabetic patient, although repeated rejection episodes can potentially result in subtotal destruction of islets and reduction in beta cell mass (Sutherland, Chinn, Elick, & Najarian, 1984). Because a whole graft yields a greater beta cell mass, a whole pancreas may be better able to withstand the rejection process. Most transplant centers currently procure whole-pancreas cadaver grafts with or without a patch, or segment of duodenum. Using a segmental or whole cadaver pancreas graft is commonplace, although a few programs use segmental grafts from living-related donors as well as segmental or whole grafts from cadavers (Sutherland, Goetz, & Najarian, 1979; Sutherland, Goetz, & Najarian, 1984).

Living Donors

The rationale for the use of living-related donors is the same as for kidney grafts: a shortage of suitable donors and the immunologic advantage of less tendency for rejection in using a genetically similar graft. Also, patients who have received a previous kidney transplant from the pancreas donor have a particularly strong immunologic advantage in that they have not rejected a kidney and are already immunosuppressed. Living-related pancreas donors must meet strict criteria indicating that they are not at increased risk to develop diabetes and are medically able to tolerate surgery without risk. The criteria that must be met by the potential pancreas transplant donor are summarized in Table 10–2 (Sutherland, Goetz, & Najarian, 1987). If the criteria are applied in the selection of living-related donors, the risk of inducing a significant metabolic change by hemipancreatectomy should be low.

Other components of the living-related donor evaluation include metabolic studies, laboratory determinations, x-rays, and psychiatric and psychosocial evaluation. Of 60 patients used as living-related pancreas donors in the University of Minnesota series since 1979, most have experienced only a temporary hyperglycemia and hyperamylasemia in the immediate postoperative period. Long term, two donors who did not meet the criteria above developed type II diabetes after hemipancreatectomy (Sutherland, Goetz, & Najarian, 1984b), whereas the others have remained nondiabetic. All who met the criteria above have had normal oral glucose tolerance tests when tested after donation. Complications of the surgery have occurred in eight donors (13%). These complications have included leakage from the pancreatic duct in one case, splenectomy in two cases, abscess formation in two cases, and intra-abdominal fluid collections in three cases (Sutherland, Goetz, & Najarian, 1987). Accord-

TABLE 10–2. CRITERIA FOR SELECTION OF LIVING-RELATED PANCREAS DONORS

Preevaluation Criteria
1. Recipient and donor discordant for diabetes for at least 10 years
2. Donor at least 10 years older than age of onset of diabetes in recipient
3. In cases of sibling donation, no family members, other than the proband, are diabetic

Postevaluation Criteria
1. Normal oral glucose tolerance test (OGTT) result by criteria of Fajans and Conn and of the National Diabetes Data Study Group
2. a. Delta insulin >90 uU/ml for sum of 0-, 60-, 120-, and 180-minute values during cortisone-stimulated OGTT minus sum during standard OGTT according to technique of Fajans and Conn
   b. Sum of one- and three-minute insulin values during intravenous glucose tolerance test >80 uU/ml
3. No islet cell antibodies
4. Other metabolic parameters normal

From the University of Minnesota Hospital, Minneapolis, MN.

ing to Sutherland, Goetz, & Najarian (1984b), the risk of living-related pancreas donation appears to be acceptably low, with the surgical complication rate no higher than reported from living-related donors of kidney grafts; however, most centers still prefer to use cadaver donors (Weiland, Sutherland, Chavers, Simmons, Ascher, & Najarian, 1984).

Cadaver Donors

Pancreas grafts may be procured from virtually any cadaver donor who is suitable as a liver, heart, or kidney donor, unless the donor has diabetes or has had direct pancreatic trauma. Also, a cadaver donor who may not be suitable for liver donation, for example, because of elevated liver enzyme levels, may be suitable for pancreas donation. Many cadaver donors have elevated serum amylase levels or elevated glucose levels, or both. Neither of these conditions appears to be a reliable indicator of pancreatitis, pancreatic injury, or endocrine insufficiency (Hesse, Najarian, & Sutherland, 1985). During the procurement process it is important to administer exogenous insulin to restore euglycemia. Viable pancreas grafts procured from these cadaver donors will establish a euglycemic state in the recipient after transplantation without the need for additional insulin administration.

Donor Operation

The techniques for whole or segmental pancreatectomy from cadaver and living-related donors are described in detail elsewhere (Sutherland, Ascher, & Najarian, 1984). Briefly, segmental grafts are procured by dividing the neck of the pancreas and removing the tail and body based on a vascular pedicle of the splenic artery and vein, the splenic vessels alone for living-related donors or cadaver liver donors, and in continuity with the portal vein and celiac axis for non-liver cadaver donors. Whole-pancreas grafts are procured from cadaver donors by excising the entire pancreas. Either a button of the duodenum encompassing both the papilla of Vater and the duct of Santorini (patch technique), or the intact duodenum (pancreaticoduodenal graft) is excised in the donor operation. The vascular component includes taking the portal vein and a Carrel patch of aorta encompassing the celiac axis and superior mesenteric artery, unless the procurement is from a liver donor. In this case most of the portal vein and celiac axis are retained for the liver. The pancreatic portion of the portal vein can be lengthened by an iliac vein graft if necessary, and either the proximal splenic artery of the graft is anastomosed to the superior mesenteric artery of the donor pancreas, or the donor internal and external iliac arteries with the common iliac in continuity can be used as a Y-graft anastomosed to the splenic and superior mesenteric arteries of the pancreas (Sutherland, Moudry, Elick, Goetz, & Najarian, 1987).

Hemodynamic monitoring is an important component for optimal maintenance of the cadaver donor for pancreas procurement. Postoperative function of the pancreas graft is reflective of procurement and preservation techniques. In situ flushing of the pancreas graft is usually not performed unless a whole-organ graft is procured from a liver donor, in which case the liver is flushed. Removal of the pancreas graft is done with the heart beating or concomitant with cardiectomy.

Organ Preservation

After procurement of the pancreas is completed the cadaver organ is intra-arterially flushed ex vivo and preserved by cold storage. Historically, a variety of solutions have been used, ranging from Collins' solution to the more recent hyperosmolar solutions, including silica gel–filtered plasma and ViaSpan solution (Florack, Sutherland, Heil, Squifflet, & Najarian, 1983; Heise, Sutherland, Heil, & Najarian, in press; Wahlberg, Southard, & Belzer, 1986).

Pancreas grafts are removed from the preservation solution and immediately vascularized in the recipient. Preservation times vary in most centers, but all agree that minimal cold ischemia time is ideal. Successful pancreas transplants have been performed with grafts preserved for as long as 28 hours (Florack, Sutherland, Heise, & Najarian, 1987).

PREPARATION OF THE RECIPIENT

Immunologic evaluation of the recipient is important before living-related or cadaver pancreas transplantation takes place. The use of pretransplant deliberate blood transfusions, believed to be beneficial in the past in kidney transplantation (Opelz & Mickey, 1973), is now questioned with utilization of new immunosuppressive drugs such as cyclosporine, and monoclonal antibody (Groth, 1987; Opelz, 1987). Donor-specific or random blood transfusions can be used. Although the benefits of each are generally accepted, the risk of antibody formation (sensitization) is always present. Some transplant centers give deliberate blood transfusions with concomitant immunosuppressive agents to provide the therapeutic advantage of transfusions while hoping to prevent sensitization (Anderson, Tyler, Rodey, Etheredge, & Anderman, 1987; Norman, Fletcher, & Barry, 1987).

Preparation of the pancreas transplant patient depends on the immunologic status of both recipient and donor. For example, if a recipient obtains a living-related pancreas transplant from a human leukocyte antigen (HLA)-identical donor or from the same living-related donor who previously donated a kidney and is already immunosuppressed, the recipient may not benefit from deliberate transfusions before pancreas transplant. If a nonuremic recipient, however, obtains a pancreas transplant from a cadaver donor, the recipient may be more immunocompetent than a uremic pancreas-kidney recipient, and this recipient may benefit greatly from deliberate random blood transfusions before the transplant and, possibly, even pretransplant splenectomy. Preparation of these patients includes immunologic assays to identify HLA-A, -B, -C, and -DR transplant antigens as well as specific cytotoxic antibodies. Clinically, prospective tissue-matching between donor and recipient remains debatable (Hardy, 1987; van Rood, 1987), although most centers require a prospective negative T lymphocyte crossmatch before transplantation.

An essential component of preparation for the recipient includes an understanding of the surgical procedure, immunosuppressive medications and their possible side effects, and the likelihood of success or failure of the pancreas transplant procedure. Patients must be made aware of the possibility of complications and given statistical evidence of such. The data must be presented in a variety of ways so that patients believe that they are informed.

Support groups facilitated by a social worker, transplant coordinator, or both are invaluable in regard to sharing information. Often patients who have undergone pancreas transplantation are willing to speak with prospective candidates about their experiences. Both positive and negative experiences related to prospective candidates will allow potential recipients to make the best decision for themselves.

IMPLANTATION PROCEDURE

Graft Placement

In the recipient operation the pancreas is placed heterotopically into either the right or left iliac fossa after a midline or groin incision is made. The right iliac fossa is the preferred site because there is less chance of kinking of the portal vein after the venous anastomosis is completed. Also, absorption of residual enzyme secretion is best in this position. The pancreas has been placed either intraperitoneally or extraperitoneally, with or without a vent into the peritoneum.

Oftentimes when using a cadaver donor the pancreaticosplenic graft is left intact until the recipient vascular anastomosis is completed; then, before closing the incision, the spleen is removed. This maneuver allows the surgeon to observe revascularization in order to decide whether the pancreatic graft is positioned correctly. Any firmness, distention, or blue discoloration of the spleen can indicate impairment of the venous runoff (Sollinger, Stratta, Kalayoglu, Belzer, et al., 1987). If the spleen looks viable, indicating adequate blood flow, it will then be removed (Sollinger et al., 1987).

It was previously thought that leaving the spleen as part of the pancreas graft would preserve the normal blood flow and allow an immunologic advantage. However, this technique was abandoned because of frequently occurring graft-versus-host disease (Corry et al., 1986).

Implantation Approaches

There are three basic approaches used to implant pancreas tissue: whole gland, segmental gland, and islet cell infusion. Each approach has distinct advantages and disadvantages.

One advantage to transplanting the whole gland versus the segmental gland is that there is an increased number of islet cells transplanted. Another advantage is that transplanting the whole pancreas along with the duodenum into the bladder provides a clinical marker by which to monitor for rejection.

If a successful islet cell technique is perfected, it may be the preferred implantation approach. After islet cells are isolated from the whole donor pancreas they can be injected into the renal capsule, liver, or spleen. These areas are the preferred sites because of their rich blood supply. The advantages of this type of procedure are many: less surgical time, decreased cost, decreased hospitalization, and fewer complications.

A disadvantage of this approach is the difficulty in monitoring for rejection, since the only parameter used can be the serum glucose level, which has been shown to be a late indicator of rejection.

Vascular Anastomoses

The first step of vascular anastomosis of a whole pancreas graft is an end-to-side connection between the portal vein and the side of the external iliac vein (Mittal & Toledo-Pereyra, 1986). It is important that the pancreas be correctly positioned to avoid twisting of the portal vein. After the venous anastomosis is completed the arterial anastomosis is performed by connecting the Carrel patch of the aorta, which contains the origin of the celiac axis, and the superior mesenteric artery end-to-side to the external iliac artery (Fig. 10–4). Once the venous and arterial anastomoses are completed, the surgeon removes the vascular clamps to perfuse the whole organ; it should become pink. Oftentimes there are small vessels that ooze from the head of the pancreas; these vessels must be ligated to prevent postoperative bleeding.

Methods of Exocrine Drainage

The most important technical issue in pancreas transplantation is provision for management of exocrine secretions (Sutherland, Kendall, Goetz, & Najarian, 1986). Several methods have been used to control pancreatic exocrine secretions; the following surgical techniques represent some of the methods used.

Duct Injection

Occlusion of the pancreatic duct with synthetic polymer or other agents has been used for segmental and whole-organ pancreas transplants (Land, 1980). Polymer agents used have included neoprene, prolamine, polyisoprene, and alphacyanoacrylate. One of these agents is injected into the pancreatic duct, and the open end of the duct is ligated. Ideally, complete occlusion of the ductal system suppresses exocrine function (Fig. 10–5).

A problem that may occur from duct injection is residual enzyme leakage from the pancreatic surface. To circumvent this problem after

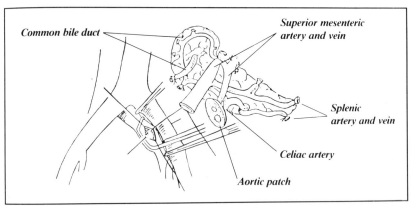

FIGURE 10–4. Recipient vascular anastomoses. (Redrawn with permission from *AORN Journal, 43*, p. 625, March 1986. Copyright © AORN Inc., 10170 East Mississippi Avenue, Denver, CO, 80231.)

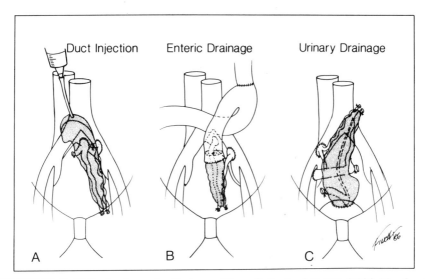

FIGURE 10–5. Methods of exocrine Drainage. (From Sutherland, D.E.R. (1986, May-June). *Clinical Diabetes, 61.* Reproduced with permission from the American Diabetes Association, Inc.)

duct injection the pancreatic graft is usually implanted intraperitoneally. Residual secretions may then be absorbed by the peritoneum. Although this procedure has been accepted, extensive fibrosis of the pancreatic graft, pancreatitis from direct injection, and even polymer extravasation into the abdominal cavity have occurred. Cessation of function of some technically successful grafts has occurred abruptly in a pattern consistent with either acute rejection or chronic pancreatitis (Mittal & Toledo-Pereyra, 1986).

Open Duct

Another method used to control exocrine secretions is placement of the pancreatic graft with the duct draining directly into the peritoneal cavity. Draining enzymes remain inactive because the enzyme enterokinase, found in the duodenum, is not released. This approach is the simplest technique but has not been successful in most patients, although the longest surviving pancreas recipient did undergo transplantation using this procedure. In some patients the exocrine secretion rate exceeds the peritoneal absorption rate; the result is massive ascites or peritonitis secondary to infection (Mittal & Toledo-Pereyra, 1986).

Duct Ligation

Ligating the pancreatic duct does not necessarily reduce the volume of the pancreatic secretions because the peripancreatic lymphatics connect at accessory ducts, and a fistula or fluid accumulation can occur (Mittal & Toledo-Pereyra, 1986). This approach has not proved to be successful. Patients may experience pancreatitis, pseudocyst, or peritonitis.

Enteric Drainage

The Roux-en-Y procedure is probably the most physiologic approach to the management of pancreatic exocrine secretions. The Roux-en-Y placement involves anastomosis of the distal divided end of the small bowel. The proximal end is anastomosed to the small bowel below the anastomosis. For segmental grafts intussusception of the pancreatic neck into the end of the Roux-en-Y limb of the recipient jejunum is performed. In whole-pancreas grafts the donor duodenum is anastomosed into the side of the Roux-en-Y limb of the recipient's jejunum (Fig. 10–5).

Some of the complications patients have experienced with this technique include fistula or abscess formation, jejunal loop necrosis, vascular thrombosis, infection, and anastomotic leaking. Pancreaticojejunostomy can result in microbial contamination followed by activation of the pancreatic enzymes (Mittal & Toledo-Pereyra, 1986). If anastomotic breakdown occurs, the complications in an immunosuppressed patient can be serious and sometimes fatal.

Bladder Drainage

Becoming the most widely used approach to the management of pancreatic exocrine secretions is the anastomosis of the pancreatic duct to the bladder. During procurement of the whole pancreas a duodenal patch, or segment, is left, including the ampulla of Vater. This segment, or button, of duodenum is anastomosed to the dome of the bladder to allow pancreatic secretions to drain into the bladder.

There are several advantages to this approach. First and foremost, it allows for the measurement of the urine amylase level. This has been shown to be an early marker for pancreas rejection. Second, there is a decreased risk of infection, since the bladder is usually free of pathogens, whereas the intestinal tract is not. Because of these factors, more pancreas transplant centers are using this technique.

Disadvantages include possible leakage from the pancreaticocystostomy anastomosis, pancreatitis, infection, abscess formation, and urinary extravasation. The major disadvantage of the bladder drainage technique is the urinary loss of bicarbonate, which cannot be compensated for by the kidney graft during periods of dysfunction (Ngheim, Gonwa, & Corry, 1987). Acidosis is not a problem if the recipient has adequate renal function; however, because of diabetic nephropathy in conjunction with cyclosporine, which decreases creatinine clearance, most patients require oral bicarbonate supplements.

One advantage in using a duodenal segment instead of a duodenal button is that the difficult separation of the duodenum from the pancreatic head can be avoided. This minimizes the potential for bleeding from small vessels in the pancreatic head and reduces the risk of injuring accessory ducts. Another advantage is that it includes both pancreatic ducts and, therefore, decreases complications that might be caused by ligating accessory ducts or leaving them to drain freely.

There is, however, evidence of an increased risk of metabolic acidosis related to the increased bicarbonate loss if more length of duodenum is transplanted, since the duodenum stimulates increased exocrine activity from the pancreas. Another disadvantage is that lymphoid tissue may be simultaneously transplanted, which may possibly lead to sloughing of the duodenal mucosa and hematuria during rejection episodes.

Placement of Simultaneous Kidney Graft

If a simultaneous pancreas and kidney graft is performed, the kidney is placed in either the right or the left iliac fossa and the pancreas placed on the opposite side. Vascular anastomosis is as previously described (Fig. 10–6).

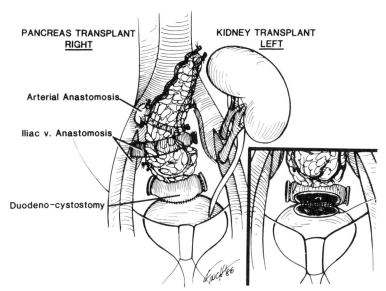

FIGURE 10–6. Placement of simultaneous kidney graft. (Reprinted with permission from Prieto, M., et al. (1987). Surgery, *102*, 682.)

POSTOPERATIVE MANAGEMENT

Monitoring of Metabolic Changes

Different protocols are used to monitor carbohydrate control after transplantation. After the initial surgical recovery, patients undergo glucose tolerance tests and a metabolic profile consisting of measurement of serum glucose levels both before and one to two hours after meals for a 24-hour period. These values serve as the baseline for comparison with fasting and postprandial serum glucose levels measured at home.

Glycosylated hemoglobin A (or hemoglobin A_{1C}) is used as a measure of long-term glucose control. Hemoglobin A_{1C} is a stable glycosylated hemoglobin formed through a nonenzymatic glycosylation of hemoglobin A. This glycosylation is entirely dependent on the level of serum glucose (Corry et al., 1986). It measures the average glucose level attained over the preceding two to four months.

Although glucose control may be normal in patients who receive a pancreas transplant, it is still too early to evaluate objectively whether the diabetic complications are reversed or halted.

Nutritional Management

Postoperatively, patients are unable to eat and drink until bowel function returns, generally in three to five days. A nasogastric tube is placed to suction intermittently, and intravenous fluids are used during this time.

Hyperalimentation is administered if oral feedings cannot be resumed within one week. Because hyperalimentation consists of glucose-containing solutions, insulin should be administered in a separate infusion to maintain normoglycemia. Insulin requirements should also be monitored.

IMMUNOLOGIC REGIMENS

A variety of immunosuppressive regimens have been used in pancreas transplantation. Some authors report the use of no immunosuppression in recipients of three identical-twin pancreas transplants (Sutherland, Sibley, Chinn, Michael, Srikanta, et al., 1984). Although the use of immunosuppressive drugs to prevent rejection in these recipients was not warranted, these patients later presented with recurrence of diabetes, documented histopathologically (Sibley, Sutherland, Goetz, & Michael, 1985). One subsequent twin treated with azathioprine has maintained a functioning graft for more than three years, and another treated with cyclosporine and azathioprine was functioning one year later. Other protocols include the use of triple therapy—cyclosporine, azathioprine, and prednisone (Sutherland, Goetz, & Najarian, 1986)—and quadruple therapy—cyclosporine, azathioprine, prednisone, and antilymphocyte globulin—to prevent rejection (Sollinger et al., 1987).

Accepted immunosuppression protocols used by pancreas transplant centers depend on multiple factors: (1) the donor source, (2) the recipient's uremic status, (3) the presence or absence of a functioning kidney transplant, (4) the recipient's renal tolerance of cyclosporine, (5) the recipient's history of chronic immunosuppression, and (6) the specific surgical technique used for graft placement. A patient receiving a pancreas graft from the same living-related donor who donated a previous kidney may simply be treated with maintenance immunosuppression, whether it be azathioprine with prednisone or cyclosporine with prednisone. A patient receiving a simultaneous cadaver kidney-pancreas graft who has never before been immunosuppressed may be given an induction dose of prednisone, azathioprine, and/or cyclosporine with prophylactic antilymphocyte globulin or OKT3, depending on the presence of immediate or delayed kidney graft function, tissue-matching, and the recipient's uremic status. Rejection episodes can usually be treated by an increase in corticosteroids. However, corticosteroids seem to be the only drugs that aggravate associated hyperglycemia. When this occurs, patients are placed on exogenous insulin for an indeterminate time. Resolution of rejection can be confirmed by C-peptide determinations in conjunction with glucose levels and urine amylase concentrations in bladder-drained grafts.

The maintenance dose of immunosuppressive drugs at one year post transplant in a patient without a history of rejection episodes should be minimal. Attention should be given to the long-term effects of cyclosporine nephrotoxicity, the effect of azathioprine therapy in its relation to bone marrow suppression, the variety of side effects of prednisone therapy, and the incidence of infections, as well as the patient's overall well-being after transplantation.

COMPLICATIONS OF PANCREAS TRANSPLANTATION

Vascular Thrombosis

Vascular thrombosis remains a major problem during the immediate postoperative period. The cause is unclear, but there are many potential causes of thrombosis, including mechanical obstruction, poor blood flow through the gland, intraglandular microthrombi, traumatic removal of the gland during donor procurement, pancreatitis, prolonged cold ischemic time, and the possible thrombogenic effect of cyclosporine and antilymphocyte globulin (Soon-Shiong, White, De Mayo, Koyle, & Danovitch, 1988).

Graft thrombosis is manifested by a sudden, sharp decrease in urine amylase level, a simultaneous rapid increase in serum glucose level, and, usually, gross hematuria. The patient may complain of severe pain in the iliac fossa, and on physical examination a tender graft may be palpable. The absence of blood flow noted by a nuclear imaging scan or angiography confirms the diagnosis. Treatment for vascular thrombosis is a total graft pancreatectomy.

Rejection

Rejection is the major cause of graft loss, with a reported incidence of 40 per cent to 50 per cent (Sutherland & Kendall, 1985). Pancreas rejection is oftentimes subtle and difficult to differentiate from other causes of graft failure, such as pancreatitis, vascular thrombosis, and recurrence of disease (Sollinger et al., 1987).

Before the development of the bladder technique the only way to monitor rejection was to measure serum glucose and serum amylase levels. Once hyperglycemia occurred, there was minimal chance for reversal. The widespread use of the bladder technique for exocrine management has greatly improved graft survival rates. Based on urine amylase levels, which are monitored daily (or more frequently) during hospitalization, a diagnosis of rejection can be made if there is a 25 per cent to 50 per cent decrease in the urine amylase level from posttransplant baseline. Studies have indicated that the exocrine pancreas is more sensitive to rejection than the endocrine pancreas, with the reduction in exocrine function preceding the onset of hyperglycemia (Prieto, Sutherland, Fernandez-Cruz, Heil, & Najarian, 1987; Schulak & Drevyanko, 1985).

The urine pH can also be used as a parameter to identify rejection, although it is not as reliable. Pancreatic juices secreted into the bladder are alkaline; therefore, normal urine pH in these patients ranges from 7.0 to 8.5. If there is a consistent decrease in the urine pH, it may be indicative of a decrease in exocrine function, possibly suggesting rejection. Another possible cause can be closure of the pancreatic duct. This can be confirmed by cystoscopy.

Serum C-peptide levels can be measured but are not useful. The results are not readily available for several days and can only be used retrospectively.

Radionuclide imaging (i.e., DPTA, technetium 99m, indium 111–labeled white blood cells and platelets, and 75 selenomethionine) has provided useful information regarding the physiologic status of the pancreas. With refinements, these techniques may prove to be more useful in diagnosing rejection. Characteristics of rejection demonstrated by nuclear scanning include platelet sequestration, diminished visualization and perfusion, graft swelling, and loss of border resolution (Sollinger et al., 1987).

Sutherland, Goetz, & Najarian (1984a) have recommended open biopsy (wedge or needle) under direct vision as the only definitive method of diagnosing rejection. This procedure, however, carries an increased risk, since a laparotomy needs to be performed, which increases the chance of infection and bleeding. Fine-needle biopsy of the pancreas has proved unreliable, and percutaneous needle biopsy has resulted in bleeding and fistula formation; therefore, pancreatic allograft biopsy is seldom used routinely.

The simultaneous kidney and pancreas transplant has proved beneficial in diagnosing rejection. Numerous studies have demonstrated that kidney allograft rejection precedes pancreas rejection (Baumgartner, Largiader, Uhlschmid, & Binswanger, et al., 1983; Florack, Sutherland, Sibley, Najarian, & Squifflet, 1985; Traeger, Dubernard, Piatti, Bosi, Gelet, et al., 1984). Kidney transplant rejection can occur independently and without concomitant detectable pancreas rejection; however, studies indicate that isolated pancreas rejection in combined grafts from the same donor is rare (Dubernard, Traeger, Touraine, Betuel, & Malik, 1980; Tyden, Lundren, Ost, Gunnarsson, Ostman, & Groth, 1986). The delay in pancreas allograft rejection may be due to an inherent difference in organ susceptibility to rejection, anatomical differences in vascularization (lower flow), larger functional reserve, or the sensitivity of currently available tests of pancreatic function (Sollinger et al., 1987).

Nursing assessment in the postoperative period is a critical factor in the diagnosis of rejection. The nurse must monitor the urine pH and the urine amylase and serum glucose levels closely; this will aid in early diagnosis and prompt implementation of therapy. Pancreas transplant rejection is easily reversed if diagnosed early. Vital signs should be monitored every four hours, or more frequently, depending on the patient's condition. A fever may be indicative of rejection or infection, and either possibility must be ruled out (Table 10–3).

TABLE 10–3. DIAGNOSIS OF REJECTION

1. Decreased urine amylase level
2. Decreased urine pH
3. Increased serum glucose level
4. Decresed C-peptide levels
5. Nuclear scanning
6. Increase serum creatinine level if simultaneous kidney transplant

Infection

Infection remains the major cause of morbidity and mortality in the kidney transplant population (Chmielewski, 1987). The same is true for the pancreas transplant population, since similar immunosuppressive regimens are used. Strict aseptic technique is important in nursing management to prevent infection.

Graft and wound infection can occur as a complication of the surgical procedure. Residual enzyme secretions, swelling of the transplanted graft, and edema of the peritoneal tissues cause temporary ascites, adding to the increased risk of infection. The patient should be monitored for such signs as fever, purulent wound drainage, erythema at the incision site, and graft tenderness. Prophylactic antibiotics can be administered post-operatively to help prevent infection.

A bladder infection in a pancreas or kidney transplant recipient is a potentially serious complication. Sterility must be maintained at all times when catheterizing a patient or changing the tubing. Nursing care should include frequent urinary meatal and perianal care to reduce the possibility of infection. When using the bladder drainage technique the length of time in which an indwelling catheter is used varies. It should be left in place long enough to relieve incisional stress, provide visual monitoring of sediment and blood clot, and prevent residual urine, and yet be removed quickly enough to prevent infection.

Cardiovascular Problems

Because of pre-existing and often asymptomatic cardiovascular disease in patients with type I diabetes, the possibility of postoperative cardiovascular problems exists. These may include myocardial infarction and even death in the immediate postoperative period. Appropriate nursing assessment and monitoring are critical.

Other Complications

Many other complications can occur, such as sepsis, intestinal fistula, graft pancreatitis, bladder anastomotic leak, and hematuria. Oftentimes during the immediate postoperative period, transient elevated serum amylase levels are noted that are thought to be due to procurement and preservation injury.

Sloughing or necrosis of the duodenal mucosa has been noted and is thought to be due to rejection of the duodenum; this causes the delicate lymphatic tissue to become friable and bleed, resulting in hematuria. Cystoscopy can be used to identify the bleeding site. Three-way bladder irrigation has been used to encourage healing.

DISCHARGE AND FOLLOW-UP

The patient who receives a pancreas transplant must indicate a commitment to self-care and follow-up procedures. Education in self-care and monitoring tasks is mandatory before the patient is discharged from the hospital. Information regarding medication, diet, symptoms of graft failure, laboratory and clinic routines, and mechanism of communication with the transplant center is imperative for patient self-care.

Meticulous monitoring and record keeping by the patient enable both the patient and the care provider to have a knowledgeable data base on which to make informed decisions about ongoing care. Monitoring parameters include daily weight, twice-daily temperatures, frequent blood pressure and pulse readings, and serial blood determinations in order to assess organ function. Plasma glucose levels are monitored in all patients. Because of individual variation in glucose levels, records of a 24-hour glucose profile obtained during hospitalization will provide a baseline for comparison studies when the patient returns home. An approximate increase in glucose of 25 per cent over a baseline fasting or postprandial glucose level may indicate rejection, which can be treated. Progression of hyperglycemia may necessitate the use of exogenous insulin.

For enteric-drained, open duct, duct-ligated, or duct-injected grafts the only available parameter for diagnosis of rejection is the plasma glucose level. A rise in the fasting plasma glucose level may be an indicator of rejection, although Groth and associates (1980) found that postprandial glucose levels rose before fasting glucose levels in some pancreas transplant recipients undergoing rejection. A decrease in C-peptide concentration has also been associated with rejection (Groth, Lundgren, Gunnarsson, Hardstedt, & Ostman, 1980). Unfortunately this test cannot be done quickly or frequently enough to monitor day-to-day functioning of the pancreas graft. When the endocrine function alone is used to monitor for rejection, rejection is diagnosed late and reversal may not be achieved (Sutherland, Casanova, & Sibley, 1987). Ideally, a pancreas graft biopsy should be performed to confirm a diagnosis of rejection (Sutherland, Casanova, & Sibley, 1987).

Serum amylase levels are also monitored and remain elevated in some patients. In these patients a precipitous decline may precede hyperglycemia as a manifestation of rejection. In general, however, serum amylase levels are difficult to interpret in relation to pancreas graft function. It is important to realize that signs of rejection usually become evident relatively late in the rejection process. By the time these signs appear, significant graft damage may have occurred. For this reason increased benefit has been demonstrated by using the bladder drainage technique, which allows for monitoring of the urine amylase level (Sollinger, Cook, Kamps, Glass, & Belzer, 1984). A decrease in exocrine function of the pancreas as exhibited by a decrease in the urine amylase level may be an indicator of rejection before an increase in the plasma glucose level is seen. Frequent urine collections for urine amylase determinations are commonly performed in bladder-drained pancreas transplant recipients after transplantation.

Patients who are at home also monitor urine pH after transplantation. The urine pH in pancreas recipients with bladder-drained grafts is commonly above 7.0, a reflection of alkalinization of the urine by bicarbonate that is secreted directly into the bladder by the pancreas graft. A decrease in urine pH may be an indicator of graft dysfunction.

Other parameters commonly monitored are electrolytes, hemoglobin, white blood cell count, and serum creatinine, blood urea nitrogen, cyclosporine, and bicarbonate levels. These results are used to adjust immunosuppressive medications and assist the care provider in making clinical decisions. Patients with functioning grafts are required to monitor themselves for a lifetime with monthly laboratory determinations, yearly examination, and periodic visits to the transplanting institution.

Long-Term Follow-up of Secondary Diabetic Complications

Patients with long-term functioning grafts are asked to participate in investigative studies to document the prevention or progression of secondary complications of diabetes. These observations will ultimately provide researchers with answers to the question of whether the establishment of euglycemia will have an effect on secondary complications.

Commonly, detailed studies of eye, nerve, and renal function or morphology performed before the transplant will be performed at one year post transplant and serially thereafter. In regard to the effect of pancreas transplantation on secondary complications, preliminary studies show improvement in neuropathy in nonuremic patients and no improvement in retinopathy once it is in the preproliferative or proliferative phase (Ramsay, Rice, Sutherland, Goetz, & Najarian, 1986; Sutherland, Goetz, Hesse, Kennedy, Ramsey, Mauer, Steffes, Kendall, & Najarian, 1986). Of utmost importance is the fact that patients who had a previous kidney transplant did not develop diabetic lesions in the kidney graft (Bohman, Tyden, Wilezek, Lundgren, Jaremko, Gunnarsson, Ostman, Gross, et al., 1985). The patient with the longest pancreas graft function (10.5 years) and kidney graft function (16 years) has been observed to have regression of diabetic kidney lesions.

More follow-up is needed to document stabilization of the disease process in recipients of pancreas transplantation, especially those who are nonuremic, non–kidney transplant recipients. Prevention or regression of these lesions in the kidney is an impetus to provide pancreas transplantation to selected patients with early renal lesions of diabetes.

ROLE OF THE NURSE AND CLINICAL TRANSPLANT COORDINATOR IN PANCREAS TRANSPLANTATION

Nursing management of the pancreas transplant recipient is an essential ingredient to successful pancreas transplantation. Tables 10–4 and 10–5 outline the various responsibilities of the nurse in all phases of the transplant process. From the initial evaluation through the care given after hospitalization, the transplant nurse and transplant coordinator are integral members of the multidisciplinary health care team. They must be proficient in diagnosis, assessment, and implementation of established protocols.

In addition to providing information to the candidate and family, the transplant coordinator usually assesses the patient's knowledge base of the disease process and assists with review of the objective data accumulated in the evaluation process. The transplant coordinator is the key figure in facilitating the transplant process for the patient and family, and is responsible for assuring that appropriate information is transmitted to the referring physician (Schanbacher & Hasselman, 1986).

Financial Consideration

A substantial impediment to offering pancreas transplantation to large numbers of medically qualified candidates is the difficulty in securing funding for the procedure. The benefits of successful heart and liver transplantation are obvious; however, there is still a paucity of data documenting the efficacy of pancreas transplantation. Many third-party payers consider the procedure experimental, and their policies do not

TABLE 10–4. ROLE OF THE NURSE IN PANCREAS TRANSPLANTATION

I. Facilitator
   A. Receive initial referral.
   B. Organize evaluation.
   C. Accumulate data and records from local physician(s).
   D. Present pretransplant data to transplant physicians and surgeons for disposition.
   E. Implement protocols.
   F. Organize posthospitalization education and preparation for home care.
   G. Assess patient and family with flow-through posthospital system.

II. Educator
   A. Arrange for orientation conference for candidate and family.
   B. Provide information to candidate and family throughout the evaluation process.
   C. Prepare and deliver public and professional education programs regarding pancreas transplantation.
   D. Explain clinical and research protocols.
   E. Educate patient and family for posthospital care.

III. Evaluator
   A. Assess patient's knowledge base of diabetes and renal failure.
   B. Assess candidacy for transplantation.
   C. Evaluate patient's understanding of transplant information.
   D. Review medical data.
   E. Assess patient's adaptation to posttransplant status.
   F. Evaluate patient and family knowledge of posthospitalization routine (follow-up).
   G. Evaluate effectiveness of education methods and tools.

IV. Counselor
   A. Evaluate patient's support system.
   B. Act as patient advocate.
   C. Assure the delivery of the appropriate psychosocial intervention.
   D. Provide setting for patient and family to share concerns in posttransplant phase.
   E. Assist with development of pretransplant and posttransplant support groups.
   F. Prepare public and professional education relative to organ donation and transplantation.
   G. Inform referring physician about posttransplant care.

cover experimental therapy. Federal and state programs follow similar guidelines. Therefore, it is imperative that a thorough financial investigation precede the transplant evaluation.

Most third-party payers who fund the procedure require a prior approval process, which includes documentation of the medical condition of the candidate, expected outcome of the procedure, documentation of determination of candidacy by the transplant center, and other information that will support the rationale for proceeding with the transplant. The clinical transplant coordinator participates in this process by assuring that accurate information is presented to the prospective payer(s). Most transplant centers do not have the capabilities of performing pancreas transplantation on a gratis basis.

Occasionally representatives of local community resources offer to initiate fund-raising for organ transplant procedures. Although the gesture is noble, these efforts notoriously fall far short of reaching their goal. Therefore, one must exercise caution in relying solely on community fund-raising for organ transplantation.

**TABLE 10–5. NURSING CARE PLAN
FOR PANCREAS TRANSPLANT RECIPIENT**

Nursing Diagnosis	Outcome Criteria	Nursing Interventions
Potential for alteration in cardiac output: decreased, related to surgical procedure	Patient will have normal cardiac output as evidenced by: 1. Stable BP	1. Monitor BP supine and standing q 2 h. 2. Auscultate apical pulse q 2 h for rate and regularity of rhythm.
	2. No jugular vein distention	1. Inspect neck for internal jugular venous distention.
	3. Strong peripheral pulses	1. Observe skin over extremities for color, pallor, rubor, hair distribution. 2. Inspect for superficial vessels. 3. Palpate skin over extremities to note temperature. 4. Palpate pulses (radial, femoral, posterior tibial, and dorsalis pedis), comparing symmetry from side to side. 5. Palpate skin over tibia for edema.
	4. No cyanosis	1. Observe earlobes, fingernail beds, palms, and buccal mucous membranes for color changes. 2. Palpate for sweaty, cold, clammy, warm, or dry skin.
Potential for injury of transplanted organ related to rejection	Patient will not reject transplanted pancreas as evidenced by: 1. Serum glucose level between 60 and 110 mg/dl	1. Monitor serum glucose level q 2 h for 48 h and then q 6 h. (May use Accu-check TID). 2. Notify M.D. of upward trend.
	2. No significant drop or downward trend in urine amylase level	1. Collect urine at 6-h intervals. 2. Send specimen to lab for measurement of urine amylase level. 3. Monitor results. 4. Notify M.D. of downward trend.
	3. Urine pH between 7.0–8.5	1. Monitor urine pH q 6 h with dipstick. 2. Notify M.D. of downward trend.
	4. Afebrile	1. Monitor temp q 4 h and PRN. 2. Notify M.D. of increased temp.

Table continued on following page

**TABLE 10–5. NURSING CARE PLAN
FOR PANCREAS TRANSPLANT RECIPIENT** *Continued*

NURSING DIAGNOSIS	OUTCOME CRITERIA	NURSING INTERVENTIONS
	5. No pain, edema, or tenderness at graft site	1. Assess complaints of pain for onset, duration, location, quality, and degree of relief from pain meds. Compare with previous relief from pain. 2. Palpate graft site for pain, edema, and tenderness. 3. Notify M.D. of significant changes.
Potential for injury of transplanted organ related to graft thrombosis	Patient will not thrombose graft as evidenced by: 1. Serum glucose level remains between 60 and 110 mg/dl 2. No significant drop in urine amylase level	1. Administer anticoagulants per M.D. to decrease plt aggregation. 2. Maintain bed rest for 48–72 h to allow surgical anastomoses sites to heal. 3. Review nuclear scan results with M.D. to assess for evidence of thrombosis. 4. Monitor serum glucose level q 2 h for 48 h and then q 6 h for sudden increase. 5. Monitor urine amylase level q 6 h for a sudden drop.
Potential for infection related to immunosuppression and invasive surgery	Patient will be free of infection as evidenced by: 1. WBC <10,000	Obtain and monitor WBC and differential as ordered.
	2. Afebrile	Monitor V.S. q 4 h and PRN for increase in temp and heart rate.
	3. Absence of redness and purulent drainage from wound and invasive sites	1. Maintain aseptic and sterile technique for dressing and tubing changes. 2. Inspect wounds and invasive sites for S/S of infection (erythema, edema, purulent drainage, tenderness) q shift and PRN. 3. Assess urine color, clarity, and odor. Obtain UA and C&S QOD and monitor culture results. 4. Provide Foley and meatal care with soap and water q shift. 5. Inspect skin and mucous membranes for breakdown areas and bacterial and fungal overgrowth q shift and PRN.

**TABLE 10–5. NURSING CARE PLAN
FOR PANCREAS TRANSPLANT RECIPIENT** *Continued*

Nursing Diagnosis	Outcome Criteria	Nursing Interventions
		6. Provide mouth care q shift and PRN.
		7. Provide nutritional support as needed.
		8. Maintain clean and safe environment.
	4. Lungs clear	1. Assess and monitor resp status q 2–4 h and PRN for character, rate, and quality. Auscultate for breath sounds. ABG's as ordered
		2. Provide vigorous pulmonary toilet q 2–4 h and PRN. (TC&DB, incentive spirometer, chest physiotherapy). Encourage ambulation as ordered.

BP, Blood pressure; WBC, white blood cells; S/S, signs and symptoms; UA, urinalysis; C&S, culture and sensitivity; QOD, every other day; ABG, arterial blood gases; TC & DB, turn, cough and deep-breathe.

RESEARCH

Islet Cell Transplantation

Only whole-organ or segmental pancreas transplantation has been effective in reversing diabetes in humans. Researchers are diligently working on methods to extrapolate islet cells from the whole pancreas. By isolating only the insulin-producing cells of the pancreas it may be possible to avoid a major surgical procedure as well as the dangers of the exocrine secretions.

There are several obstacles to islet cell transplantation. First, it is difficult to get sufficient numbers of islet cells out of the pancreas without destroying them. Second, it is difficult to isolate pure islet cells from the pancreas; therefore, acinar cells are also removed in the process. Finally, long-term viability of functioning islets has not been attained. A few centers have reported islet cell function for two to four weeks before rejection occurs. Function has been defined as either free from exogenous insulin or decreased insulin requirements.

Separating islets from the human pancreas is a difficult task. The human pancreas consists of tissue that is fibrous and tough, requiring skillful processing to free the islets interspersed throughout the gland. During this process the digestive enzymes from the acinar cells within the pancreas are released and begin to autodigest the pancreas tissue. The process of isolating islets is delicate, time-consuming, and inefficient.

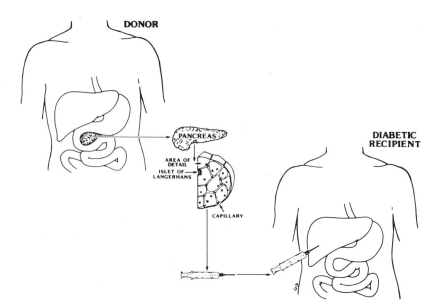

FIGURE 10–7. Islet cell separation from the human pancreas. (Used with permission from the artist, Linda Leib, Wadsworth VA Medical Center. From Soon-Shiong, P. (1987). *UCLA Health Insights, 5,* 1–5. © 1987 by the Regents of the University of California.)

It may require three to five technicians working eight to ten hours each to isolate islets from a single pancreas (Fig. 10–7).

Difficult as this task may seem, success may soon be a reality. With advances in technology, efficiency of islet cell separation will clearly be improved by mechanical automation or by immunologic purification using monoclonal antibodies to remove damaging, autodigestive acinar cells (Soon-Shiong, 1987). Alternative sources of islet tissue that are being explored include human fetal islet cells and animal (pig) cells.

Microencapsulation of Islet Cells

Once islet cells are separated and injected into the liver, spleen, or renal capsule, the problem of rejection remains. Researchers are exploring ways to prevent this. One method of preventing rejection is to envelop the islet cell in a protective capsule to prevent antibodies from reaching the islet cells. Such a microcapsule is currently being tested. By coating islets with two polymers a semipermeable membrane is formed that allows insulin to be secreted through the pores but prohibits antibodies from entering and causing rejection. Should these studies prove successful, a remarkable self-regulating artificial pancreas may be a viable solution to the problem of treating diabetes (Soon-Shiong, 1987).

References

American Diabetes Association. (1987). Diabetes: Facts you need to know. *Fact Sheet.*

Anderson, C.B., Tyler, J.D., Rodey, G.E., Etheredge, E.E., Anderman, C.K., Flye, M.W., Jendrisak, M.D., & Sicard, G. A. (1987). Preoperative immunomodulation of renal allograft recipients by concomitant immunosuppression and donor-specific transfusions. *Transplantation Proceedings, 19*(1), 1494–1497.

Baumgartner, D., Largiader, F., Uhlschmid, G., & Binswanger, U. (1983). Rejection episodes in recipients of simultaneous pancreas and kidney transplantation. *Transplantation Proceedings, 15*(1), 1330–1331.

Bohman, S.O., Tyden, G., Wilezek, A., Lundgren, G., Jaremko, G., Gunnarsson, R., Ostman, J., & Gross, C.G. (1985). Prevention of kidney graft diabetic nephropathy by pancreas transplantation in man. *Diabetes, 34*(3), 306.

Chmielewski, C. (1987). Early recognition of infection after renal transplantation. *ANNA Journal, 4*(6), 389–408.

Christman, C. & Bennett, J. (1987). Diabetes: New names, new tests and new diet. *Nursing '87, 17*(1), 34–41.

Conway, P.M. & Davis, C.P. (1987). The diabetic transplant patient: Nursing considerations. *ANNA Journal, 14*:379–383, 410.

Corry, R.J. (1987). The University of Iowa experience in pancreatic transplantation. *Transplantation Proceedings, 19*(4), 37–39.

Corry, R.J., Ngheim, D.D., Schanbacher, B.A., & Gonwa, T.A. (1987). Critical analysis of mortality and graft loss following simultaneous renal/pancreatic duodenal transplantation. *Transplantation Proceedings, 19*(1), 2305–2306.

Corry, R.J., Ngheim, D.D., Schulak, J.A., Beutel, W.D., & Gonwa, T.A., (1986). Surgical treatment of diabetic nephropathy with simultaneous pancreatic duodenal and renal transplantation. *Surgery, Gynecology and Obstetrics, 162*, 547–555.

Davidson, M.B. (1978). The case for control in diabetes mellitus. *Western Journal of Medicine, 129*, 193–200.

Dubernard, J.M., Traeger, J.L., Touraine, H., Beutel, H., & Malik, M.C. (1980). Rejection of human pancreatic allografts. *Transplantation Proceedings, 12*(4), 103–106.

Florack, G., Sutherland, D.E.R., Heil, J., Squifflet, J.R., & Najarian, J.S. (1983). Preservation of canine segmental pancreatic autografts: Cold storage versus pulsatile machine perfusion. *Journal of Surgical Research, 34*, 493–504.

Florack, G., Sutherland, D.E.R., Heise, J., & Najarian, J.S. (1987). Successful preservation of human pancreas grafts for up to twenty-eight hours. *Transplantation Proceedings, 19*:3882–3885.

Florack, G., Sutherland, D.E.R., Sibley, R., & Najarian, J.S. (1985). Combined kidney and segmental pancreas allotransplantation in dogs. *Transplantation Proceedings, 17*(1), 374–377.

Grenfell, A. & Watkins, P. (1986). Clinical nephropathy: Natural history and complications. *Clinics in Endocrinology and Metabolism, 15*(4), 783–805.

Groth, C.G. (1987). There is no need to give blood transfusions as pretreatment for renal transplantation in the cyclosporine era. *Transplantation Proceedings, 19*(1), 153–154.

Groth, C.G., Lundgren, J., Ostman J., Gunnarsson, R. (1980). Experience with nine segmental pancreas transplantations in pre-uremic diabetic patients in Stockholm. *Transplantation Proceedings, 12*, (4, Suppl 2), 68–72.

Hardy, M.A. (1987). Prospective HLA typing is helpful in cadaveric renal transplantation—maybe? *Transplantation Proceedings, 19*(1), 144–148.

Heise, J., Sutherland, D.E.R., Heil, J., & Najarian, J.S. (in press). Comparison of two colloidosmotic solutions in 72 hour preservation of pancreatic segments in a dog autotransplant model. *Transplantation Proceedings.* In press.

Hesse, U.J., Najarian, J.S., & Sutherland, D.E.R. (1985). Amylase activity and pancreas transplantation. *The Lancet, 2*(8457), 726.

Holleroroth, H.J. (1986). *Diabetes Teaching Guide.* Boston, Joslin Diabetes Center.

Kelly, W.D., Lillehei, R.C., Merkel, F.K., Idezuki, Y., & Goetz, F.C. (1967). Allograft transplantation of the pancreas and duodenum along with the kidney in diabetic nephropathy. *Surgery, 61*(6), 827–837.

Land, W. (1980). Simultaneous kidney and pancreas transplantation using prolamine for duct obstruction. *Transplantation Proceedings, 12*, 76–77.

Mauer, S.M., Steffes, M.W., Sutherland, D.E.R., Najarian, J.S., Michael, A.F., & Brown, D.M. (1975). Studies of the rate of regression of the glomerular lesions in diabetic rats treated with pancreatic islet transplantation. *Diabetes, 24*, 280–285.

Memmler, R.L. & Wood, D.L. (1987). *Structure and Function of the Human Body* (4th ed.). Philadelphia: J.B. Lippincott.

Mittal, V.K. & Toledo-Pereyra, L.H. (1986). Pancreatic transplantation: The surgical process. *AORN Journal, 43*(3), 620–629.

Ngheim, D.D., Gonwa, T.A., & Corry, R.J. (1987). Metabolic monitoring in renal-pancreatic transplants with urinary pancreatic exocrine diversion. *Transplantation Proceedings, 14*(1), 2350–2351.

Norman, D.J., Fletcher, L., & Barry, J. (1987). A randomized study of buffy coat transfusions in cadaveric renal transplantation. *Transplantation Proceedings, 19*(1), 1967–1970.

Opelz, G. (1987). Improved kidney graft survival in nontransfused recipients. *Transplantation Proceedings, 19*(1), 149–152.

Opelz, G. & Mickey, M.R. (1973). Identification of unresponsive kidney transplant recipients. *Transplantation Proceedings, 5*, 1149.

Prieto, M., Sutherland, D.E.R., Fernandez-Cruz, L., Heil, J., & Najarian, J.S. (1987). Experimental and clinical experience with urine amylase monitoring for early detection of rejection in pancreas transplantation. *Transplantation, 43*(1), 73–79.

Ramsay, R.C., Rice, S.W., Sutherland, D.E.R., Goetz, F.C., & Najarian, J.S. (1986). Visual status following pancreas transplantation for type 1 diabetes mellitus. *Transplantation Proceedings, 18*(6), 1774.

Schanbacher, B.A. & Hasselman, E. (1986). Management of the diabetic transplant recipient. *ANNA Journal, 13*, 187–190.

Schulak, J.A., & Drevyanko, T.S. (1985). Experimental pancreas allograft rejection: Correlation between histologic and functional rejection and the efficacy of antirejection therapy. *Journal of Surgery, 98*(2), 330–336.

Sibley, R.K., Sutherland, D.E.R., Goetz, F., & Michael, A.F. (1985). Recurrent diabetes mellitus in the pancreas iso- and allograft: A light and electron microscopic and immunohistochemical analysis of four cases. *Laboratory Investigation, 53*, 132–144.

Smith, J.L., Wright, F.H., Schanbacher, B.A., & Corry, R.J. (1988). Improving patient and graft survival rates in pancreatic transplantation. *Transplantation Proceedings, 20*(1), 866–867.

Sollinger, H.W., Cook, K., Kamps, D., Glass, N.R., Stratta, R.J., Kalayoglu, M., & Belzer, F.O. (1984). Clinical and experimental experience with pancreaticocystostomy for exocrine pancreatic drainage in pancreatic transplantation. *Transplantation Proceedings, 16*(3), 749–751.

Sollinger, H.W., Stratta, R.J., Kalayoglu, M., & Belzer, F.O. (1987). The University of Wisconsin experience in pancreas transplantation. *Transplantation Proceedings, 14*(4), 48–54.

Sollinger, H.W., Stratta, R.J., Kalayoglu, M., Pirsch, J.D., & Belzer, F.O. (1987). Pancreas transplantation with pancreaticocystostomy and quadruple immunosuppression. *Surgery, 102*, 672–676.

Soon-Shiong, P. (1987). Transplant research—diabetes: New cures in the offing? *Health Insights, UCLA 5*(12), 1, 5.

Soon-Shiong, P., White, G., DeMayo, E., Koyle, M., & Danovitch, G. (1988). Mechanical obstruction of the portal vein as a cause of vascular thrombosis after pancreatic transplantation in man. *Transplantation Proceedings, 20*(5), 399–402.

Sutherland, D.E.R. (1986). Current status of pancreas transplantation. *Clinical Diabetes*, 55–70.

Sutherland, D.E.R., Ascher, N.L., & Najarian, J.S. (1984). Whole pancreas donation from a cadaver donor, distal pancreas donation from a living relative, and pancreas transplantation. In R.L. Simmons, M.E. Finch & N.L. Ascher (Eds.). *Manual of Vascular Access, Organ Donation and Transplantation*. New York: Springer-Verlag (pp. 144–164).

Sutherland, D.E.R., Casanova, D., & Sibley, R.K. (1987). Monitoring and diagnosis of rejection. *Transplantation Proceedings, 19*(1), 2329–2331.

Sutherland, D.E.R., Chinn, P.L., Elick, B.A., & Najarian, J.S. (1984). Maximization of islet mass in pancreas grafts by near total or total whole organ excision without the duodenum from cadaver donors. *Transplantation Proceedings, 16*(1), 115–119.

Sutherland, D.E.R., Goetz, F.C., Hesse, U.J., Kennedy, W.R., Ramsey, R.C., Mauer, S.W., Steffes, M.W., Kendall, D.M., & Najarian, J.S. (1986). Effect of multiple variables on outcome in pancreas transplant recipients at the University of Minnesota and preliminary observations on the course of pre-existing secondary complications of diabetes. In E.A. Friedman & F.A. L'Esperance (Eds.). *Diabetic Renal Retinal Syndrome 3: Therapy* (pp. 481–499). Orlando: Grune & Stratton.

Sutherland, D.E.R., Goetz, F.C., & Najarian, J.S. (1979). Intraperitoneal transplantation of immediately vascularized segmental pancreatic grafts without duct ligation. *Transplantation, 28*:485–491.

Sutherland, D.E.R., Goetz, F.C., & Najarian, J.S. (1984a). One hundred pancreas transplants at a single institute. *Annals of Surgery, 200*(4), 414–440.

Sutherland, D.E.R., Goetz, F.C., & Najarian, J.S. (1984b). Pancreas transplants from related donors. *Transplantation, 38*(6), 625–633.

Sutherland, D.E.R., Goetz, F.C., & Najarian, J.S. (1986). Improved pancreas graft survival rates by use of multiple drug combination immunotherapy. *Transplantation Proceedings 18*, 1770–1773.

Sutherland, D.E.R., Goetz, F.C., & Najarian, J.S. (1987). Pancreas transplantation at the University of Minnesota: Donor and recipient selection, operative and postoperative management outcome. *Transplantation Proceedings, 19*(4, suppl. 4), 63–74.

Sutherland, D.E.R. & Kendall, D.M. (1985). Pancreas transplantation: Registry report and a commentary. *Western Journal of Medicine, 143*(6), 845–852.

Sutherland, D.E.R., Kendall, D., Goetz, F., & Najarian, J. (1986). Pancreas transplantation. *Surgical Clinics of North America, 66*(3), 557–582.

Sutherland, D.E.R., Moudry, K.C., Elick, B.A., Goetz, T.C., & Najarian, J.S. (1984). Selected issues of importance of clinical pancreas transplantation. *Transplantation Proceedings, 16*(1), 661–669.

Sutherland, D.E.R., Moudry, K.C., Elick, B.A., Goetz, F.C., & Najarian, J.S. (1988). Pancreas transplant protocols at the University of Minnesota: Recipient and donor selection, operative and postoperative management and outcome. In P. Teraski (Ed.). *Clinical Transplants 1987.* Los Angeles: UCLA Tissue Typing Laboratory (pp. 109–126).

Sutherland, D.E.R., Sibley, R.K., Chinn, P.L., Michael, A., Srikanta, S., Taub, F., Najarian, J.S., & Goetz, F.C. (1984). Twin to twin pancreas transplantation: Reversal and recurrence of pathogenesis in type I diabetes. *Clinical Research 32*(2), 561A.

Traeger, J., Dubernard, J.M., Piatti, E., Bosi, E., Gelet, A., Elyafi, S., Betuel, H., Secchi, A., Touraine, J.L., & Possa, G. (1984). Clinical aspects of pancreatic rejection in pancreatic and pancreaticorenal allotransplants. *Transplantation Proceedings, 16*(3), 718–719.

Tyden, G., Lundgren, G., & Ost, L. (1986). Are pancreatic grafts prone to rejection? *Transplantation Proceedings, 18*(1), 27–29.

van Rood, J.J. (1987). Prospective HLA typing is helpful in cadaveric renal transplantation. *Transplantation Proceedings, 19*(1), 139–143.

Wahlberg, J.A., Southhard, J.H., & Belzer, F.O. (1986). Development of a cold storage solution for pancreas preservation. *Cryobiology, 23*, 447–482.

Weiland, D., Sutherland, D.E.R., Chavers, B., Simmons, R.L., Ascher, N.L., & Najarian, J.S. (1984). Information on 628 living-related kidney donors at a single institution with long-term followup in 472 cases. *Transplantation Proceedings, 16*, 5–7.

Weintrauch, L.A. (1977). Coronary angiography and acute renal failure in diabetic azotemic nephropathy. *Annals of Internal Medicine, 86*, 56.

11
Corneal Transplantation

Mary Beth Danneffel

Corneal transplantation, when compared with organ transplants, has always enjoyed a greater success rate, thought to be due to the normally avascular state of the cornea, which protects the donor graft from immunologic surveillance of the recipient. The first successful human-to-human penetrating corneal transplant was reported in 1906 by Edward Zirm (Zirm, 1906).

Since that time the success rate has increased because of such factors as the introduction of the operating microscope; new and improved surgical instruments, suture materials, and microsurgical techniques; and improved preoperative and postoperative management. Donor cornea processing, which includes donor evaluation, tissue retrieval, storage, and handling, has become more sophisticated, and has also contributed to the greater success rate of penetrating keratoplasty. At the same time an increasingly older population with greater longevity and expansion of the reasons for performing corneal transplants have increased the number of penetrating keratoplasties done annually in the United States (Buxton & Norden, 1986). The number of corneal transplants performed in 1976 was approximately 6,500 (T.J. Moore, personal communication, December 9, 1987), compared with 31,000 in 1986 and 35,930 in 1987 (Eye Bank Association of America, 1987; Eye Bank Association of America, 1988).

Penetrating corneal transplant, or penetrating keratoplasty, is the surgical procedure whereby an abnormal full-thickness cornea is removed from the host recipient and replaced with full-thickness donor corneal tissue. Lamellar keratoplasty refers to the removal and replacement of a partial thickness of the cornea. This chapter focuses on the more commonly performed procedure, penetrating keratoplasty.

ANATOMY AND PHYSIOLOGY

The human cornea is normally a transparent, avascular, dime-sized tissue, measuring approximately 11 mm in diameter and ranging in thickness from 0.6 mm at the periphery to 0.5 mm centrally. It is continuous with the white sclera of the eye and is situated anteriorly over the iris (the pigmented or colored portion of the eye) and the pupil (Fig. 11–1). The cornea acts as a refractive "window" through which light passes to the retina. The cornea has five layers (Fig. 11–2):

1. The epithelium is five to six cell layers thick and serves as a barrier to microorganisms such as bacteria and fungi, which, along with the tear film, provides a "smooth refracting surface at the front of the eye" (Friend, 1983). It is richly supplied with sensory pain fibers; this is why a corneal abrasion or injury is so painful. However, damage to the epithelium causes only slight, transient swelling that clears when the epithelial cells regenerate (Vaughan & Asbury, 1986).

2. Bowman's layer lies immediately beneath the epithelium and is a clear acellular layer.

3. The stroma accounts for 90 per cent of the corneal thickness and is composed of intertwining lamellar fibers running almost the full diameter of the cornea and parallel to the surface (Vaughan & Asbury, 1986).

4. Descemet's membrane is a collagen layer adjacent to and believed to be secreted by the endothelium.

5. The endothelium, a single layer of cells that lines the inner

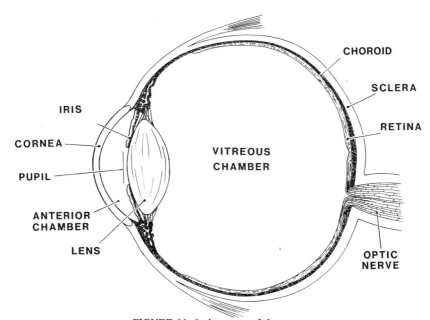

FIGURE 11–1. Anatomy of the eye.

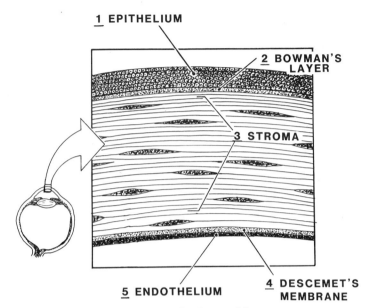

FIGURE 11–2. The five layers of the cornea.

surface of the cornea, performs several vital functions, the most important of which is corneal dehydration. It has been identified as the layer across which excess water from the stroma is transported. The actual water-pumping mechanism of the corneal endothelium is unclear. The cornea depends on an intact, viable endothelial layer in order to keep the stroma from swelling (Dohlman, 1983). Endothelial cells do not regenerate.

INDICATIONS FOR PENETRATING KERATOPLASTY

Any injury, infection, disease, inherited dystrophy, or other disorder that damages the corneal endothelium may result in corneal edema or swelling, and loss of clarity. An injury that penetrates the stroma may result in a permanent scar, which, if large enough, would also interfere with vision. The most common indication for penetrating keratoplasty is bullous keratopathy or corneal swelling (Musch, Meyer, Sugar, & Soong, 1985) (see Table 11–1). Aphakic bullous keratopathy indicates corneal decompensation after cataract extraction; pseudophakic bullous keratopathy refers to corneal edema after implantation of an intraocular lens. Numerous other disorders, listed in Table 11–1, may also lead to the need for corneal transplantation.

**TABLE 11-1. PRIMARY DIAGNOSIS
OF CORNEAL TRANSPLANTATION PATIENTS**

DIAGNOSIS	No. OF PATIENTS (n = 1054)	(%)
Pseudophakic bullous keratopathy	215	(20.4)
Aphakic bullous keratopathy	190	(18.0)
Fuchs' corneal dystrophy	152	(14.4)
Keratoconus	131	(12.4)
Interstitial keratitis	118	(11.2)
Herpes simplex keratitis	74	(7.0)
Failed corneal graft	31	(2.9)
Other corneal dystrophies	31	(2.9)
Traumatic scarring	28	(2.7)
Corneal ulceration	24	(2.3)
Other corneal scarring	15	(1.4)
Bullous keratopathy	12	(1.1)
Chemical burn	12	(1.1)
Varicella zoster keratitis	4	(0.4)
Other causes	17	(1.6)

From Musch, D. C., et al. (1985). Michigan Corneal Transplant Patient Registry: Summary Project Report, 1984-1985. Ann Arbor: University of Michigan Medical Center, W. K. Kellogg Eye Center.

PATIENT SELECTION

The decision to have a corneal transplant, when it is clearly indicated for the improvement or restoration of sight, should be a joint one between patient and surgeon. The patient should carefully assess the extent of visual impairment versus personal needs. These needs may be social or work- or autonomy-related. Alteration in comfort or pain may impact on the decision for transplant. Impaired tissue integrity, such as a corneal perforation or impending perforation resulting from infection or disease, may necessitate an emergent decision for transplant in order to save the eye. The recipient patient's age is not a primary consideration; corneal transplants have been performed on a 9-day-old baby and a 103-year-old great, great grandfather (Eye Bank Association of America, 1987). The important question to answer is, what degree of visual improvement can be achieved through penetrating keratoplasty? The patient should decide whether an anticipated improvement is worth the risk and whether to accept the posttransplant responsibilities.

PREOPERATIVE EXAMINATION AND MEASUREMENTS

A careful history should be obtained from the patient. Assessment should include histories of the course of the visual loss, trauma, and any ophthalmic medications taken to control intraocular pressure or inflammation. A systemic medical evaluation is important for the planning of anesthesia and postoperative care. A careful medical history for illness, medications, and drug allergies should be elicited. The preoperative evaluation is used to diagnose the corneal alteration and determine whether corneal transplantation would be beneficial.

The preoperative evaluation and examination may be done jointly by the ophthalmic nurse or technician and the surgeon. Visual acuity measurements in both eyes are taken, with and without pinhole (which sharpens vision without the need for squinting). Tear function is evaluated with a Schirmer test and rose bengal staining (Forstot, 1986). Intraocular pressure is measured by applanation tonometry using an instrument such as the Goldmann or MacKay-Marg tonometer or a pneumotonometer. Glaucoma must be well controlled before corneal transplantation (Buxton & Norden, 1986).

A careful slit-lamp biomicroscopic examination is performed to assess the lids, conjunctivae, and cornea. The extent of the opacity is observed to help determine graft size. Presence or absence of corneal vascularity may indicate the propensity for rejection (Forstot, 1986). The anterior chamber is carefully examined for signs of iritis and the presence of anterior synechiae, particularly in patients who have had a cataract extraction with intraocular lens implantation. In an aphakic patient the anterior chamber is assessed for the presence, position, type, and stability of an intraocular lens.

Corneal thickness is measured by a pachymeter. Corneal irregularity is assessed by a corneoscope, which is useful in checking scarring and irregularity in keratoconus (Forstot, 1986). The retina is examined by indirect or direct ophthalmoscopy, or both. Ultrasound may be needed to rule out retinal detachment. It is particularly important to assess eyes with aphakic or pseudophakic bullous keratopathy for cystoid macular edema. Although the presence of cystoid macular edema may not rule out corneal transplant, the patient should be informed of limited visual prognosis (Sugar, A., 1986). Corneal endothelial cell density may be determined by specular microscopy. A very low cell count (less than 600 cells per millimeter) along with beginning decompensation indicates that the cornea will probably become more edematous over time (Sugar, A., 1986).

The prognosis for postoperative visual outcome is based on many factors, including psychosocial considerations. The patient should be presented with the diagnosis, prognosis, and options for surgery. Careful assessment of the patient's understanding of the transplant process and capacity for self-care is made. The patient should be aware that complete postoperative visual rehabilitation may take a year or more, and that the best visual acuity may require contact lenses or spectacles. The patient should also understand that graft rejection may occur at any time in the postoperative period. Diligent surveillance for the earliest detection of posttransplant complications will be crucial to graft survival (Buxton & Norden, 1986).

Preoperative Patient Teaching and Care

Once the decision for corneal transplantation has been made, the nurse initiates patient teaching on an outpatient basis. This teaching will be continued during the immediate preoperative admission period.

Nursing Assessment and Outpatient Teaching

Careful nursing evaluation and teaching are required to prepare the patient for surgery. The nurse will have participated in the patient's initial examination and should assess the patient for the presence of the preoperative nursing diagnoses in Table 11–2.

Information regarding the surgical procedure and postoperative care is conveyed to the patient. Printed information may be given to the patient for later reinforcement. Diagrams such as that shown in Figure 11–3 may be helpful. The patient is told that her name will be placed on the eye bank's waiting list. When a cornea becomes available the surgeon is notified and contacts the patient for immediate admission (within 24–48 hours) for surgery. Because the cornea is normally avascular, tissue-typing is usually not performed, and there is no matching based on sex or race. However, in selected high-risk cases, such as in patients with a history of rejection or those with vascularized corneas, histocompatibility antigen matching, crossmatch testing, or both may be beneficial. Because only a portion of the clear cornea is transplanted, the color of the donor's eye (iris) is irrelevant. Reassurance that the donor tissue has been screened for acquired immunodeficiency syndrome and hepatitis may also be given.

Corneal transplants may be performed on an outpatient basis. A one- or two-day hospital stay is occasionally required. The decision for outpatient or inpatient surgery is determined by the needs of the patient, available resources, and assessment of the patient's individual circumstances.

Similarly, the patient should be informed about options for anesthesia. Corneal transplantation is generally performed under local anesthesia with a regional block by retrobulbar injection. General anesthesia may be indicated for a very young patient or one who is extremely anxious or restless.

Success of the corneal transplant will depend, to some extent, on

TABLE 11–2. PREOPERATIVE NURSING ASSESSMENT AND DIAGNOSES FOR CORNEAL TRANSPLANT RECIPIENT

Nursing Diagnosis	Risk Factors	Signs/Symptoms	Nursing Implications
Alteration in visual sensory-perception	Corneal edema, or scarring	Decreased visual acuity, with blurred or cloudy vision; patient may have light perception only	Patient may be unable to read, drive, or move around home to perform activities of daily living without assistance.
Self-care deficits	Impaired vision	Poor personal hygiene, i.e., dirty, uncombed hair	Patient's visual loss may be great enough to require assistance with bathing, grooming, and dressing.
Alteration in nutrition	Depression resulting from increasing dependence on others for assistance	Loss of appetite with weight loss and other signs of nutritional deficiency, including obesity	Assess nutritional status for any deficits; explore with patient a plan of care to correct any nutritional deficiencies.
Alterations in self-concept; disturbances in body image or self-esteem	Loss of independence	Anger, increased anxiety, or depression as indicated by lack of interest in environment	Assess for existing support from family members until time of transplant.
Alterations in comfort	Extreme corneal swelling (bullous keratopathy)	Pain, photophobia	Determine what medications may be prescribed to decrease discomfort; what other measures may increase comfort, such as ophthalmic drops with high concentration of balanced salt solution, bandage contact lens, or patching of the eye.
Impaired tissue integrity	Impending or existing corneal perforation owing to corneal infection, trauma, or persistent epithelial defects in patients with rheuematoid arthritis, erythema multiforme, vitamins A and B complex deficiencies	Extreme thinning of the anterior surface with possible leakage of aqueous fluid; patient with history of dry eye may experience some pain with sudden "tearing"	Patient will require immediate referral to a surgeon for treatment.

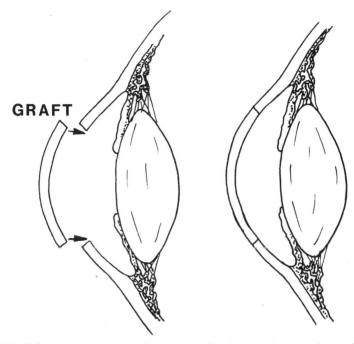

GRAFT

FIGURE 11–3. Segment of the cornea that is removed and replaced in corneal transplantation.

the patient's understanding of the postoperative treatment. Because of the cornea's lack of blood supply, healing will be slow and the restoration of vision will be gradual. Sutures may not be removed for a year or more, and some may remain indefinitely. Vision may be blurred until final suture removal, when glasses or contact lenses are prescribed.

It is imperative that the patient understand the need for frequent postoperative visits at weekly, biweekly, and then monthly intervals, so that the corneal surgeon can assess the status of the graft, eye pressure, and signs of inflammation or infection. The patient also should plan ahead for postoperative restrictions. Assistance may be needed with transportation and activities of daily living.

The patient should be informed that there is potential for rejection. Signs and symptoms of rejection include redness of the eye, pain, decreased vision, and increased light sensitivity, all or any of which must be reported to the nurse or surgeon. Graft success or failure hinges on diligent observation and care by the patient.

Patient Preparation and Teaching in the Immediate Preoperative Period

On admission either to an outpatient surgical unit or to a hospital inpatient unit important aspects of the immediate postoperative care are reviewed by the nurse. The patient is instructed to remain in bed or in an easy chair and to lie supine or on the unoperated side immediately after surgery. She is cautioned not to lift, stoop, strain, or bend for approximately one month to avoid increasing intraocular pressure and placing stress on the sutures (Tooke, Elders, & Johnson, 1986). The patient should notify the nurse when feeling nauseated, so that medication can be prescribed to avoid vomiting, which would stress the wound. Showering, shampooing the hair, and sexual activity may be limited during the first postoperative week. The eye should be kept covered and a metal shield worn at night when sleeping. Strenuous activity such as heavy housework and athletics is discouraged for three months (Tooke et al., 1986). Swimming, which would risk contamination, is also not advised. Reading, writing, and watching television are allowed as tolerated by the patient.

The patient will be visited by the anesthesiologist before surgery. Electrocardiography and blood tests as ordered will have been done to determine general health. The patient is advised to shower and shampoo the hair the night before surgery. Her face will be washed with an antibacterial soap, the eyelashes will be clipped, and antibiotic eye drops, such as gentamicin, may be instilled the night before and again just before surgery. The patient should be instructed to take nothing by mouth after midnight the day before surgery. A medication for sleep may be prescribed for the patient who has a high level of anxiety. If outpatient surgery is scheduled, most of these procedures will have been done before admission.

OPERATIVE CONSIDERATIONS

Donor Tissue Quality Assurance

The increased availability and improved quality of donor corneal tissue are the result of organized eye-banking efforts in the United States. The first eye bank in the United States was the Eye Bank for Sight Restoration in New York, which was formed in 1945 under the direction of Dr. R. Townley Paton (Farge, 1986). Many of the early eye donations came from recently executed prisoners. In 1961 the Eye Bank Association of America (EBAA) was established. It developed policy and procedures, including membership requirements and a code of ethics that continues to guide eye bank practices.

As the number of eye banks and corneal transplantation procedures increased, the first reports of disease transmission from donor tissue to recipients began to appear. In 1978 the EBAA established its Medical Standards Committee (Mannis, 1986). In 1981 the process for site visit inspection and certification of eye banks was initiated. The site visit encompasses a detailed review of eye-banking procedures. Recertification is required with a repeat site visit every three years.

Corneal donor tissue selection is based on the EBAA's medical standards. The acceptable age of the donor tissue varies among eye banks, ranging from 6 months to 70 years. Surgeons prefer younger donor tissue in the belief that it will provide a greater endothelial cell density. This may compensate for the expected cell loss that accompanies removal from the donor and transplantation into the recipient (Koenig, 1986). In general, the sooner the retrieval of the donor eyes or corneas after death, the better the condition of the tissue.

Until the middle to late 1970s whole globes were stored in a sterile moist chamber for up to 78 hours after the donor's death. The corneo-scleral rim was not excised from the whole eye until surgery. A new era in corneal preservation dawned in 1974 with the introduction of Mc-Carey-Kaufman (M-K) tissue culture medium (Brightbill, 1986). Within 8 to 12 hours of a donor's death the corneoscleral rim was removed and placed in M-K medium. It could be stored in this manner for 72 to 84 hours. Newer tissue culture media such as CSM and K-Sol, which contain chondroitan sulfate, allow for corneal storage for up to 14 days.

EBAA medical standards currently mandate that all donor tissue offered for corneal transplant be tested and found non-reactive for hepatitis B surface antigen and human immunodeficiency virus antibody. Careful screening of the donor's medical history is also done to rule out any other potentially transmissible diseases. Cultures of the corneoscleral rim are obtained at the time of initial corneoscleral rim removal or at the time of transplant. Slit-lamp biomicroscopy of the donor tissue is routinely performed, and the tissue is assigned a rating based on its microscopic appearance.

Specular microscopy may be performed; this allows visualization of the corneal endothelium (see Fig. 11–4). The endothelial cells are assessed for such characteristics as morphology and density. Although there is no agreement on an absolute minimum cell count, the goal is to transplant as many viable donor endothelial cells as possible (Bourne, 1986).

Care and Handling of Donor Tissue

Donor tissue is sent to the operating room where the transplant will be performed. The donor cornea is stored in a vial or storage chamber containing a tissue culture medium with an antibiotic, such as gentamicin, at 4°C. (normal household refrigerator temperature). It is then packed inside a Styrofoam transport canister with wet ice and labeled "Human

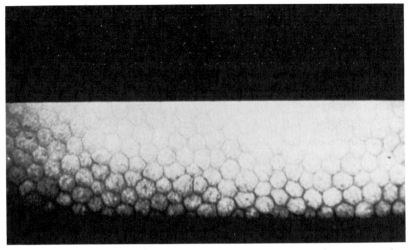

FIGURE 11–4. Corneal epithelial cells visualized under the specular microscope.

Eye Tissue." The eye tissue is shipped by commercial airline, bus, taxi, or courier. On arrival at the hospital it should be taken immediately to the operating room refrigerator. It is the responsibility of the transplanting surgeon to check the donor medical information and quality of the tissue before its surgical use.

Intraoperative Patient Care and the Surgical Procedure

The patient is given a preoperative medication. In the operating room the patient may be placed on an egg-crate mattress for comfort. An intravenous line is established, and leads are placed for cardiac monitoring. Many surgeons prefer to use local anesthesia because it allows for more rapid postoperative patient mobility (Sugar J., 1986). It may also reduce the possibility of postoperative nausea and vomiting, which may compromise graft integrity. A short-acting drug may be given to avoid the pain associated with the periorbital injections for regional or local anesthesia (Tooke et al., 1986).

The patient's head is positioned and fixed, and the operative eye draped. The procedure begins with exposure of the anterior segment with lid speculums. A fixation ring is sutured to the superficial sclera for stability and support. The donor cornea is removed from its storage chamber and placed endothelial side up on a firm cutting surface, such as a Teflon block. The surgeon uses a trephine to trim the corneal button to the preferred diameter. The corneal button is temporarily left in the well of the block with the addition of a balanced salt solution.

The recipient bed is likewise prepared under an operating microscope. A trephine of similar size is used to cut either three-fourths of the way or completely through the anterior chamber. If trephination is three-fourths of the way, the surgeon will use scissors to complete the cutting and remove the damaged host cornea. If the patient has a cataract, it is removed at this time and an intraocular lens may be implanted. The donor cornea is then placed onto the recipient bed and sutured. There are many variations in suture techniques, including multiple interrupted, single running, double running, or a combination of these sutures. Through-and-through suturing generally is avoided because of the potential for endothelial cell damage. Knots are buried beneath the surface to block formation of new blood vessels, which may increase the likelihood of rejection. Wound integrity is assessed for leakage. Local instillation of antibiotic ointment or injection of subconjunctival antibiotics may be used. Subconjunctival steroids may also be injected, although the benefit of this is unclear (Sugar J., 1986).

Intraoperative Surgical Complications

The following complications may occur during surgery:

1. Hemorrhage from the retrobulbar block. This should be identified, immediately followed by cancellation of the procedure. Hemorrhage from a highly vascularized cornea when these vessels are cut at trephination, or abnormal vessels in the anterior chamber angle require cauterization or topical epinephrine to vasoconstrict. The most serious ocular emergency is expulsive hemorrhage of the choroid (Cowden, 1987). This is treated by immediate tamponade with aspiration of the blood and immediate closure of the corneal wound.

2. Problems in trephination, leading to donor-recipient disparity. This may require another donor cornea immediately.

3. Trauma to the iris or lens from the trephine. This may require a partial excision of the iris, or lensectomy.

4. Loss of vitreous from the eye. This may occur if there is positive vitreous pressure from collapse of the sclera or choroidal hemorrhage. It requires immediate recognition and treatment by vitrectomy.

5. Flattened anterior chamber that does not adequately reform. This may be due to sutures that are too loosely tied, or not enough sutures, resulting in wound leakage. The anterior chamber will need to be reformed and deficiencies in wound closure corrected (Cowden, 1987).

The eye is patched with two eye pads taped to the skin, and a metal shield is taped over these for additional protection (see Figs. 11–5 through 11–10 showing the preoperative and postoperative eye, and the transplant procedure).

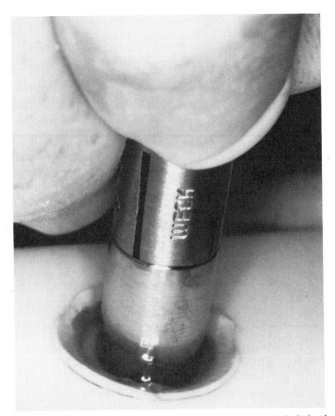

FIGURE 11–5. Punching of the donor button from the endothelial side.

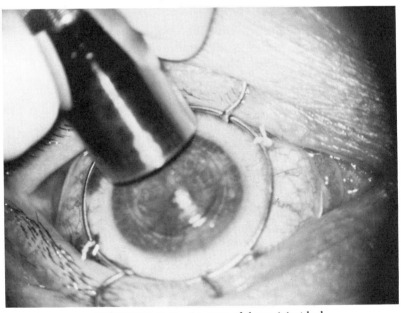

FIGURE 11–6. Trephination of the recipient bed.

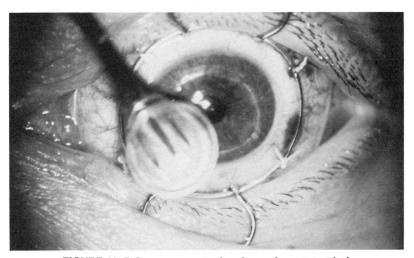

FIGURE 11–7. Donor cornea is placed over the recipient bed.

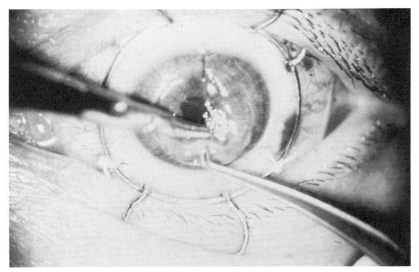

FIGURE 11–8. Placement of initial interrupted fixation suture at 12 o'clock position.

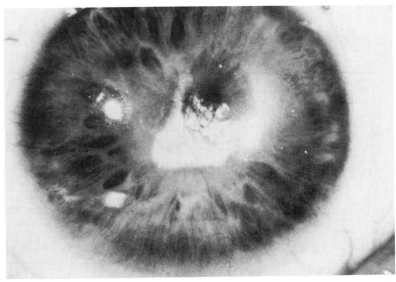

FIGURE 11–9. Preoperative view of patient with corneal decompensation secondary to pseudophakic bullous keratopathy (PBK).

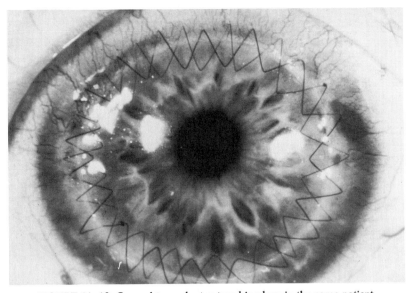

FIGURE 11–10. Corneal transplant sutured in place in the same patient.

**TABLE 11–3. POSTOPERATIVE RESTRICTIONS IN ACTIVITY
FOR CORNEAL TRANSPLANT RECIPIENT**

Postoperative Day 1
Bed rest or easy chair, lie supine or on
  unoperated side
Control nausea and vomiting with
  medications if necessary
Operated eye should remain shielded at
  all times

First Month
No lifting, stooping, straining, or bending
  that would increase intraocular
  pressure and place stress on sutures

First Week
Limit showering and shampooing of hair
Limit sexual activity
Cover eye with metal shield at night
  when sleeping
Reading, writing, and watching TV as
  tolerated

First 3 Months
No strenuous activity such as athletics or
  heavy housework
No swimming owing to risk of
  contamination

POSTOPERATIVE MANAGEMENT

Tables 11–3 and 11–4 outline the postoperative restrictions in
activity and the postoperative assessment and frequency of follow-up
office visits. Immediate postoperative assessment and care center around
assessing the patient for level of comfort and tissue integrity; this will
be followed by an assessment of the patient's understanding regarding
postoperative care, possible noncompliance owing to incomplete knowl-

**TABLE 11–4. POSTOPERATIVE ASSESSMENT OF
CORNEAL TRANSPLANT RECIPIENT**

Frequency of Office Visits
Weekly for 3–4 weeks
Biweekly for 6–8 weeks
Monthly through year 1
Biyearly or yearly for remainder of patient's life
More frequently in presence of problems or symptoms

Usual Examination Procedure
1. Review of history; ask patient to repeat signs indicating possible graft
   rejection (RSVP); review medications; review instillation technique for
   ophthalmic drops to ensure safety and effectiveness

2. Visual acuity check with pinhole; reading vision check; refraction of
   current prescription lenses; astigmatism measurement with keratometer

3. External examination of lids, conjunctivae, and anterior segment

4. Slit-lamp examination to assess for signs of infection, inflammation,
   edema, problem sutures, epithelial defects, or keratitic precipitates, which
   indicate graft rejection

5. Intraocular pressure check with tonometer

6. Fluorescein applied to assess integrity of the corneal epithelium

7. Funduscopic examination with ophthalmoscope to detect retinal
   problems

8. Pachymetry to measure corneal thickness

9. Recording of impressions; advise patient; schedule next visit

edge, and making sure the patient is able to adequately provide self-care or has family members who are able to assist.

During the first postoperative day topical steroid drops may be applied hourly, and then the frequency decreased to once or twice a day through the first three months. Prophylactic topical antibiotics may be started the day after surgery with twice-daily application and then once or twice daily for three weeks, or until the epithelium appears intact and infection is not suspected.

It is important for the patient to understand that, especially in the first year after corneal transplantation, frequent and regular visits to the surgeon will need to be made (see Table 11–4). In the absence of complications, visits are scheduled at more widely spaced intervals. Because most complications are successfully treated with early intervention, the patient should be advised to immediately report any problems.

The signs and symptoms of infection and rejection should be reviewed during each postoperative visit; use of the mnemonic RSVP may be helpful:

R = redness,
S = sensitivity to light,
V = vision loss, and
P = pain (Tooke et al., 1986).

Treatment of Rejection Episodes

The patient must be made aware that surveillance for signs of rejection should be a daily, lifelong practice. The earlier that rejection episodes are detected, the greater the success in treatment and reversal. The patient should be instructed to telephone the office or clinic immediately on suspicion of any of the cardinal signs.

The patient should realize that the incision site will remain the weakest part of the eye and could be ruptured by direct trauma at any time; for that reason she should avoid contact sports and other risky activities. The most important postoperative care instructions should be printed for the patient to take home. These include instruction in the instillation of drops or ointment and patching of the eye:

1. Instillation of drops
   a. The patient should begin with careful handwashing.
   b. The lower lid should be pulled down to form a pouch.
   c. The patient should look up.
   d. One drop is placed in the pouch. (More than one drop is not helpful, as the conjunctival sac is incapable of holding more.)
   e. The eye should be closed for at least one full minute.

  f. If more than one type of drop has been prescribed, wait two to three minutes between instillation of the drops.
  g. Advise patients not to touch the dropper tip with the fingers or to the eye. Some patients find that steadying the dropper on the bridge of the nose makes it easier to aim the drops. If the eye drops are refrigerated, their cool temperature may help the patient to determine whether the drop has reached its intended target (Tooke et al., 1986). Ointment is applied in a similar manner, except that about 1/4 inch of ointment is squeezed into the pouch.
2. Patching of the eye
  a. Two pieces of tape, either paper or plastic, are placed sticky side up on a flat surface.
  b. Two oval eye pads are secured to the tape.
  c. The pad with tape is brought to the closed eye and adhered with three or four more pieces of tape to give a secure, snug fit.
  d. The metal shield is then taped over the pad with two or more pieces of tape.

If an elderly or significantly sight-impaired patient has difficulty with these procedures, the assistance of a family member may be required.

Possible Complications

Early postoperative medical complications of corneal transplantation include primary graft failure, infection, healing disorders, and glaucoma. A primary graft failure is a hazy, thickened graft from the first postoperative day that fails to improve in the absence of other complicating factors. It is thought to be due to an inadequate number of endothelial cells needed to keep the cornea deturgesced or clear. The causes may be poor donor tissue owing to excessive time between death and preservation or transplantation, and diseased or aged donor endothelium. Poor handling techniques or surgical trauma may cause endothelial cell loss, leading to primary graft failure. Treatment is regrafting (Cowden, 1987).

An infection, such as endophthalmitis, or corneal ulceration is a serious complication. Although careful eye-banking practices reduce the chance for donor-transmitted infections, they will still occasionally occur. Treatment of endophthalmitis may include emergency vitrectomy with intraocular infusion of antibiotics and graft replacement. Systemic broad-spectrum antibiotics are administered until culture and sensitivity reports identify the most appropriate drug. Delayed healing or reepithelialization of the corneal graft leads to increased risk of infection and corneal scarring. Antibiotics may be applied and the eye patched. Glaucoma or elevated intraocular pressure is controlled with antiglaucomatous medications.

Late medical complications include the following:

1. Corneal decompensation (edema) from defective donor tissue, surgical trauma, inflammation, rejection, or glaucoma.

2. Allograft rejection. This may occur approximately two weeks after the transplant, when the patient may miss the symptoms of decreased vision, light sensitivity (photophobia), and redness. Most rejection reactions (90%) occur within the first year of surgery, and half within the first three months (Cowden, 1987). Early treatment (within the first three days of onset) with systemic and concentrated topical steroids can successfully suppress rejection, which is why it is so important for the patient to be able to recognize the symptoms.

3. Graft vascularization, in which blood vessels are attracted and grow in toward the graft. These vessels grow toward irritated or edematous areas, such as exposed and irritated sutures.

4. Recurrence of the patient's original corneal disease, such as herpes simplex keratitis.

Suture Removal

Broken sutures are removed as soon as detected. Time tables for suture removal vary, depending on the thickness and composition of suture material used. Removal is done on an outpatient basis and may begin as early as three months, although some sutures may be left in place indefinitely. Topical anesthetic drops are instilled before suture removal. The patient may experience discomfort (foreign body sensation) for up to 48 hours afterward, and antibiotic drops may be used to prevent infection. Vision changes may occur, with a change in refractive error after suture removal.

CORRECTION OF POSTOPERATIVE ASTIGMATISM AND VISUAL REHABILITATION

Final visual acuity (20/40 or better) is usually achieved with spectacles or contact lenses after suture removal. Fitting of contact lenses is usually done four to six weeks after the sutures are removed and the wound has stabilized. Types of contact lenses that may be prescribed include hard, soft daily wear, soft extended wear, and silicone soft/hard lenses (Brightbill & Laux, 1986). Correction of high amounts of residual postoperative astigmatism may require surgical intervention. Techniques such as relaxing incisions or wedge resections are used. These are usually performed on an outpatient basis.

OTHER KERATOPLASTY PROCEDURES

Two other types of keratoplasty procedures, less often performed, are as follows:

1. Lamellar keratoplasty, a partial-thickness corneal transplant in which only the outer layers of the donor cornea are used. Consequently good donor endothelium is not important. Tissue from older donors may be used in this procedure.

2. Refractive keratoplasty procedures, developed to correct high degrees of myopia (near-sightedness) and as an alternative to intraocular implantation after cataract extraction.

The two basic procedures are known as keratomileusis and epikeratophakia (keratophakia). Keratomileusis involves removal of part of the patient's cornea, freezing it, cryolathing it to a desired correction, and then suturing it back into the patient. Epikeratophakia involves freeze-drying a donor cornea and cryolathing it according to various prescriptions. The surgeon then reconstitutes the donor lenticule in sterile saline solution, prepares the recipient bed, and sutures this "living contact lens" in place. This procedure has been used particularly in very young aphakic patients who cannot wear contact lens and in patients after cataract extraction (Vaughan & Asbury, 1986).

FUTURE CONSIDERATIONS

Considerations for the future of corneal transplantation include increasing the already high success rate of penetrating keratoplasty through improvements in surgical technique. Technique is improved through the development of better suture material and instrumentation, which leads to fewer postoperative complications and possibilities for graft rejection. Improvements in postoperative care are continually being made, as well as those involving the preparation and storage of donor tissue. Development of newer tissue culture media may extend the life of the tissue, providing even greater flexibility in scheduling for both patient and surgeon. More penetrating keratoplasties will be done on an outpatient basis. The overall success rate, already high, ranges from 85 per cent to 90 per cent. However, in high-risk cases, such as in those patients with a history of rejection or in patients with vascularized corneas, the graft success rate is much lower. In these high-risk cases histocompatibility antigen matching, crossmatch testing or both may be beneficial. A national six-center study, called the Collaborative Corneal Transplantation Studies, is investigating this issue and will report their findings sometime in the 1990s.

SUMMARY

It has been the intent of this chapter to cover nursing considerations of the patient undergoing penetrating keratoplasty or corneal transplantation. A brief overview of anatomy and physiology of the cornea has been provided in order to give a clearer understanding of the indications for PKP. The preoperative assessment of the patient has been reviewed, along with important nursing diagnoses. An outline, with illustrations, of the surgical procedure has been provided. Issues surrounding eye banking and selection of donor tissue have been presented. Finally, the postoperative management has been outlined.

It is hoped that this chapter will assist nurses in the teaching and care of the patient undergoing corneal transplantation. This chapter is dedicated to the thousands of patients whose quality of life has been enhanced by restoration or improvement of sight through corneal transplantation.

Acknowledgments: I thank the following people: Mary Nehra Waldo, BSN, RN, and the nursing staff at the W. K. Kellogg Eye Center at the University of Michigan; the three medical directors of the Michigan Eye-Bank and Transplantation Center; Dr. John Cowden, head of the Cornea Service at Kresge Eye Institute, Wayne State University; Dr. Roger Meyer, head of the Cornea Service at W. K. Kellogg Eye Center, University of Michigan, and Dr. Joel Sugar, head of the Cornea Service at the University of Illinois, Chicago. Also, special thanks to Csaba L. Martonyi, CRA, FOPS, and the ophthalmic photography department at the University of Michigan; and to Anthony J. Tyrer (my spouse) for the excellent drawings as well as moral support. Finally, and very importantly, thanks to Thomas Moore, President of the Eye Bank Association of America, and to the Michigan Eye Bank and Transplantation Center.

References

Bourne, W. M. (1986). Endothelial cell loss after keratoplasty. In F. S. Brightbill (Ed.). *Corneal Surgery: Theory, Technique, and Tissue* (pp. 352–355). St. Louis: C. V. Mosby.

Brightbill, F. S. (1986). Tissue storage: Short term comparison of methods and results. In F. S. Brightbill (Ed.). *Corneal Surgery: Theory, Technique, and Tissue* (pp. 75–77). St. Louis: C. V. Mosby.

Brightbill, F. S., & Laux, D. J. (1986). Contact lens fitting. In F. S. Brightbill (Ed.). *Corneal Surgery: Theory, Technique, and Tissue* (pp. 344–351). St. Louis: C. V. Mosby.

Buxton, J. N. & Norden, R. A. (1986). Adult penetrating keratoplasty: Indications and contraindications. In F. S. Brightbill (Ed.). *Corneal Surgery: Theory, Technique, and Tissue* (pp. 129–140). St. Louis: C. V. Mosby.

Cowden, J. W. (1987). Corneal transplantation: Medical and surgical complications. In L. H. Toledo-Pereyra (Ed.). *Complications of Corneal Transplantation* (pp. 379–397). New York: Marcel Dekker.

Dohlman, C. H. (1983). Physiology of the cornea: Corneal edema. In G. Smolin & R. A. Thoft (Eds.). *The Cornea* (pp. 3–15). Boston: Little, Brown.

Eye Bank Association of America. (1987). Activity Report. Washington, D.C.: EBAA.

Eye Bank Association of America. (1988). 1987 Eye Banking Activity. Washington, D.C.: EBAA.

Farge, E. J. (1986). The Eye Bank Association of America: History and development. In F. S. Brightbill (Ed.). Corneal Surgery: Theory, Technique, and Tissue (pp. 673–678). St. Louis: C. V. Mosby.

Forstot, S. L. (1986). Adult penetrating keratoplasty: Preoperative evaluation. In F. S. Brightbill (Ed.). Corneal Surgery: Theory, Technique, and Tissue (p. 141). St. Louis: C. V. Mosby.

Friend, J. (1983). Physiology of the cornea: Metabolism and biochemistry. In G. Smolin & R. A. Thoft (Eds.). The Cornea (pp. 17–28). Boston: Little, Brown.

Koenig, S. B. (1986). Donor selection: B. Donor age. In F. S. Brightbill (Ed.). Corneal Surgery: Theory, Technique, and Tissue (pp. 15–23). St. Louis: C. V. Mosby.

Mannis, M. J. (1986). Medical standards for eye banks. In F. S. Brightbill (Ed.). Corneal Surgery: Theory, Technique, and Tissue (pp. 3–5). St. Louis: C. V. Mosby.

Musch, D. C., Meyer, R. F., Sugar, A., & Soong, H. K. (1985). Michigan Corneal Transplantation Patient Registry: Summary Project Report, 1984–1985. Ann Arbor: University of Michigan Medical Center, W. K. Kellogg Eye Center.

Sugar, A. (1986). Aphakic and pseudophakic eyes. In F. S. Brightbill (Ed.). Corneal Surgery: Theory, Technique, and Tissue (pp. 145–149). St. Louis: C. V. Mosby.

Sugar, J. (1986). Phakic keratoplasty. In F. S. Brightbill (Ed.). Corneal Surgery: Theory, Technique, and Tissue (pp. 194–199). St. Louis: C. V. Mosby.

Tooke, M. C., Elders, J., & Johnson, D. E. (1986). Corneal transplantation. American Journal of Nursing, 86, 685–687.

Vaughan, D., & Asbury, T. (1986). General Ophthalmology (10th ed). Los Altos, Calif.: Lange Medical Publications.

Zirm, E. (1906). Eine erfolgreiche totale keratoplastik. Albrecht von Graefes Arch. Ophthalmol., 64, 580–593.

12

Bone Marrow Transplantation

Patricia F. Jassak and Nancy L. Porter

TRANSPLANT OVERVIEW

History of Bone Marrow Transplantation

Bone marrow transplantation (BMT) has changed dramatically in the past 25 years. Initially regarded as an experimental treatment approach, BMT currently is recognized as a curative treatment modality for malignant and nonmalignant hematologic diseases. The earliest BMT research was undertaken in mice; studies began after the atomic bombs were dropped on Japan. In 1949, Jacobson and co-workers reported that when the spleens of mice exposed to lethal doses of radiation were shielded, the mice survived (Jacobson, Marks, & Gaston, 1949). Lorenze and associates (1951) demonstrated that guinea pigs and mice exposed to lethal irradiation doses could be protected by infusion of bone marrow (Lorenzo, Uphoff, Reid, & Shelton, 1951). Lindsley and colleagues (1955) found that this protection stemmed from the growth of the donor bone marrow cells (Lindsley, Odell, & Tausche, 1955).

Over the next ten years BMT was attempted in humans who, in the terminal stages of their illness, did not live long enough to provide sufficient data to evaluate the procedure. During the 1950s and 1960s successful BMTs were performed, but major complications of graft-versus-host disease (GVHD) and lethal viral and fungal infections were problems (Bortin, 1970).

Other early problems that were faced in human BMT included the (a) inability to select donors, (b) absence of preventive infection control measures, (c) lack of effective antimicrobial agents, and (d) unavailability of adequate blood products to support the prolonged pancytopenic period (Doney & Buckner, 1985).

280

Technical improvements in human leukocyte antigen (HLA) testing during the mid-1960s and early 1970s aided the search for perfecting BMT (Santos, 1983; see Chapter 3). HLA typing made it feasible to match the recipient's tissue type with that of the donor. In addition, advances in blood support made it feasible to support patients through prolonged periods of aplasia. Throughout the years clinical research has focused on alleviating the complications first associated with BMT.

Indications for Bone Marrow Transplantation

BMT allows intensive chemotherapeutic and radiation doses to be administered without regard to hematopoietic toxicity. Also, it potentially provides the leukemic patient with a changed immunologic response that may subsequently protect the patient from residual tumor cells (Santos & Kaizer, 1982). BMT is currently the treatment of choice for adult patients with acute myelogenous leukemia in first remission, chronic leukemias, children in a second remission of acute lymphocytic leukemia, myelodysplastic diseases, lymphomas, multiple myeloma, neuroblastoma, and selected solid tumors (Doney & Buckner, 1985). This procedure is also used in the treatment of nonmalignant hematologic diseases, such as aplastic anemia, Fanconi's anemia, and sickle cell anemia, and in selected immunodeficient states.

Types of Bone Marrow Transplants

There are three types of donor bone marrow: allogeneic, syngeneic, and autologous. The type of BMT undertaken depends on two factors: (1) the disease being treated and (2) the availability of an HLA-matched donor.

The most common type of BMT is allogeneic. In such cases the donor is usually the sibling with the most similar HLA tissue-typing. In rare instances an unrelated person may be the donor. The use of an unrelated donor is made possible by the initiation of tissue donor banks in the United States and Europe. Clinical practice and research have demonstrated that the more closely matched the donor and recipient HLA, the less likely the recipient will be to develop GVHD. It should be noted that it is feasible for the donor to have matched HLA typing, be mixed lymphocyte culture–nonreactive, and yet possess a different ABO type. Steps will then be taken to correct the ABO incompatibility before proceeding with the bone marrow infusion.

Syngeneic transplantation uses bone marrow from an identical twin donor. This marrow is genetically identical to the marrow of the recipient, and the risk of GVHD is substantially decreased. Autologous transplantation is the use of the patient's own marrow that may be harvested at an earlier date and stored for later use.

Patient Selection and Eligibility

In allogeneic transplants patient selection is determined by the stage of disease, the patient's overall clinical status, and the availability of an acceptable donor. The critical factor in syngeneic transplant is the presence of an identical twin.

Cogliano-Shutta and co-workers (1985) identify several distinct eligibility criteria for autologous transplantation: (1) the patient's bone marrow must be free of detectible tumor or, if involved, be capable of an in vitro purging response; (2) the disease is responsive to therapy (i.e., there is reasonable likelihood that more effective tumor eradication can be achieved by a higher intensity of chemotherapeutic agents, radiation therapy, or both); (3) the patient is physiologically able to withstand bone marrow harvesting (i.e., the use of general anesthesia and removal of 10 ml of marrow per kilogram of body weight); and (4) the patient is free of major risk factors (e.g., active infection, advanced age, any organ or system dysfunction, or central nervous system disease) (Cogliano-Shutta, Broda, & Gress, 1985). Other general eligibility criteria considered include a comprehensive history and physical assessment, baseline and laboratory studies, and psychological assessment of the patient, donor, and family.

Conditioning Regimens

Once the patient has met the eligibility criteria for BMT and the type of transplant is decided on, the recipient is prepared for transplant. A protocol or treatment regimen for immunosuppression is determined. This plan is referred to as the conditioning regimen.

Conditioning regimens generally last between one and eight days and are directly influenced by the patient's underlying disease and the previous chemotherapy and radiation therapy used. The conditioning regimen serves three purposes: (1) it provides a state of immunosuppression, (2) it eradicates malignant cells, and (3) it creates space in the bone marrow for engraftment of the new marrow.

Generally, protocols combine total-body irradiation in multiple fractionated doses with supra lethal doses of chemotherapeutic agents. Common chemotherapeutic agents used in conditioning regimens include cyclophosphamide, busulfan, etoposide, cisplatin, carmustine (BCNU), and cytarabine (cytosine arabinoside). Currently, aziridinlybenzoqui-none, a phase I National Cancer Institute investigational agent, is also being used with autologous transplants.

The high doses of cyclophosphamide that are administered mandate the use of continuous bladder irrigation to prevent the development of hemorrhagic cystitis. Generally a three-way Foley catheter is inserted for a two- to three-day interval.

Complications of the conditioning regimen are directly related to the individual toxicities of the chemotherapeutic agents used. The most common side effects experienced are nausea, vomiting, diarrhea, skin reactions, nutritional alterations, stomatitis, sterility, hormonal dysfunction, and alopecia. Many of these side effects can be diligently managed with astute nursing interventions that provide symptomatic relief and patient comfort. Nursing care of the BMT recipient in this phase and all further phases is summarized in Table 12–1.

Total-body irradiation may cause low-grade fevers, parotid gland tenderness and swelling, skin changes, nausea, vomiting, mucositis, and diarrhea. These toxicities generally diminish once treatment is completed.

BONE MARROW TRANSPLANT PROCESS

The BMT process is initiated with patient selection and eligibility. The pretransplant assessment phase is critical in helping to determine eligibility and the patient and family understanding of the complex process they will embark on. Autologous transplants are harvested before the patient receives the conditioning regimen.

Bone Marrow Harvest

Three essential components of patient teaching are the harvest procedure, expected presurgical and postsurgical routines, and donor recovery. Preharvest critical laboratory tests are listed in Table 12–2. For the nonautologous bone marrow harvest, donor evaluation and counseling by the social worker, nursing staff, or primary physician are essential to determine the donor's perceptions or attitudes toward the transplant process, the relationship between the patient and family members, availability of support systems, and effects of an interrupted life-style.

The donor is usually admitted to the hospital the evening before or early on the morning of the bone marrow harvest. The marrow harvesting is done in the operating room under general or spinal anesthesia. Approximately 500 to 800 ml of bone marrow is obtained through

TABLE 12–1. CARE OF THE BONE MARROW TRANSPLANT PATIENT

Nursing Diagnosis	Predisposing Factors	Signs and Symptoms	Interventions/Nursing Implications
Knowledge deficit related to transplant process	Components and potential complications of the bone marrow transplant	Questions from patient and family	Assess patient and family knowledge. Provide accurate and consistent information. Document teaching provided for patient and family.
Potential for activity intolerance	Anemia, fatigue, infection	Inability to sustain prescribed activity levels	Structure balanced periods of rest and activity. Correct anemia. Treat infection. Coordinate nursing activities to promote rest.
Disturbance in self-concept related to temporary alopecia	Conditioning regimen	Patient statements reflecting feelings about alopecia Refusal to permit visitors Alteration in coping	Inform patient that alopecia is likely to occur. Provide resource for purchase of wigs or scarves. Provide emotional support. Inform patient that regrowth of hair will occur.
Alteration in comfort related to pain, nausea, and vomiting	Conditioning regimen GVHD Mucositis	Open, red, raw areas in mouth Irritation around anus Facial grimacing Fist clenching Withdrawal Verbal complaints of pain	Perform frequent oral hygiene. Apply topical anesthetics as ordered. Administer antiemetics and antidiarrheals as ordered. Administer pain medications as ordered. Assess pain relief. Perform skin care as ordered. Provide emotional support.
Alteration in fluid volume—excess	Veno-occlusive disease Excessive fluid administration related to total parenteral nutrition,	Weight gain Ascites Edema Respiratory distress Intake and output	Administer spironolactone as ordered. Obtain weight measurement twice daily. Measure and record

TABLE 12–1. CARE OF THE BONE MARROW TRANSPLANT PATIENT *Continued*

Nursing Diagnosis	Predisposing Factors	Signs and Symptoms	Interventions/Nursing Implications
Alteration in fluid volume—excess *Continued*	maintenance IVs, frequent antibiotics, patient oral intake, blood products	Cough Shortness of breath	abdominal girth daily. Maintain strict intake and output. Maintain fluid restriction as ordered. Administer diuretics as ordered.
Potential for injury	Conditioning regimen–induced thrombocytopenia	Petechiae Prolonged bleeding Nosebleeds Bleeding from gums, urine, stool Altered neurologic status	Transfuse platelets as ordered. Avoid use of razors and toothbrushes. Monitor platelet counts. Instruct patient on safety measures to be followed. Monitor patient for change in visual acuity or neurologic status. Administer vitamin K as ordered.
Potential for infection	Conditioning regimen–induced immunosuppression	Fever Pain, redness, swelling at right atrial catheter site Altered respiratory status Change in vital signs Lethargy, listlessness	Administer antipyretics as ordered. Observe catheter site for signs and symptoms of infection. Monitor WBC count and differential. Follow prescribed isolation techniques. Encourage activity to diminish pulmonary secretion stasis. Culture patient as ordered. Monitor culture results. Follow sterile technique as indicated for procedures. Administer antibiotics as ordered. Observe temperature pattern—steroids may mask signs and symptoms of infection.

TABLE 12–2. PREHARVEST CLINICAL LABORATORY TESTS

Complete blood count with differential and reticulocyte count
Chemistry profile
Hepatitis screen
HIV antibody status
ABO and Rh grouping
CMV antibody status
EKG
Chest x-ray
Coagulation studies
HSV$_1$ antibody test titers
HSV$_2$ antibody titers
Pregnancy test

multiple aspirations from multiple sites of the posterior and anterior iliac crests and the sternum.

The marrow is then mixed with heparinized saline solution and filtered for removal of fat and possible bone particles. It is then transferred into a transfusion bag. If the transplant is syngeneic or allogeneic, the bone marrow is sent directly from the operating room to the area where the patient is located. It is immediately administered intravenously. The day of transplantation is commonly referred to as day 0. Marrow is infused, unirradiated, and without a blood filter, over a three- to four-hour period, depending on the volume.

If the marrow is to be cryopreserved, it is transferred into a transfusion bag and immediately transported to the bone marrow research laboratory. When the harvested marrow is without evidence of malignant disease, a nonpurged method of storage is used. If malignant disease is present in the harvested marrow, the marrow is treated with monoclonal antibodies or chemotherapeutic agents in vitro, in an effort to purge the marrow of the residual tumor cells. The autologous marrow is then frozen and stored until its use is clinically warranted.

Bone Marrow Infusion

Major side effects of any type of marrow infusion include fluid overload, development of micropulmonary emboli causing chest tightness or pain, sensitivity reactions to the white cells in the marrow, and, rarely, bacterial contamination of the marrow. Nursing interventions include monitoring for changes in vital signs and observing for chills, urticaria, fever, dyspnea, orthopnea, and complaints of chest pain. The marrow infusion may be slowed to assist in alleviating these complaints.

If the bone marrow has been stored, a garlic odor may be present on reinfusion. This is due to the preservative agent dimethyl sulfoxide (DMSO), which is used to protect marrow viability. Bone marrow has recently been cryopreserved with DMSO and hydroxyethyl starch with minimal, if any, symptoms on infusion (Stiff, Koester, Weidner, Dvorak, & Fisher, 1987).

Preengraftment Period

The next phase of the process is the preengraftment period. In the allogeneic or syngeneic BMT patient this is a two- to four-week period during which time the marrow cannot produce any cells. In the autologous BMT patient preengraftment is usually a one- to two-week period of limited marrow development.

The patient's preengraftment course can be difficult and complicated. The patient is pancytopenic for a minimum of ten days. It generally takes 10 to 20 days before the donor stem cells can begin to proliferate and mature; therefore, preengraftment is a critical period, and supportive care is essential for survival. The primary complications during this period are bleeding, malnutrition, infection, and psychosocial adaptation.

During the preengraftment period patients are encouraged and required to participate in their own care. Daily activities, including sitting up in a chair and riding a stationary bike, are mandatory. Patients must also adhere to hygiene requirements designed by the nursing staff, including twice-daily baths and scrupulous mouth care.

Engraftment

Engraftment should occur after a period of profound pancytopenia for the autologous BMT patient and aplasia for the allogeneic or syngeneic BMT recipient. Engraftment is described as a rise in the patient's granulocyte and platelet count and demonstrates that the donor marrow is starting to function and produce new marrow. Because of the severe immunosuppression that occurs with the conditioning regimen, allogeneic as well as syngeneic and autologous BMT patients will have a deficient immune system for up to a year post transplant.

General criteria for discharge are listed in Table 12–3. Depending on the patient's disease stage and clinical status, the benefits of transplant

TABLE 12–3. CRITERIA FOR DISCHARGE

Granulocyte count >100/mm^3
Platelet count >20,000/mm^3
Oral calorie intake >1500 calories per day
Absence of signs and symptoms of infection
Competency in self-care behaviors

when cure is the goal outweigh the risks. The risks, however, cannot be minimized because potentially fatal complications do occur.

POST-TRANSPLANT COMPLICATIONS

Graft-Versus-Host Disease

In all organ transplants the new organ is in danger of being rejected by the body's immune system. In BMT the new immune system may attack cells that carry the foreign HLA antigens found in the patient's body. This results in the development of graft-versus-host disease (GVHD).

GVHD is often difficult to diagnose. The symptoms are similar to those that occur with drug reactions, infection, and radiation toxicity. The diagnosis is generally made from clinical, laboratory, and x-ray data (Ford & Ballard, 1988). The opportunity of obtaining a biopsy for diagnosis must be carefully evaluated in view of the risks of infection and bleeding.

GVHD involves donor T cells. After the patient has received high doses of chemotherapy, radiation therapy, or both, her own immune systems, including the T cells, are suppressed. Because of this suppression, the body's T cells cannot recognize the donor's bone marrow as foreign. Therefore, the recipient's T cells will not attack the donor's marrow. But T cells in the donor's marrow may recognize the cells in the recipient's body as foreign and attack them.

Symptoms of acute GVHD can occur as early as one to three weeks after transplantation, with the median time of onset at approximately post-transplant day 25 (Champlin & Gale, 1984; McDonald, Shulman, & Sullivan, 1986). Chronic GVHD generally appears after post-transplant day 100. GVHD may occur in one or more organ systems, most commonly the skin, gastrointestinal tract, and liver. When GVHD involves the skin, a faint red rash can erupt over the center of the face, forehead, palms, and soles. It then spreads and may involve the arms, legs, and trunk. Dryness and peeling may occur with a deepening of the skin's color. Patients may complain of itching and burning of the skin. If the disease progresses, there may be a reddening of the skin over the entire body. Blistering and sloughing of the skin may result. GVHD of the skin may progress to scleroderma and contractures, although early diagnosis and treatment decrease the development of these complications (Sullivan, 1986).

When GVHD involves the gastrointestinal tract the major symptom is green, watery stool that may contain blood. In mild cases the diarrhea may amount to 300 to 500 ml per day. In severe cases the stool may total between 6000 and 7000 ml per day as the intestines are denuded. Other signs and symptoms may include loss of appetite, nausea, vomiting, and abdominal pain. Acute intestinal GVHD may lead to a paralysis of the bowel with an accumulation of fluid in the abdomen.

GVHD of the liver produces signs and symptoms that are similar to those of hepatitis. These include fatigue, weakness, jaundice, fever, itching, and altered liver function tests. Table 12–4 depicts the grading system of GVHD.

Approximately 40 per cent to 50 per cent of BMT patients develop acute GVHD; of these about 8 per cent die of this condition and the associated infections (Storb & Thomas, 1985). High-risk patients include those over age 30; those who receive marrow from opposite-sex donors; and those who demonstrate various degrees of mismatched HLA antigens with their donors.

Several measures are used to prevent and treat acute GVHD. Prevention includes irradiation of transfused blood products. This destroys any T cells that are present in the blood product that could interact and cause GVHD. Other measures include administration of cyclosporin A, methotrexate, steroids, antilymphocyte globulin, monoclonal antibodies or a combination of these therapies. These medications work in various ways to suppress the immune response (see Chapter 4). It must be noted that cyclosporin A (also called cyclosporine or Sandimmune) is used to suppress T cells. Patients may begin receiving the drug several days before transplant, depending on the protocol being followed. Intravenous cyclosporine may be administered continuously or intermittently. It is likely that the patient will take the drug for only about 180 days after transplant, unlike other organ transplant recipients, who must take the drug for the rest of their lives.

Methotrexate may be given to reduce the incidence or severity of GVHD. It suppresses all rapidly growing cells, including the T cells responsible for GVHD development. The use of methotrexate can also

TABLE 12–4. CLINICAL GRADES OF GVHD

GRADE	ORGAN INVOLVEMENT
1	Mild rash; no gut or liver involvement; no alteration in performance of activities of daily living
2	Mild to moderate rash; mild gut and liver involvement; mild alteration in ability to perform activities of daily living
3	Moderate to severe rash; moderate to severe gut and liver involvement; marked alteration in ability to perform activities of daily living
4	Extreme constitutional symptoms

Adapted from Thomas, Storb, Clift, Fefer, Johnson, et al. (1975). Bone marrow transplantation. N. Engl. J. Med., 292:832–843, 895–902.

result in delayed engraftment of the bone marrow. Moderate to severe mucositis may be seen in patients who receive methotrexate.

If skin GVHD develops, topical steroids are applied to reduce the itching, burning, and inflammation. Side effects from topical steroids are usually minimal because the steroids are not absorbed into the body.

Nursing Implications

GVHD is a potentially fatal condition. Prophylaxis and treatment are essential in the total care of the BMT patient. Nursing care and medical management of the patient are often complex and challenging. Nursing assessments need to be thorough and accurate. Inspection of the patient's skin can be invaluable in early diagnosis of GVHD. Essential nursing interventions include strict monitoring of intake and output, assessment of stools, and continued evaluation of liver function tests. Consistent evaluation of fluid, electrolyte, and nutritional status is also necessary. Managing skin care, nausea, vomiting, and diarrhea provides the nurse with multiple challenges related to symptom management and patient comfort.

Patients who develop GVHD require additional psychological support. Although GVHD may have some potential antileukemic effects, the difficulties arising from the development of this condition are often disturbing to patients and family members. Nurses need to be aware of the many implications of GVHD and the treatment of this condition.

Veno-occlusive Disease

One of several potentially fatal complications of transplantation is the development of veno-occlusive disease (VOD) of the liver. Veno-occlusive disease was unrecognized as a separate disease process until 1977 because of the number of liver problems that are commonly seen in the post-transplant period (Schulman, McDonald, Matthews, Doney, Kopecky, et al., 1980).

The development of VOD may be seen in approximately 21 per cent of patients who undergo BMT. The incidence of VOD is apparently dependent on several factors, including age, underlying disease, history of hepatitis, and the type of conditioning regimen administered (McDonald, Sharma, Matthews, Shulman, & Thomas, 1985).

Pathophysiology and Clinical Features

Intrahepatic hypertension with ascites, encephalopathy, and hepatic enlargement results from the obstruction of blood flow from the sinusoids of the liver (Ford, McClain, & Cunningham, 1983; Schulman et al., 1980). Under normal circumstances blood from the portal vein and hepatic artery flows through the liver by way of the sinusoids. The sinusoids empty into the central veins that lead into the hepatic veins. In VOD this flow is obstructed by occlusion of the central vein with collagen-like fibers. The endothelial lining of the central vein is disrupted. Sinusoidal pore narrowing by subendothelial fibrosis, trapped cellular debris, and exfoliated hepatocytes cause centrilobular congestion and stasis of blood. Necrosis of hepatocytes from compression and ischemia leads to bile stasis and elevated levels of serum liver enzymes. As the vein walls fragment and thicken, fibrin, collagen fibers, foamy cells with lipofuscin, bile, red cells, and hemosiderin-laden macrophages occlude the lumen in a concentric pattern. The obstruction of blood flow causes the fluid content of the blood to enter the lymphatics and drop off the liver surface into the peritoneal cavity. This results in the development of ascites.

Symptoms of VOD of the liver typically develop within 7 to 21 days post transplant. Approximately one-half of patients who develop VOD will die (Ford et al., 1983). Clinical characteristics of this disease include sudden weight gain, hepatomegaly, right upper quadrant abdominal pain, ascites, jaundice, hyperbilirubinemia, and encephalopathy (Ford et al., 1983; McDonald et al., 1985; Schulman et al., 1980). All of the symptoms can be associated with pathologic changes within the liver. Evaluation of the above as well as for pericardiac tamponade and right heart failure; analysis of peritoneal fluid for infection, tumor cells, and amylase; and ruling out intra-abdominal infection or other liver pathologies are necessary to differentiate VOD from other pathologic processes such as GVHD (Ford et al., 1983).

Nursing Implications

Management of the patient with VOD is aimed at resting the liver and supporting the patient through the acute phase of the disease. It is hoped that resolution of this condition will result from these interventions. Sodium restriction, while maintaining adequate intravascular volume and perfusion of the renal system, is essential. Fluid restriction lessens the degree of third-spacing, improves blood flow, enhances patient comfort, and decreases pulmonary congestion. All intravenous lines not in use should be heparin locked. Physicians need to carefully determine antibiotic usage because certain antibiotics have a high sodium content. The administration of 25% normal human albumin is used to maintain serum albumin levels and plasma oncotic pressure.

The administration of spironolactone to patients with ascites can be helpful; however, because there is about a four-day lag period before diuresis begins, spironolactone administration should be initiated as soon as VOD is suspected. Spironolactone, available only in 25-mg tablets, is usually administered in doses of 200 to 400 mg. Patients with mucositis in addition to VOD may experience difficulty complying with this medication regimen. Evaluation of urine sodium levels is a useful indicator of the effectiveness of spironolactone. Dose modifications may be based on the results of urine sodium levels.

It is tempting to administer diuretics like furosemide and thiazides to patients with VOD. This must be avoided because a maximum of 1 liter of fluid per day can be mobilized from the abdominal cavity. If a patient with VOD does not have this amount of ascites, the remaining fluid will be drawn from the intravascular space. When this occurs renal blood flow is diminished and the creatinine and blood urea nitrogen levels rise, resulting in prerenal azotemia. Prerenal azotemia is treated by the administration of sodium and water, which may add to the ascites.

The patient's weight and abdominal girth should be measured and recorded twice a day. Strict intake and output records are maintained. Monitoring the central venous pressure may be of assistance in evaluating intravascular fluid status.

Abdominal paracentesis may be used to relieve discomfort and difficulty in breathing. The paracentesis carries a risk of infection and bleeding. The use of a side-to-side portacaval shunt has recently been tried for the treatment of VOD (Murray, LaBrecque, Gingrich, Pringle, & Mitros, 1987).

Because of the liver's role in drug metabolism, patients who develop VOD may have unpredictable drug levels. The levels may be either subtherapeutic or toxic. For pain management, short-acting narcotics administered intravenously are the drugs of choice, although meperidine is contraindicated because of the complications associated with its metabolite, normeperidine. Also, narcotic effects can be reversed by the administration of naloxone if toxicity occurs. Sedatives that do not require liver metabolism are preferred.

Hepatic encephalopathy resulting from VOD is probably related to the accumulation of ammonia when venous blood is not detoxified in the liver. Lactulose may be effectively used, although management of this drug's side effects can be a nursing challenge. Decreasing protein intake by 0.5 g/kg of body weight may be helpful in treating hepatic encephalopathy.

Adequate caloric intake is essential for minimizing catabolism. This can be difficult to achieve because of fluid restriction requirements. The administration of lipid emulsions in patients with VOD is controversial. Nutritional support for patients with VOD is often difficult to achieve but is essential to the management of this condition.

In summary, VOD of the liver after BMT is a potentially fatal condition. It is associated with the immunosuppressive conditioning regimen used to prepare patients for transplant. Astute nursing assessment of the patient is essential if this condition is to be recognized in its early stages. Aggressive nursing care of the patient is critical in preventing further complications while minimizing the effects of those that are present.

Infection

Infections in BMT patients are life-threatening and yet a fairly common occurrence. Wide ranges of viral, bacterial, protozoan, and fungal infections may be seen separately or concomitantly in this patient population.

The signs and symptoms of infection in BMT patients do not always follow the classic pattern that nurses have been taught to recognize. Pancytopenia often makes it impossible to see localized inflammation and elevated white blood cell counts. Similarly, the use of steroids may mask signs of an infection. In addition, fever, which may accompany blood product transfusion or drug reaction, complicates detection of infection.

Meyers and Atkinson (1983) and van der Meer, Guiot, van den Brock, and van Furth (1984) define the risk factors that BMT patients have for infection. These risks include prolonged neutropenia, GVHD, hematologic malignancy, extensive use of antibiotics, radiation therapy, organism colonization, and older age. The goal of prophylaxis and therapy in the transplant patient is to provide optimal treatment until the patient's immune system has recovered and body defense lines are normalized.

Ford and Ballard (1988) list some of the measures that attempt to provide the transplant patient with protection from infection. These measures include protective isolation, laminar airflow rooms, prophylactic systemic antibiotics, trimethoprim-sulfamethoxazole, acyclovir, oral nonabsorbable antibiotics, passive immunization with antibodies, cytomegalovirus screening of blood products, granulocyte transfusions, low-bacteria sterile diet, and routine mouth care.

The role of the nurse in preventing infection cannot be minimized. Surveillance cultures, medication administration, and ongoing assessment are vital. Monitoring the patient's physical condition to assess for early changes associated with infection is critical. Encouraging the patient to maintain appropriate activity levels, personal hygiene, and mouth care is the responsibility of the nurse (see Chapter 5).

The destruction of the patient's old immune system and the lag time involved before the new immune system is functional place the patient at risk. Approximately 40 per cent to 50 per cent of patients will experience localized varicella zoster infections in the first year after transplant (Locksley, Flournoy, Sullivan, & Meyers, 1985).

Pneumonias are the single greatest cause of death during the first 100 days after transplant. Those associated with cytomegalovirus account for about 50 per cent of pneumonias seen in transplant patients, or 13 per cent of all transplant deaths (Buckner, Meyers, & Springmayer, 1984; Press, Schaller, & Thomas, 1987). Patients who develop interstitial pneumonias present with nasal flaring, dry cough, dyspnea, tachypnea, diffuse chest x-ray infiltrates, and alterations in blood gas measurements. Adenovirus, herpes simplex, fungi, and bacteria account for about 15 per cent of pneumonias in this population. Historically, *Pneumocystis carinii* pneumonia caused significant mortality in transplant patients; however, the use of trimethoprim-sulfamethoxazole has significantly lowered the morbidity and mortality of patients exposed to this protozoan.

Once an infectious process is suspected and identified, it is the nurse's responsibility to act promptly in carrying out medical orders. The initiation of antibiotics is crucial to the management of the patient. Assisting in diagnostic procedures and providing the patient and family with emotional support are essential. Infections occur in transplant patients with surprising rapidity and may result in acute physiologic changes. Evidence of sepsis and septic shock may appear without warning. It is the keen assessment skill of the nurse that may make a difference in patient survival.

Relapse and Oncogenesis

Unfortunately relapse or recurrence of the malignancy may occur after BMT. Studies involving patients who have relapsed after transplant demonstrate that most recurrences have been in host cells. This demonstrates a failure to eradicate malignant cells with the pretransplant conditioning regimen and a high degree of tumor resistance to chemotherapy, radiation therapy, or both. (Sullivan, Deeg, Sanders, Shulman, Witherspoon, et al., 1984). Recurrent malignancies are most likely to occur within several years after transplant, especially if the patient was initially transplanted while in relapse. One of the difficulties in transplanting patients in relapse is eradicating a sufficient number of tumor cells in order to prevent relapse after transplant.

Relapse rates are also affected by the timing of the transplant. Cells that are resistant to conditioning regimens are likely to become more numerous with each passing relapse-remission cycle. For example, leukemic patients transplanted in an initial remission are less likely to relapse than those treated in subsequent remissions or in relapse (Dinsmore & O'Reilly, 1982; Gale, Kersey, Bortin, Dicke, Good, et al., 1983;

Quinn, 1985; Sarna, Feiq, Opelz, Young, Langdon, et al., 1977; Thomas, 1983).

Oncogenesis is the production of a second malignancy. The development of a second malignancy after chemotherapy, radiation therapy, or both has increased as survivors of cancer therapy live longer. Small numbers of second malignancies have been observed in BMT patients (Deeg, Sanders, Martin, Fefer, Neiman, et al., 1984). These second malignancies appear to be a late sequela of treatment. They have also been reported in recipients of solid organ transplants who receive long-term immunosuppressive therapy. It is thought that reactivation of or exposure to the Epstein-Barr virus might predispose patients to the development of second malignancies after transplantation. Continued study and accurate data collection in this area are necessary to determine risk patterns.

Nursing Implications

The nurse's primary role in dealing with relapse or oncogenesis is to provide patient and family education and emotional support. In most instances the patient undergoes BMT as curative therapy for an existing disease state. When relapse or oncogenesis occurs emotions ranging from anger to disappointment and disbelief may result. The donor may feel guilty and responsible for the relapse in the mistaken belief that her bone marrow was not "strong" enough, therefore believing that she is responsible for the relapse. When patients and family members are considered for BMT, physicians inform them of the potential for relapse to occur. Sometimes this information can be overshadowed by the potential for cure. Thus anger and disbelief can be seen when the disease recurs. Finally, once it appears that the BMT has been successful, there may be a tendency for patients and family members to forget about the potential for oncogenesis, especially when it occurs years after transplant.

Nurses may present information about relapse and the potential for oncogenesis to patients and family members after determining the optimal time for this teaching to occur. The nurse should be cautious in presenting this information. Patients and family members should not become so acutely attuned to the potential for disease recurrence and oncogenesis that other important teaching is neglected.

If relapse becomes evident after transplant, the hope for a permanent cure is dashed. The nurse needs to support the family as they work through their disbelief and grief. While providing emotional support it is important for the nurse to guide the patient and family toward a realistic understanding of what has happened and its potential impact. The family may not understand the treatment options that have been presented by the health care team. It is up to the nurse to assess the understanding of the family and to structure teaching and emotional support at this level.

Because of the serious and potentially fatal consequences if a second malignancy should occur, the nurse plays a significant role. The nurse must carefully assess the patient and determine a plan of care that will assist the patient and family to cope with the possibility of relapse or oncogenesis.

Cataracts

Sullivan and co-workers (1984) reported that approximately 75 per cent of BMT patients will develop cataracts within six years of transplant. The incidence of cataracts is associated with the use of radiation in the pretransplant conditioning regimens. In Sullivan's work cataracts were reported as early as one year after transplant. Their incidence can be reduced by as much as 25 per cent if fractionated irradiation is used in the preparative regimen (Nims & Strom, 1988). Shielding the lens during therapy may also reduce the incidence of cataracts. However, it must be remembered that shielding of the lens in leukemic patients may increase the potential for relapse because the eyes are usually a secondary site for leukemic infiltrates. Sullivan and colleagues (1981) note that patients with chronic GVHD treated with corticosteroids developed cataracts more frequently than did other BMT recipients (Sullivan, Shulman, Storb, Weiden, Witherspoon, et al., 1981).

Nursing Implications

Cataracts that develop after BMT may be visible on examination or may be detectable only by a slit-lamp examination performed by an ophthalmologist (Ruccione & Fergusson, 1984). If the cataracts are detected, surgical removal and use of corrective lenses are advised for patients with pronounced visual impairment.

Nurses play a significant role in pretransplant counseling. Patients should be counseled about the potential for cataract development and taught what visual changes should be reported. A baseline vision screening, assessment, and visual acuity test should be performed.

In the posttransplant period nurses should evaluate patient knowledge about the potential for cataract development. Information should be provided as needed. Nurses should continue to test vision and visual acuity throughout the transplant hospitalization. The detection of unusual findings should be reported to the physician for follow-up evaluation and treatment.

The development of cataracts at some point after syngeneic or allogeneic BMT is likely. Nurses need to be aware of this complication and include thorough vision screenings and patient education in their assessment of patients post BMT.

Infertility and Hormonal Dysfunction

The use of chemotherapeutic agents and radiation therapy can cause infertility and hormonal dysfunction in adults. The drugs most commonly associated with gonadal dysfunction are cyclophosphamide, chlorambucil, and busulfan (Kumar, McEvoy, Biggart, & McGeown, 1972). The use of supralethal doses of radiation therapy and chemotherapeutic agents in the conditioning regimens used for BMT increases the probability of infertility and hormonal dysfunction. However, this depends on the age of the patient, the conditioning regimen used, and prior therapy. Both males and females may develop infertility and hormonal dysfunction that can be either temporary and reversible or permanent and severe.

The female who receives treatment before puberty may demonstrate absence of secondary sexual development, elevated serum gonadotropin level, and low serum estradiol concentration (Shalet, Beardwell, Jones, Pearson, & Ornell, 1976; Stillman, Schinfield, Schiff, Gelber, Greenberger, et al., 1981). In the postpubertal female, chemotherapy and radiation therapy may cause amenorrhea, oligomenorrhea, and menopausal symptoms (Baker, Morgan, Peckham, & Smithers, 1972; Li & Jaffe, 1974; Luschbaugh & Casarett, 1976). It appears that women who receive both radiation therapy and chemotherapy have an increased incidence of ovarian failure compared with women who receive only one treatment modality.

In males the degree of testicular damage is directly related to the radiation dose (Luschbaugh & Casarett, 1976; Rowley, Leach, Warner, & Heller, 1974; Speiser, Rubin, & Casarett, 1973). Testosterone levels remain normal; however, both follicle-stimulating hormone (FSH) and luteinizing hormone (LH) levels may be elevated (Byrd, 1983). When radiation injury to the testes does occur recovery of spermatogenesis is unlikely (Waxman, Terry, Wrigley, Malpas, Rees, et al., 1983; Whitehead, Shalet, & Blackledge, 1982). The effects of alkylating agents on the gonads of postpubertal males are manifested by germinal aplasia. They also demonstrate oligospermia, aspermia, loss of libido, and decreased sexual functioning.

Nursing Implications

Nurses must assess the knowledge level of the patient and family regarding the potential for infertility and hormonal dysfunction. The patient and family are then educated in those areas in which a clear understanding was not demonstrated. Patients and their family members are likely to have misconceptions about the difference between infertility and impotence. Such misunderstandings need further clarification.

Depending on the age of the patient undergoing BMT, an evaluation of gonadal function may be suggested. Measurement of LH, FSH, estrogen, and testosterone levels may be made at the time of treatment and then periodically post transplant. The nurse must make sure that test results are available. The nurse should also know the implications of the test results. If sperm count evaluations are ordered, it may be the responsibility of the nurse to educate the patient about the procedure. These instructions should be provided in a simple, clear, and unembarrassed way.

Education and counseling about normal sexual and reproductive function are the nurse's responsibility. Ideally, these tasks should be completed before therapy is initiated. Patients should be advised not to assume that they are sterile until tests to determine this are carried out and the physician has the results. The nurse can also advise the patient about sperm banking, if a number of healthy sperm exist before the preparative regimen is initiated. Sperm banking must be done before the cytoreductive therapy is initiated.

Although it may be an uncomfortable subject area, nurses need to realize that sexual, reproductive, and hormonal functions may be areas of concern for the transplant patient. Without open discussion and correct information patients may not realize the implications of beginning supralethal therapy. The patient may not be comfortable in initiating these conversations. Therefore, it is up to the nurse, as the patient advocate, to ensure that the patient remains informed.

PATIENT AND FAMILY PSYCHOLOGICAL SUPPORT AND EDUCATION

Undergoing BMT requires a great deal of thought on the part of patients and their families. The implications of transplant are many, and informed consent is essential before the process begins. Once the conditioning regimen is initiated, there is no turning back. Patients and family members require psychological support throughout all phases of BMT. Such support ideally begins at the initial pretransplant discussion stage. The success for BMT may suddenly be devastated by complications that prove fatal to the patient. Nurses must be able to effectively cope with the multitude of challenges that patients and families present.

Stages of Bone Marrow Transplantation

Brown and Kelly (1976) have divided BMT into eight stages. Although the stages enable practitioners to identify specific issues that usually occur, it must be realized that often the stages overlap and clear-cut delineation may not be possible. In addition, it must be remembered that not all patients will follow the stages as outlined.

Stage 1: The Decision to Accept Treatment

BMT often provides hope to the patient and the family for cure of the identified disease. The decision to undergo a BMT usually occurs after consultation with the patient's primary physician and the physician in charge of the transplant program. The patient and family are informed of the potential risks and benefits. The type of BMT to be undertaken is decided on. The amount of information presented to the patient and family at this time is often overwhelming. Yet it is during this stage that the patient and family are asked to decide if they want to proceed. The volume of information may inhibit the ability of the patient and family to supply an informed consent.

Patients in this stage may or may not exhibit symptoms of their illness. For example, patients with aplastic anemia may be relatively asymptomatic. Therefore, the patient and family may experience disbelief when told that a life-threatening transplant may cure the disease. The intensity of treatment and recovery may make the patient apprehensive about proceeding. Patients with leukemia, on the other hand, have usually been symptomatic and have already faced chemotherapy. Frequently such therapy has failed to produce a sustained remission. This may encourage the leukemic patient to accept a transplant because she is "willing to try anything" to achieve a cure. Both types of patients may feel pressured by time to make a decision regarding transplantation.

Family members face the anxieties of the unknown. They may question whether any other form of treatment is available and wonder how they will cope if permanent disability or death results. For patients undergoing a syngeneic or allogeneic transplant, donor selection occurs during this stage. For donors, there may be questions about whether they have truly volunteered to donate bone marrow, or if pressure of an external or internal source has played a role in their decision.

While in this stage patients and family members become acquainted with the potential long-term complications of transplant, as discussed earlier. Certainly the patient and the family must consider these risks when giving an informed consent. Yet, because of the voluminous amount of information, the patient and family members may not fully recognize the seriousness of these long-term problems.

Finally, the patient and family members must realize that BMT is expensive. Insurance carriers may require prior approval before agreeing to pay for the transplant. Even then, funding may be limited or nonexistent. This may require the patient and family to find alternate sources of money to pay for the transplant. Some patients may find this unacceptable, yet realize that without funding, the transplant cannot proceed. This places additional stress on the patient and family.

The nurse's primary role during this stage is to provide information and clarify issues of concern. This will assist the patient and the family in the decision-making process.

Stage 2: Initial Admission Evaluation and Care Planning

During this stage the patient has been admitted for transplantation. Patient and family anxieties may become more pronounced as final testing is completed and the routines for care are established.

Nurses should evaluate the patient and family for their understanding of the illness, the transplant procedure, and previous coping strategies. Social and emotional assessments should also be undertaken.

The patient and family will probably be introduced to the members of the transplant team during this time. Nurses need to schedule these introductions in a timely manner, taking care not to overwhelm the patient and family.

It is helpful for the nurse to begin introducing the patient and family to the activities and procedures that the patient is expected to comply with throughout hospitalization. Such activities and procedures may include special dietary modifications, physical activity schedules, hygiene routines, and daily care patterns. The nurse should also begin to establish a relationship with the patient and family and help them to identify questions or concerns that arise.

Stage 3: Immunosuppression and Entry into Isolation

The initiation of the conditioning regimen is viewed as the "point of no return." Most patients feel psychologically vulnerable as they realize that there is no turning back. They also feel worse during this stage than they did on admission to the hospital because of the multiple side effects of the conditioning regimen.

When patients are put on isolation precautions family members may be hesitant to participate in their usual means of affection. They may feel that hugging or touching the patient may cause contamination and increase the patient's vulnerability to infection. The patient often experiences a heightened feeling of aloneness because of the strictness of isolation procedures. Tension, fear, and somatic complaints may intensify, partly because of the preparative regimen and partly because of the isolation.

During this stage nurses need to evaluate the patient and family for any changes in coping that may become evident as a result of isolation or that may be related to treatment side effects. Team conferences help to inform the transplant team about how the patient and family are coping, both physically and emotionally.

Stage 4: The Transplant Day

Infusion of the bone marrow is usually brief, uncomplicated, and anticlimactic for the patient and family when compared with the stresses they have faced during the preparative phase. If the bone marrow has been donated by someone other than the patient, the patient and family members may express concern for the donor. There may also be concern on the part of the patient and family that something is wrong because the patient does not feel any different after the marrow has been infused.

On the day of transplant the nursing staff can help the family by communicating information about the donor's condition, if such information is requested. The nurse can also explain to the patient and family that their lack of feeling different is normal and expected. At the same time, the nurse can assist the patient and family in understanding why the infusion seems anticlimactic after the preparative regimen. It is important that families and patients realize that the most difficult time of the process is yet to come.

Stage 5: Engraftment or Graft Rejection

While waiting for the new bone marrow to begin functioning the days in isolation mount, and patients and families may find it increasingly difficult to tolerate isolation. Support from transplant team members and well-structured activity plans are essential in helping the patient and family during this stage. If the patient feels well physically, boredom can be a significant problem.

Infections and mucositis are common during this stage. The physical condition of the patient may make coping difficult. Pain from mucositis may require the administration of narcotics. Such alterations in comfort may predispose the patient to the development of apathy toward self-care activities. Altered rest patterns are not unusual.

The role of the nurse requires astute physical and emotional assessments. It is a challenge to promote patient compliance with activities designed to promote recovery and prevent physical and emotional deterioration. Allowing the patient control in care decisions can be helpful in promoting compliance. Informing the patient about signs of bone marrow recovery can be helpful in alleviating the stresses experienced during this stage.

Family members also need support because sometimes patients feel too ill to appreciate their presence. It can also be difficult for family members to help pass the time until engraftment occurs. Stress on the relationship between patient and family may become evident. The nurse can assist in helping everyone involved to realize that this is not unusual and to determine new ways to assist in coping.

Stage 6: Graft-Versus-Host Disease

Successful engraftment of the bone marrow can result in the development of GVHD. Patients and family members may express anger and depression when GVHD develops because of the numerous side effects that are very uncomfortable.

The donor may express feelings of guilt, thinking that her marrow led to the development of GVHD. The donor may also feel that something in the past may have contributed to the development of this condition. The nurse needs to clarify these concerns and provide appropriate reassurance to the donor.

The patient and family members often need assistance in coping with their anger and depression when GVHD occurs. They also require education about the treatment of GVHD. An evaluation of the level of knowledge the patient and family have about GVHD is essential if they are to understand the implications of this condition and participate in its management.

Stage 7: Preparation for Discharge

Once the bone marrow has engrafted and is adequately functioning, preparation for discharge is initiated, although, ideally, teaching has been under way since admission. Patients and family members may display a great deal of anxiety about leaving the hospital, which has been a safe environment. Entering the home environment may provoke a great deal of fear, especially related to the potential for the development of infection and family inadequacies in managing care. The nursing staff needs to recognize that these uncertainties exist and begin to increase patient self-care. This provides the opportunity for the patient and family to be comfortable with the patient's care needs long before discharge. Any concerns can be dealt with as they arise.

The patient and family will usually have numerous questions related to sexual activity, employment, diet, body image, and participation in social activities. The nurse should evaluate patient and family understanding of the discharge instructions. Reinforcement of instructions should occur until the transplant team is satisfied that the patient can be safely discharged.

Stage 8: Adaptation Out of the Hospital

Once the patient has been discharged, it may be difficult for the nursing staff to evaluate the psychological condition of the patient and family. The patient and family are changed by the transplant process because of the necessary restrictions. They require a great deal of assistance in successfully managing their return to the community.

After discharge, the patient and family members may become more acutely aware of their financial indebtedness. The patient may also require assistance in realizing how dependent she may have become on the family, the donor, and the nursing and medical staff. Some patients return to the transplant unit to visit. Others may choose not to visit. In either case, the nursing staff must support the patient and family in their decision.

Death of the Transplant Patient

The death of the transplant patient is difficult for the family. The donor may feel a great deal of guilt and wonder if there was something wrong with her marrow if relapse, rejection, or GVHD is the cause of death. Family members may be angry or feel guilty. Questions may be raised about whether the transplant should have been done, or if the patient should have been allowed to live in relative comfort without the transplant. Most of these questions are not answerable to any satisfactory degree. Family members may require counseling and support in order to facilitate successful grieving.

ISSUES IN BONE MARROW TRANSPLANT NURSING

Care of the BMT patient is challenging. It requires the nurse to care for a chronically ill patient who has the potential to develop acute complications during the transplant process. The nurse must demonstrate expert assessment and care-planning skills. The length of hospitalization and the depth of family involvement can be taxing. In addition, the ever-present potential for death and fatal complications can be difficult for the nurse. BMT nurses require a great deal of ongoing support from their peers, managers, medical staff, families, and transplant team members.

Acknowledgments: The authors wish to acknowledge the support and assistance of Patrick J. Stiff, M.D., in the preparation of this chapter.

References

Baker, J. W., Morgan, R. L., Peckham, M. J., & Smithers, D. W. (1972). Preservation of ovarian function in patients requiring radiotherapy for para-aortic and pelvic Hodgkin's disease. *Lancet, 1,* 1307–1308.

Bortin, M. (1970). A compendium of reported human bone marrow transplants. *Transplantation, 9,* 571–587.

Brown, H. N. & Kelly, M. J. (1976). Stages of bone marrow transplantation: A psychiatric perspective. *Psychosomatic Medicine, 38*(6), 439–446.

Buckner, C. D., Meyers, J. D., & Springmayer, S. C. (1984, Suppl. 15). Pulmonary complications of marrow transplantation. *Experimental Hematology, 12*(6), 450–460.

Byrd, R. L. (1983). Late effects of treatment of cancer in children. *Annals of Pediatrics, 12*(6), 450–460.

Champlin, R. E. & Gale, R. P. (1984). Role of bone marrow transplantation in the treatment of hematologic malignancies and solid tumors: Critical review of syngeneic, autologous and allogeneic transplants. *Cancer Treatment Reports, 68*(1), 145–161.

Cogliano-Shutta, N. A., Broda, E. J., & Gress, J. S. (1985). Bone marrow transplantation. *Nursing Clinics of North America, 20*(1), 49–66.

Deeg, H. J., Sanders, J., Martin, P., Fefer, A., Neiman, P., Singer, J., Storb, R., & Thomas, E. D. (1984). Secondary malignancies after marrow transplantation. *Experimental Hematology, 12,* 660–666.

Dinsmore, R. B. & O'Reilly, R. J. (1982). Bone marrow transplantation: Current status. *Annals of Pathobiology, 12,* 212–231.

Doney, K. C. & Buckner, C. D. (1985). Bone marrow transplantation: Overview. *Plasma Therapy Transfusion Technology, 6,* 149–161.

Ford, R. & Ballard, B. (1988). Acute complications after bone marrow transplantation. *Seminars in Oncology Nursing, 4*(1), 15–24.

Ford, R., McClain, K., & Cunningham, B. A. (1983). Venoocclusive disease following marrow transplantation. *Nursing Clinics of North America, 18*(3), 563–568.

Gale, R. P., Kersey, J. H., Bortin, M. M., Dicke, K. A., Good, R. A., Zwaan, F., & Rimm, A. (1983). Bone marrow transplantation for acute lymphoblastic leukemia. *Lancet, 2,* 663.

Jacobson, L. O., Marks, E. K., Gaston, E. O., Robson, M. J., Gaston, E., & Zirkle, R. E. (1979). Effect of spleen protection on mortality following x-irradiation. *Journal of Laboratory and Clinical Medicine, 34,* 1538–1543.

Kumar, R., McEvoy, J., Biggart, J. D., & McGeown, M. G. (1972). Cyclophosphamide and reproductive function. *Lancet, 1,* 1212–1214.

Li, F. P. & Jaffe, N. (1974). Progeny of childhood-cancer survivors. *Lancet, 2,* 707–709.

Lindsley, D. L., Odell, T. T., Jr., & Tausche, F. G. (1955). Implantation of functional erythropoietic elements following total-body irradiation. *Proceedings of the Society of Experimental Biological Medicine, 90,* 512–515.

Locksley, R. M., Flournoy, N., Sullivan, K. M., & Meyers, J. D. (1985). Infection with varicella-zoster after marrow transplantation. *Journal of Infectious Disease, 152,* 1172–1181.

Lorenze, E., Uphoff, D. E., Reid, T. R., & Shelton, E. (1951). Modification of irradiation injury in mice and guinea pigs by bone marrow injection. *Journal of the National Cancer Institute, 12,* 1538–1543.

Luschbaugh, C. C. & Casarett, G. W. (1976). The effects of gonadal irradiation in clinical radiation therapy: A review. *Cancer, 37,* 1111–1120.

McDonald, G. B., Sharma, P., Matthews, D. E., Shulman, H. M., & Thomas, E. D. (1985). The clinical course of 53 patients with venocclusive disease of the liver after marrow transplantation. *Transplantation, 39*(6), 603–608.

McDonald, G. B., Shulman, H. M., & Sullivan, K. M. (1986). Intestinal and hepatic complications of human bone marrow transplantation. *Gastroenterology, 90*, 460–477.

Meyers, J. D., & Atkinson, K. (1983). Infections in bone marrow transplantation. *Clinics in Hematology, 12*, 791–811.

Murray, J. A., LaBrecque, D. R., Gingrich, R. D., Pringle, K. C., & Mitros, F. A. (1987). Successful treatment of hepatic venocclusive disease in bone marrow transplant patient with a side-to-side portacaval shunt. *Gastroenterology, 92*, 1073–1077.

Nims, J. W. & Strom, S. (1988). Late complications of bone marrow transplant recipients: Nursing care issues. *Seminars in Oncology Nursing, 4*(1), 47–54.

Press, O. W., Shaller, R. T., & Thomas, E. D. (1987). Bone marrow transplant complications. In L. H. Toledo-Pereyra (Ed.). *Complications of Organ Transplantation.* New York: Marcel Dekker.

Quinn, J. J. (1985). Bone marrow transplantation in the management of childhood cancer. *Pediatric Clinics of North America, 32*(3), 811–833.

Rowley, M. J., Leach, D. R., Warner, G. A., & Heller, C. G. (1974). Effects of graded doses of ionizing radiation on the human testis. *Radiation Research, 59*, 665–678.

Ruccione, K. & Fergusson, J. (1984). Late effects of childhood cancer and its treatment. *Oncology Nursing Forum, 11*(5), 54–64.

Santos, G. W. (1983). History of bone marrow transplantation. *Clinics in Hematology, 12*, 611–639.

Santos, G. W. & Kaizer, H. (1982). Bone marrow transplantation in acute leukemia. *Seminars in Hematology, 19*, 227–239.

Sarna, G., Feig, S., Opelz, G., Young, L., Langdon, E., Juillard, G., Naiem, F., Sparkes, R., Golde, D., Territo, M., Haskell, C. M., Smith, G., Fawzi, F., Folk, P., Fancy, J., Cline, M., & Gale, R. P. (1977). Bone marrow transplantation with intensive combination chemotherapy/radiation therapy (SCARI) in acute leukemia. *Annals of Internal Medicine, 86*, 155–161.

Schulman, H. M., McDonald, G. B., Matthews, D., Doney, K. C., Kopecky, K. J., Grauvreau, J. M., & Thomas, E. D. (1980). An analysis of hepatic venocclusive disease and centrilobular hepatic degeneration following bone marrow transplantation. *Gastroenterology, 79*, 1178–1191.

Shalet, S. M., Beardwell, C. G., Jones, P. M. H., Morris Jones, P. H., Pearson, D., & Orrell, D. H. (1976). Ovarian failure following abdominal irradiation in childhood. *British Journal of Cancer, 33*, 655–658.

Speiser, B., Rubin, P., & Casarett, G. (1973). Aspermia following lower truncal irradiation in Hodgkin's disease. *Cancer, 322*, 692–698.

Stiff, P. J., Koester, A. R., Weidner, M. K., Dvorak, K., & Fisher, R. I. (1987). Autologous bone marrow transplantation using unfractionated cells cryopreserved in dimethylsulfoxide and hydroxyethyl starch without controlled-rate freezing. *Blood, 70*, 974–987.

Stillman, R. J., Schinfield, J. S., Schiff, L., Gelber, R. D., Greenberger, J., Larson, M., Jaffe, N., & Li, F. P. (1981). Ovarian failure in long-term survivors of childhood malignancy. *American Journal of Obstetrics and Gynecology, 139*, 62–66.

Storb, R., & Thomas, E. D. (1985). Graft-versus-host disease in dog and man: The Seattle experience. *Immunological Review, 88*, 215–237.

Sullivan, K. M. (1986, Suppl. 1). Acute and chronic graft-versus-host disease in man. *International Journal of Cell Cloning, 4*, 42–93.

Sullivan, K. M., Deeg, H. J., Sanders, J. E., Shulman, H. M., Witherspoon, R. P., Doney, K., Applebaum, F. R., Schumbert, M. M., Stewart, P., Springmeyers, S., McDonald, G. B., Storb, R., & Thomas, E. D. (1984). Late complications after marrow transplantation. *Seminars in Hematology, 21*, 53–63.

Sullivan, K. M., Shulman, H. M., Storb, R., Weiden, P. L., Witherspoon, R. P., McDonald, G. B., Schubert, N. M., Atkinson, K., & Thomas, E. D. (1981). Chronic graft-versus-host disease in 52 patients: Adverse natural course and successful treatment with combination immunosuppression. *Blood, 57*, 267–276.

Thomas, E. D. (1983). Marrow transplantation for malignant diseases. *Journal of Clinical Oncology, 1*, 517–531.

Thomas, E. D., Storb, R., Clift, R. A., Fefer, A., Johnson, F. L., Nieman, P. E., Lerner, K. G., Glucksberg, H., & Buchkner, C. D. (1975). Bone marrow transplantation. *The New England Journal of Medicine, 292*, 832–843, 895–902.

van der Meer, J. W. M., Guiot, H. F. L., van den Brock, P. J., & van Furth, R. (1984). Infections in bone marrow transplant recipients. *Seminars in Hematology, 21*, 123–128.

Waxman, J. H. X., Terry, Y. A., Wrigley, P. F. M., Malpas, J. S., Rees, L. H., Besser, G. M., & Lister, T. A. (1983). Gonadal function in Hodgkin's disease: Long-term follow-up chemotherapy. *British Medical Journal, 285*, 1612–1613.

Whitehead, E., Shalet, S. M., Blackledge, G., Todd, I., Crowthor, D., & Beardwell, C. G. (1982). The effect of Hodgkin's disease and combination chemotherapy on gonadal function in the adult male. *Cancer, 49*, 418–422.

13

Bone Transplantation

Patricia Piasecki

Bone transplantation, or bone allografting, has a long history in orthopedic surgery. Because of recent advances in internal fixation and cryopreservation of the grafts, bone transplantation has increased in popularity. In 1986, 200,000 bone transplant procedures were performed for various orthopedic, dental, neurosurgical, and otolaryngologic defects (American Association of Tissue Banks, personal communication, January 12, 1988).

DEFINITION OF BONE GRAFT

Bone grafts are commonly used in orthopedic surgery to fill cavities from both traumatic and surgical defects, as well as to stimulate bone healing in nonunited fractures. Bone autograft is defined as bone taken from the patient's own skeleton, usually from the ilium, fibula, or tibia. Two types of bone may be used: cortical and cancellous. Cortical bone graft is found in the shaft of long bones and is superior for fixation because of its hardness. Cancellous bone graft material is found in the pelvis and ends of bones and is preferred for osteogenesis owing to its rich blood supply. Autograft is not rejected and is the best graft material when available (Burchardt, 1983).

Autografts, however, have a number of disadvantages, including (1) additional surgical incisions; (2) risk of complications, particularly infection; (3) limited volume and shape of autograft available; and (4) absence of an articulating surface. The healing period after a bone autograft is approximately three months (Herdon & Chase, 1954).

Bone allograft is defined as bone removed from cadaveric human donors. Most often the allograft is frozen after removal and is termed fresh frozen allograft. If the articulating surface or cartilage surface is retained, the graft is called an osteoarticular graft; otherwise, it is an

307

osseous graft. The advantages of fresh frozen allografts over autografts include the ability to (1) prolong storage time, (2) provide structural stability, (3) unite to the host bone, (4) reattach host tendons and ligaments to maintain joint stability and mobility, and (5) maintain some cartilage surface, which is necessary for normal joint function.

HISTORICAL BACKGROUND

Bone allografts were first used by Lexer in 1908. He described 23 whole and 11 hemijoint transplants about the knee with a reported success rate of 50 per cent (Lexer, 1908, 1925). Herndon and Chase (1954) learned that freezing bone allografts reduced their immunogenicity. This finding spurred further clinical studies.

In the 1960s and 1970s surgeons worldwide experimented with bone allografts. They included Parrish (1966) of the United States, Volkov (1970) of the Soviet Union, and Ottolenghi (1972) of Argentina. Mankin, Doppelt, & Tomford (1982) reported on their series in the early 1980s. All of these workers used frozen allografts to replace large bony defects, usually caused by tumors. Successful results were reported in 50 per cent of patients. Complications included infection, fractures, and nonunion of the allograft. These studies concluded that the surgical procedure required improvement in order to decrease complications.

INDICATIONS FOR BONE TRANSPLANTATION

The interest in bone allografts and the indications for its use have recently increased. Current uses include skeletal reconstruction after tumor resection or traumatic bone loss, or after failed total hip or knee arthroplasty procedures. In addition, allografts may be useful in spinal fusions, bone curettages, dental procedures, mandibular reconstruction, and the repair of nonunited fractures.

Acceptable tumor patient candidates include those patients with low-grade tumors, such as giant cell tumors, adamantinomas, and chondrosarcomas. More aggressive tumors, such as osteosarcomas, can be reconstructed with an allograft if the lesion is intraosseous and nonmetastatic (Dick, Malinin, & Mnaymneh, 1985). Treatments for some of these tumors are included in Table 13–1. There is greater demand for donor tissue as the indications for bone transplantation have expanded.

BONE PROCUREMENT

Bone procurement is performed on donors who meet the standards of the American Association of Tissue Banks. Donors who have been

TABLE 13–1. KNEE RECONSTRUCTION OPTIONS

Option	Advantages	Disadvantages
Amputation	No local recurrence Fewest complications	Loss of limb and change in body image Need for prosthetic fitting Mechanical knee joint
Arthrodesis*	Durable Run stiff-legged Few complications	"Unnatural" Stiff leg for sitting Cannot be converted to arthroplasty Small chance of local recurrence
Arthroplasty†	Bendable knee Can be converted to arthrodesis	No running, heavy lifting, or high-impact activities May require revision in 10 or more years Small chance of local recurrence May have stiffness or laxity of knee joint

*Stiff knee using allograft or autograft and metal rod.
†Bendable knee using allograft or metal implant or combination of two.

clinically dead for less than 12 hours and are older than 15 years of age (to ensure closure of epiphyseal plates) and younger than 40 years of age (to minimize the risk of osteoarthritic and malignant processes) are considered (Friedlaender & Mankin, 1979). The donors are screened for the presence of the human immunodeficiency virus antibody, hepatitis, bacteremia, and syphilis. Tissue-typing is not performed. In order to minimize the risk of infection, patients who have been on a ventilator for longer than 72 hours or on steroids before their recent illness are deferred (Friedlaender & Mankin, 1981). Obtaining consent for bone donation is less productive than for other organs and tissues. Family members and hospital staff have rarely heard of bone donation and transplantation. Because patients in need of a bone transplant or allograft are not in a life-threatening condition, but rather in a limb-threatening condition, this procedure has received little media attention. There is also an unfounded fear that the donor will be disfigured after the bone procurement. Public and professional education will help allay these concerns.

Bone procurement takes place in an operating room under sterile conditions after the laboratory screening has been performed. The procedure averages four hours. The bones that are usually procured include the proximal humeri, radii, ilium, femoral heads, proximal femora, distal femora, distal tibia, patellar tendons, and Achilles tendons. Entire bones are seldom used in bone transplantation. Tendon and ligament insertions are left intact in order to permit soft tissue reconstruction. The bone segments are cultured both aerobically and anaerobically and then immersed in an antibiotic solution for five minutes. The articular surfaces are then bathed in a 10% glycerol solution for 30 minutes. Glycerol is used because it maintains cartilage viability by preventing ice crystal formation during the freezing and thawing of the bone. The specimens are then wrapped in sterile bags and labeled with a donor number and a description of the specific bone segment.

The bone is placed in a refrigerator at 4°C for 18 hours to allow the glycerol to penetrate the cartilage matrix. The specimens are later deep frozen to $-70°$. Bone tissue can be stored for five years. When it is needed, it is shipped in coolers on dry ice to requesting surgeons. Some of the procured bone is processed into small particles, blocks, and dowels. These bone pieces are freeze-dried in bottles to remove water and irradiated for secondary sterilization. This lyophilized tissue can be stored in the operating room at room temperature and is often used in acetabular reconstructions, fusions, and dental procedures.

IMMUNOSUPPRESSION

Bone is composed of a variety of cells, such as osteogenic, cartilage, and marrow cells, which have transplantation antigens on their cell surface. These cells can lead to host sensitization. Fresh bone allografts are strongly immunogenic, as are any fresh tissues or organs. Frozen and freeze-dried allografts are less immunogenic. The freezing process results in a decreased number of viable cells, thereby diminishing the graft's immunogenicity. Clinically, freeze-dried allografts show no evidence of rejection (Friedlaender, 1983).

Langer and associates (1985) noted that the implantation of frozen allograft bone in rats resulted in a positive leukocyte migration test. In animal models the result of this immune response is unknown (Langer, Czitrom, Pritzker, & Gross, 1985). Others discovered that immuno-suppression in genetically mismatched dogs improved the biological outcome of frozen bone allograft (Goldberg, Bos, Heiple, Zika, & Powell, 1984).

Despite this immunogenicity, allografts continue to heal. The mechanism for healing the allograft to host bone is by incorporation, using cells from the host bone.

In humans, frozen allografts have diminished immunogenicity. Mankin (1983) discovered that 91 per cent of his patients presented with anti-human leukocyte antibodies (HLA) without clinical significance, since the allografts do not reject or resorb in the presence of antibodies. In fact, the antibodies may actually promote revascularization of bone allografts (Mankin, 1983). Further studies regarding the significance of bone allograft–induced immune responses in humans are needed.

Neither tissue-typing nor immunosuppression is currently used in clinical practice. The results without immunosuppression are reportedly satisfactory. In Mankin's series of 91 patients 67 per cent were reported to have had an excellent or good result (Mankin, 1983). Immunosuppressive therapy could result in increased risks, such as infection. In addition, adding tissue-typing along with other sizing criteria could make it difficult to locate an allograft. Further controlled studies in this area are indicated.

SURGICAL PROCEDURE

Before the procedure is scheduled, an allograft is ordered from a bone bank. The desired segment of allograft is x-rayed and overlayed on the recipient radiograph. Size is most important for an osteoarticular allograft, since the remaining joint surface is being matched.

The surgical procedure is performed in an operating room equipped with a laminar airflow system. The staff wear personal exhaust systems to minimize bacterial contamination (Fig. 13–1). The allograft is removed from its sterile wrap and cultured again to verify its sterility (Piasecki & Rodts, 1985). The allograft is then thawed in warm saline or antibiotic solution for one hour.

In tumor surgery the surgical team changes gown and gloves after resection of the affected bone. The surgical field is redraped, and new equipment is used in an effort to prevent tumor seeding.

The surgeon cuts the allograft bone to the desired size. It is then fixed to the host bone with nails, plates, and screws. In certain cases a metallic implant is cemented into the femoral or tibial allograft to

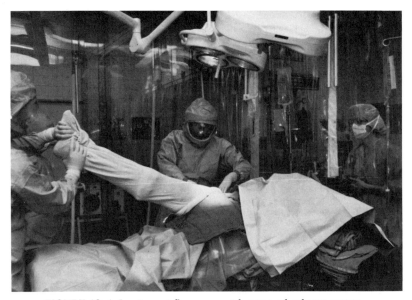

FIGURE 13–1. Laminar airflow room with personal exhaust system.

resurface the joint. This procedure is called an allograft prosthetic composite, and it is used in hip and knee revisions.

Blood loss for these procedures is significant—usually four or more units. Patients may donate four autologous units before surgery, if time permits. A cell saver is not used in patients with cancer because of the risk of seeding malignant cells. In knee surgery blood loss is reduced by placing a sterile tourniquet on the thigh during the resection of tumor and releasing it before the allograft reconstruction. The tourniquet cannot be used for more than two hours. The wound is approximated with staples. Closed-wound drainage and a pressure dressing are applied.

NURSING CARE OF THE BONE TRANSPLANT RECIPIENT

Early Postoperative Care

The patient returns to her room four to six hours after surgery is completed. The affected limb is elevated on pillows. The drain is checked and emptied every eight hours. Drainage is expected to be less than 100 ml per shift. The drain is removed 48 hours after surgery. The bulky pressure dressing is changed three days postoperatively, unless it becomes saturated with blood. If this problem occurs, the dressing is changed immediately, so that it does not become cast-like. A cast or cast brace may be applied while the tendons and soft tissues heal, usually in one month's time (Piasecki & Rodts, 1985). Surgical pain is moderate to severe, requiring strong narcotics for the first few days. Bedrest is maintained for two to four days.

Nursing interventions include assessment of the affected limb for circulation, sensation, and movement every two to four hours. Patients are encouraged to move their feet to stimulate circulation and prevent blood clots. Twice-daily physical therapy is initiated for gentle exercise and gait training. Crutches are used for four to six months, until the allograft is healed.

The patient is ready for discharge when she can ambulate independently, and is sent home with a mild narcotic analgesic. The average hospital stay is 10 to 14 days. See Table 13–2 for further discussion of nursing care.

Late Postoperative Care

The staples are removed from the incision three weeks postoperatively. Follow-up visits consisting of a physical examination and a plain

TABLE 13–2. NURSING CARE PLAN FOR BONE TRANSPLANT RECIPIENTS

NURSING DIAGNOSIS	RISK FACTOR	SIGNS AND SYMPTOMS	NURSING INTERVENTION
Knowledge deficit regarding allograft reconstruction	Anxiety regarding tumor diagnosis and surgery	Asking questions regarding surgery	Explain advantages and disadvantages of arthroplasty, amputation, and arthrodesis (Table 13–1).
			Demonstrate reconstruction techniques with x-rays.
			Allow to meet and talk with patients who have previously experienced the planned procedure to provide their perspective.
			Provide information regarding the rare possibility of AIDS and hepatitis transmission by way of the allograft. The patient needs to weigh this risk against the possibility of amputation.
			Explain surgical procedure and potential complications.
Potential fluid volume deficit	Blood loss during surgical procedure	Decreased hemoglobin	Observe for signs and symptoms of fluid volume deficit.
	Fever	Weakness	Transfuse with blood and IV fluid as needed.
		Decreased blood volume	Administer oral iron supplements as needed.
		Concentrated urine	Encourage adequate fluid intake.
		Poor skin turgor	*Table continued on following page*

313

TABLE 13–2. NURSING CARE PLAN FOR BONE TRANSPLANT RECIPIENTS Continued

Nursing Diagnosis	Risk Factor	Signs and Symptoms	Nursing Intervention
Potential for infection that can result in allograft removal or amputation	Foreign allograft Lengthy surgical procedure (4–8 h) Immunosuppression secondary to chemotherapy	Elevated white blood cell count Reddened, draining wound Fever Pain	Assess wound for signs and symptoms of infection. Administer 48 h of broad-spectrum antibiotics postoperatively as ordered. Document allograft type and donor number in patient care record in the event that there is a graft-related complication. Administer prophylactic antibiotics before dental or surgical procedures for rest of life.
Pain, alteration in comfort postoperatively	Massive resection and reconstruction	Complaints of pain Poor sleep habits Poor concentration Elevated blood pressure and pulse	Assess pain using 0–10 pain scale. Administer pain medication as ordered. Apply ice to surgical site for 15 min 4 times a day for 3 days.
Potential skin breakdown	Large skin and muscle flap Braces and casts Bed rest Preoperative irradiation	Dusky flap Necrotic wound edges	Observe for wound necrosis or dusky flaps. Assess pulses. Apply wet-to-dry dressing 3 times daily to debride necrotic tissue for 1–2 wk. Plastic surgery consult for split-thickness skin graft or other procedure to close wound as indicated.

| Impaired physical mobility | Bed rest
Crutch, brace, or cast requirements
Decreased muscle strength and range of motion due to tumor mass and pain
Allograft bone healing takes 4–12 mo or longer in conjunction with chemotherapy or radiation therapy | Limited ROM
Decreased muscle strength
Patient requires assistive devices for walking | Physical therapy twice daily for progressive exercise and restricted weight bearing with crutches.
Ensure proper fitting of braces or cast for limb immobilization.
Maintain on crutches until allograft is healed.
Assess the patient's ability to perform ADL's.
Obtain occupation and speech therapy consults as indicated.
Instruct in lifelong restriction of no lifting over 25 lb and no high-impact sports such as jogging or racquet sports.
Instruct in other lifelong exercises such as swimming and walking. |

radiograph of the operative site begin six weeks after surgery. For the first year, visits are scheduled every two months to assess for callus formation at the allograft-host junction. In patients with tumors, radiographs are checked for recurrent disease in the host bone. The treatment for a local recurrence is amputation. From years one through five twice-yearly visits occur. Subsequently yearly visits are planned.

The early complications in allograft surgery include nerve palsies (4%–7%), skin slough (2%–7%), hemorrhage (3%), and deep vein thrombosis (7%) (Gitelis, Heligman, Quill, & Piasecki, 1988; Mankin, 1983; Mankin, et al., 1982).

Late complications include local tumor recurrence (0%–3.3%), deep infection (6%–13.2%), allograft fracture (2%–16.5%), nonunion (10%–11%), and development of symptomatic degenerative arthritis (2%) (Gitelis et al., 1988; Mankin, 1983; Mankin et al., 1982). Infection can present with drainage, fever, and an elevated white blood cell count. The development of infection requires removal of the allograft and long-term antibiotic therapy. A reconstruction procedure such as arthrodesis may be performed once the infection is resolved.

Allograft fractures can occur at any time postoperatively. Allograft fractures require further surgery to replace the damaged allograft. Nonunion may also necessitate additional surgery (i.e., autogenous bone graft to allograft junction site). This surgery is performed 6 to 12 months postoperatively. Patients receiving postoperative chemotherapy do not progress to union until the chemotherapy is stopped. Degenerative arthritis in the osteoarticular allograft can occur two or more years postoperatively. Treatment may consist of nonsteroidal anti-inflammatory medications and periodic rest. As extreme a treatment as arthroplasty may be required to resurface the allograft. Patients are encouraged to call the physician or clinical nurse specialist if any problems or questions arise between scheduled visits.

Discharge Planning

Most bone allograft patients are relatively independent at discharge. Their wounds are healing uneventfully. Before discharge, patients are instructed on an appropriate physical therapy routine to be performed at home, twice daily. If indicated, a physical therapist may go to the patient's home to provide further assistance with muscle-strengthing exercises and improvement in range of motion. Visiting nurses are usually not needed. The patients are instructed to call the surgeon or the clinical nurse specialist if any signs or symptoms of infection, deep vein thrombosis, or bleeding occur. They return to the office one week after discharge for wound assessment and staple or suture removal. In tumor patients,

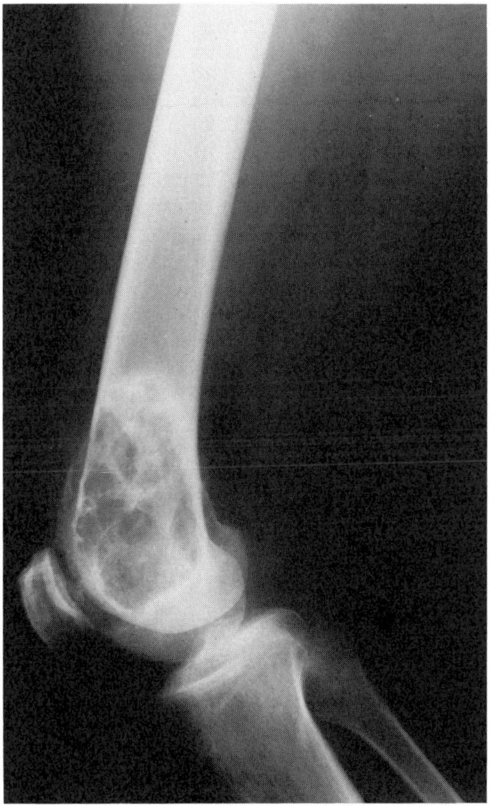

FIGURE 13–2. Giant cell tumor, right distal femur.

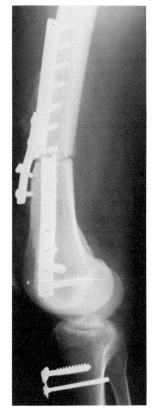

FIGURE 13–3. Nonunion of allograft, right distal femur with fractured plate.

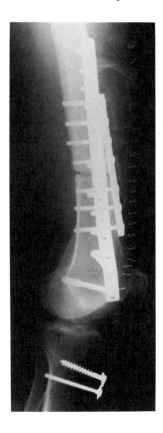

FIGURE 13–4. Postoperative autogenous bone graft with reapplication of external fixation.

FIGURE 13–5. Fully healed allograft, right distal femur.

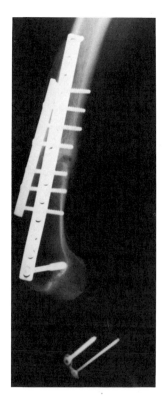

chemotherapy, radiation therapy, or both are restarted two to four weeks postoperatively.

CONCLUSION

Bone transplantation or allografting is a therapeutic alternative to amputation for patients with certain bone tumors, bony defects caused by trauma, or total hip or knee revision. The goal is to provide a functional, reconstructed limb. See Figures 13–2 through 13–5. The complication rate for bone transplantation is acceptable. Nursing care of this patient population is critical for a successful outcome.

Excellent patient satisfaction has been noted after such surgery. Nursing research in the areas of patient satisfaction and long-term rehabilitation needs to be conducted. Of additional importance is increased awareness by both health professionals and the public regarding bone donation and transplantation.

References

Burchardt, H. (1983). The biology of bone graft repair. *Clinical Orthopaedics, 174,* 28–42.

Dick, H. M., Malinin, T. I., & Mnaymneh, W. (1985). Massive allograft implantation following radical resection of high-grade tumors requiring adjuvant chemotherapy treatment. *Clinical Orthopaedics, 197,* 88–95.

Friedlaender, G. & Mankin, H. J. (1979). Guidelines for the banking of musculoskeletal tissues. *Newsletter, American Association of Tissue Banks, 3,* 2.

Friedlaender, G. & Mankin, H. J. (1981). Bone banking: Current methods and suggested guidelines. AAOS Instructional Course Lecture Series (pp. 36–55). St. Louis: C. V. Mosby.

Friedlaender, G. E. (1983). Immune responses to osteochondral allografts: Current knowledge and future directions. *Clinical Orthopaedics, 174,* 58–68.

Gitelis, S., Heligman, D., Quill, G., & Piasecki, P. (1988). The use of large allografts for tumor reconstruction and salvage of the failed total hip arthroplasty. *Clinical Orthopaedics, 231,* 62–70.

Goldberg, V. M., Bos, G. D., Geiple, K. G., Zika, J. M., & Powell, A. E. (1984). Improved acceptance of frozen bone allografts in genetically mismatched dogs by immunosuppression. *Journal of Bone and Joint Surgery, 66A,* 937–950.

Herndon, C. H. & Chase, S. W. (1954). The fate of massive autogenous and homogenous bone grafts including articular surfaces. *Surgery, Gynecology and Obstetrics, 98,* 273–290.

Langer, F., Czitrom, A., Pritzker, K. P., & Gross, A. E. (1985). The immunogenicity of fresh and frozen allogeneic bone. *Journal of Bone Joint Surgery, 57,* 271–279.

Lexer, E. (1908). Die Verwendung der Freien knochenplastic nebst Versuchen uber Gelenkversteifung & Gelenk-transplantation. *Archives Klinics Chiropract., 86,* 939–945.

Lexer, E. (1925). Joint transplantation and arthroplasty. *Surgery, Gynecology and Obstetrics, 40,* 782–809.

Mankin, H. J. (1983). Complications of allograft surgery. In G. D. Friedlaender, H. J. Mankin, & K. W. Sell (Eds.). *Bone Allografts: Current State of the Art* (pp. 259–274). Boston: Little, Brown.

Mankin, H. J., Doppelt, S. H., & Tomford, W. W. (1982). Osteoarticular and intercalary allograft transplantation in the management of malignant tumors of bone. *Cancer, 50,* 613–630.

Ottolenghi, C. E. (1972). Massive osteo and osteoarticular bone grafts: Technique and results of 62 cases. *Clinical Orthopaedics, 87,* 156–164.

Parrish, F. F. (1966). Treatment of bone tumors by total excision and replacement with massive autologous and hemologous grafts. *Journal of Bone and Joint Surgery, 48A,* 968–990.

Piasecki, P. & Rodts, M. F. (1985). Bone banking: Its role in skeletal tumor reconstruction. *Orthopaedic Nursing, 4*(5), 56–80.

Volkov, M. (1970). Allotransplantation of joints. *Journal of Bone and Joint Surgery, 52B,* 49–64.

14

Autotransplantation of the Adrenal Medulla

Elizabeth J. Buchan, Elizabeth Erb,
and Virginia Williams

The 1980s began a new era of hope for people who suffer from Parkinson's disease (PD). Research groups in several countries are currently investigating a new surgical procedure that involves the autotransplantation of the adrenal medulla to the caudate nucleus of the brain. The desired effect of this surgery is to provide the cells of the striatum with a new source of catecholamines. The first group of study patients are currently being evaluated, and plans are under way in several centers for further research. As the frequency of autotransplantation increases, the involved medical centers and their nursing staffs will need to have a more thorough understanding of PD, the operative procedure, and routines for patient management during the preoperative, operative, and postoperative periods.

The history of research concerning the autotransplantation procedure includes three studies. The first human autotransplantation of the adrenal medulla to the caudate nucleus was performed by a group of Swedish researchers in March 1982. The patient was a 55-year-old man who had an eight-year history of PD. Autotransplantation was performed on two other patients during this study. Although none of these patients suffered any adverse effects from the procedure, no clear improvement was seen in their symptoms (Backlund, Granberg, Hamberger, Knutsson, Martensson, et al., 1985).

In August 1984 Dr. Ignacio Madrazo headed a Mexican team that transplanted the adrenal medulla to the right caudate nucleus of two young patients (35 and 39 years old) with intractable PD. The researchers concluded that these autotransplantations resulted in marked improvement in the signs of PD in the patients (Madrazo, Drucker-Colin, Diaz, Martinez-Mata, Torres, & Becerril, 1987).

The autotransplantation procedure was first performed in the United States in April 1987, at Vanderbilt University Medical Center in Nashville, Tennessee. A research team headed by Drs. George S. Allen, Richard S. Burns, and Noel B. Tulipan performed autotransplantation on a 46-year-old woman. She was the first in a series of 18 patients included in a study designed to achieve the following outcomes: (1) validate the findings of the Mexican group, (2) investigate the chemical mechanisms responsible for the therapeutic effect of the surgery, and (3) examine the effect of age and disease severity on the outcomes. Preliminary data collected from this study revealed improvement in several of the younger (less than 50 years old) patients. Two of these patients showed substantial improvement in motor function. In five of the six patients between 60 and 70, postoperative confusion was a predominant side effect, lingering from several days to weeks. Postoperative confusion has also been seen in other study groups throughout the country (Penn, Goetz, Tanner, Klawans, Shannon, Commella, & Witt, 1988; Goetz, Olanow, Koller, Penn, et al., 1989). Sleep disturbances were also found in the majority of patients over 50 as well as transient depression (S. Burns, personal communication, December 1987).

The most recent studies include Penn and associates (1988), who reported the results of a study group at Rush–Presbyterian–St. Luke's Medical Center in Chicago (Penn et al., 1988). The purpose of the research project was to validate the findings of Madrazo and colleagues (1984) and to monitor patients with a standardized rating scale that would be familiar to PD study groups internationally (Madrazo et al., 1984). The mean age of PD onset was 37.8 and the mean length of levodopa treatment was 10 years. Changes in parkinsonian function were assessed over 20 weeks of follow-up using the nonparametric Friedman's one-way ANOVA. Changes were measured using a standardized activities of daily living scale and by diaries kept by the patients. Data were collected both when the patients' medications were at peak effect (on) and when they were at their nadir (off). Videotaped records using a standard protocol were obtained during both periods. Detailed psychometric tests and psychological interviews were also performed. A significant improvement was reported in the percentage of the day spent "on" with good motor function $(x^2 = 4.25; df = 5; p = 0.014)$ (Penn et al., 1988). In contrast to Madrazo and colleagues, no patient was able to stop her parkinsonian medication postoperatively.

The findings of a multicenter study was reported by Goetz and associates (1989). The surgical procedure developed by Madrazo (1984) was performed on 19 patients from three different research centers. The sample included 16 men and 3 women. Their mean age at onset of PD was 40.8 ± 10.9 years and their mean age at the time of surgery was 53.8 ± 8.0 years. The mean duration of PD was 12.9 to 17.4 years, and the mean duration of levodopa treatment 11.7 ± 4.3 years. Assessment of the extent of PD was made using two standardized rating scales. The research findings demonstrate an increase in "on" time from 48 to 78 per cent by the end of six months with a consequent reduction of "off" time to only 25 per cent of the waking day. Patients continued to have fluctuations in their motor response to antiparkinsonian medications and no patient was able to be totally withdrawn from the medications.

ETIOLOGY AND EPIDEMIOLOGY

Parkinson's disease is a chronic degenerative disorder of the extrapyramidal nervous system. The cause is unknown. Theories of PD's idiopathic development include a genetic contribution, a viral source that destroys dopamine-producing cells, and an accelerated aging process. The latter theory implies that if everyone lived long enough they would develop PD. Most patients who suffer from PD fall into the idiopathic category, but parkinsonian symptoms can develop from several other causative categories. Toxic exposure to manganese and carbon dioxide, drugs (rauwolfia alkaloids and phenothiazines), arteriosclerosis of the brain's blood vessels, and traumatic injury to the brain have been linked to parkinsonian symptoms (Garrett, 1982).

Primarily a disease of the elderly, PD's onset is usually seen between 50 and 70 years of age. The average age of onset is 65 years; however, 1.6 per cent of patients develop symptoms before age 30. There is a marked increase in prevalence and incidence with advancing age (Illson, Bressman, & Fahn, 1983). One to 1.5 million persons in the United States are estimated to be affected by PD, with 40,000 new cases diagnosed each year. The disease occurs in men slightly more often than in women, by a 3:2 ratio.

PATHOPHYSIOLOGY AND CLINICAL MANIFESTATIONS

The clinical manifestations of PD are due to pathologic changes in the basal ganglia of the extrapyramidal system (Fig. 14–1). The major functions of the extrapyramidal system are the control of body muscle tone and the refining of voluntary movements. To achieve these functions a balance must exist between the extrapyramidal and pyramidal systems. The pyramidal system uses acetylcholine for a neurotransmitter, which has an excitatory effect. Acetylcholine is secreted by the pyramidal cells of the motor cortex and by neurons in the basal ganglia (Guyton, 1986).

The extrapyramidal system is composed of the basal ganglia, which

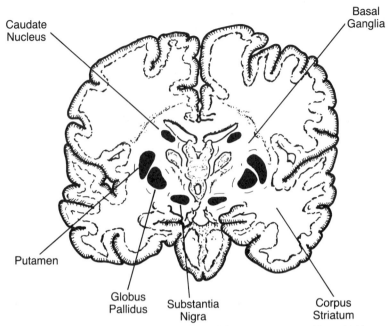

Caudate Nucleus

Basal Ganglia

Putamen

Globus Pallidus

Substantia Nigra

Corpus Striatum

FIGURE 14–1. The structures of the extrapyramidal nervous system. (From Feldman, R.G. (1985). *Hospital Practice, 20, 80B.* Copyright 1985 by Hospital Practice. Reprinted by permission.)

includes the caudate nucleus and putamen (collectively called the striatum); the globus pallidus; and several other related structures of the brain stem. Neural transmission in the basal ganglia depends on dopamine, which usually has an inhibitory effect. The highest concentrations of dopamine are normally found in the substantia nigra and the striatum. Pathologic findings in PD reveal a loss of neurons in the substantia nigra, which causes a severe reduction in the production and storage of dopamine. However, the acetylcholine-producing cells of the pyramidal system are not affected. The decrease of dopamine in relation to acetylcholine alters the neuropharmacology in the basal ganglia and creates an imbalance between the extrapyramidal and pyramidal systems. Lower levels of dopamine result in cholinergic hyperactivity related to the unopposed acetylcholine activity. The decrease in dopamine results in dysfunction of the extrapyramidal system, causing the clinical manifestations of PD, such as rigidity, tremors at rest, bradykinesia, and diminished postural reflexes (Table 14–1). The motor signs of PD can be observed when the striatal dopamine level is reduced by 20 per cent of normal. There is a direct correlation of dopamine deficiency in the striatum and the appearance of bradykinesia and rigidity. Changes in dopamine and serotonin levels probably account for the tremors.

TABLE 14–1. CLINICAL MANIFESTATIONS OF PARKINSON'S DISEASE

*Tremors at rest
*Diminished postural reflexes
*Bradykinesia
*Rigidity
 Shuffling gait
 Mask-like face
 Generalized weakness and fatigue
 Mental depression
 Autonomic dysfunction (drooling, oily skin, dysphagia, excessive
   perspiration, constipation, orthostatic hypotension, urinary hesitation and
   frequency)

*Cardinal manifestations.

MEDICAL AND SURGICAL INTERVENTION

Medical treatment of PD is directed toward the replacement of dopamine in the striatum and the inhibition of cholinergic pathways. Because dopamine cannot cross the blood–brain barrier, a precursor of the drug, levadopa, was first used in the treatment of PD. Levadopa therapy required relatively large doses to obtain therapeutic effects because of rapid liver metabolism by the enzyme dopa decarboxylase. Such doses were associated with a number of side effects, including nausea, vomiting, postural hypotension, dyskinesia, cardiac arrhythmias, and hallucinations.

Levadopa is now commonly combined with carbidopa, a peripheral dopa decarboxylase–blocking agent, which will not cross the blood–brain barrier. The action of carbidopa prevents the conversion of dopa to dopamine in the periphery, preventing the common side effects of levadopa without affecting the therapeutic effect of the drug in the extrapyramidal system. Carbidopa-levodopa therapy (Sinemet) is available in many dosage combinations expressed in a ratio of carbidopa to levadopa (e.g., 1:10 as 10/100 and 1:4 as 25/100).

Cholinergic blocking agents such as trihexyphenidyl (Artane) and benztropine (Cogentin) are also effective in reducing parkinsonian symptoms, particularly tremors. These drugs work by blocking cholinergic transmission, which is normally balanced by the inhibitory effect of dopamine. They may be prescribed in conjunction with Sinemet therapy or may be used alone, if tremors are the predominant symptom. Additionally, Cogentin has antihistaminic properties, which can be helpful if the patient also suffers from anxiety or depression. The medications commonly used in the treatment of PD are summarized in Table 14–2.

Before the adrenal-caudate autotransplant procedure was used, several types of surgical interventions were performed for patients whose conditions were refractory to medical therapy. These procedures included thalamotomy, which placed lesions in the area of the ventral

TABLE 14–2. MEDICATIONS COMMONLY USED IN THE TREATMENT OF PARKINSON'S DISEASE

AGENT	DAILY DOSAGE RANGE (mg)	SCHEDULE	SIDE EFFECTS
Indirect agonists			
Levodopa (Laradopa, Dopar)	1000–6000	100 mg four times day with meals	Nausea, vomiting, postural hypotension, dyskinesia, cardiac arrhythmias, and hallucinations
Carbidopa/ levadopa (Sinemet)	600–1200 of levodopa to 60–120 of carbidopa	25/1000 with meals and then up to every 2 to 3 hours	Dyskinesia
Direct agonist			
Bromocriptine (Parlodel)	5–50	1.25 mg every 12 hours and then increase at 1- to 2-week intervals	Nightmares, hallucinations, paranoia, nausea, hypotension
Anticholinergics			
Benztropine (Cogentin)	0.5–6.0	Start at bedtime and then after meals	Dry mouth, constipation, urine retention, confusion, and hallucinations
Trihexyphenidyl (Artane)	1–10	Start after meals and then up to three or four times a day	Dry mouth, constipation, urine retention, confusion, and hallucinations
Antihistamines			
Diphenydramine (Benadryl)	25–200	At bedtime	Dry mouth, constipation, urine retention, confusion, hallucinations, headaches, and weakness
Orphenadrine (Disipal)	25–200	At bedtime	Dry mouth, constipation, urine retention, confusion, hallucinations, headaches, and weakness

lateral thalamus, and pallidotomy, in which lesions were made in the globus pallidus. These lesions could be produced either surgically or chemically and were thought to assist in slowing the activity of neurons responsible for the symptoms.

The adrenal-caudate autotransplant places dopamine-producing cells in the caudate nucleus, a thin nuclear mass lying in the wall of the lateral ventricle. Researchers maintain that direct placement of dopamine-producing cells at this site, which is bathed in cerebrospinal fluid (CSF), will facilitate distribution of dopamine throughout the extrapyramidal system, thus decreasing the clinical manifestation of PD. Additional hypotheses to explain the improvement in the clinical manifestations include the preservation of neurons that form afferent connections and that transplanted tissue synthesizes or releases a trophic factor that has a direct effect on the neurons in this region.

ADRENAL-CAUDATE AUTOTRANSPLANT

Preoperative Period

The adrenal-caudate autotransplant candidate is admitted to a neuroscience unit usually a week before surgery. During this time a multidisciplinary team evaluates the patient. The members of this team and their roles are summarized in Table 14–3.

An abdominal computed tomography (CT) scan will demonstrate the presence or absence of the adrenal gland bilaterally. The functioning of the adrenal gland is assessed by a 24-hour urine collection for 17-ketosteroids, 17-hydroxysteroids, and free cortisol. The 24-hour urine collection is also tested for heavy metals to rule out an environmental cause for the parkinsonian symptoms. Serum cortisol levels are also measured. If the CT scan shows the absence of bilateral adrenal glands

TABLE 14–3. HEALTH CARE TEAM MEMBERS AND THEIR ROLES

Nurse
Performs a complete assessment
Identifies patient needs
Develops realistic goals with the patient and family
Communicates goals to other health team members
Coordinates activities
Implements patient education
Physical Therapist
Evaluates gait
Develops program of exercise and mobility training
Increases range of motion
Assesses changes in the patient's potential
Implements patient education
Occupational Therapist
Assesses patient's self-care skills
Teaches adaptive techniques to patient and family to maximize independence
Speech Pathologist
Evaluates communication skills
Assesses language, speech, and oral motor movement
Evaluates swallowing difficulties
Dietitian
Individualizes each patient's nutritional plan
Assists in evaluating swallowing difficulties
Respiratory Therapist
Evaluates patient's respiratory status
Assists in preoperative teaching

or if abnormally low laboratory values indicate adrenal malfunction, the autotransplantation cannot be performed.

The patient also undergoes a CT scan of the head to rule out any existing pathologic conditions and for postoperative comparison to determine the degree of swelling and the presence of air within the intracranium if these complications should occur. Patients may also have a magnetic resonance imaging (MRI) scan because many physicians believe that this scan provides a clearer picture of the intracranial contents and does not expose the patient to radiation. In addition, a positron emission transaxial tomography (PETT) scan may be performed. A PETT scan shows areas of metabolic activity, and a postoperative scan can determine an increase in activity in the region of the autotransplant.

A lumbar puncture is performed to analyze CSF for levels of epinephrine, norepinephrine, and dopamine. The results are used as a postoperative comparison to determine changes in the levels of these neurotransmitters, which may explain the improvement in the patient's clinical condition.

The patient will be evaluated both while taking her parkinsonian medications and while medication-free to determine the level of dysfunction caused by PD. The patient is evaluated using a standardized scale (i.e., the Columbia Rating Scale) (Fig. 14–2), and the information will be used for follow-up examinations. Medical treatment is restarted after the evaluation is completed until the day of surgery and is resumed immediately postoperatively during the recovery from anesthesia.

Phenytoin sodium (Dilantin), an anticonvulsant, is initiated prophylactically, since seizures may develop after intracranial surgery. Dilantin raises the seizure threshold. The patient is given an initial loading dose of 15 mg/kg until the therapeutic level is achieved, and is maintained at this level by receiving 300 to 400 mg daily.

The nurse, during the preoperative period, must complete and document an initial assessment of the candidate. An extensive history regarding the patient's PD, medical treatment, and ability to perform activities of daily living is necessary. Physiologic and psychosocial needs are identified and prioritized. Realistic goals for the hospitalization are mutually agreed on by the patient, family, and nurse. The roles of the other members of the health care team are explained. Working collaboratively with the health care team, the nurse must assess the overall plan of care to ensure that consistent, quality care is being given to meet expected patient outcomes.

Assessment Parameters and Interventions

Medical History

The history of the patient's PD includes the age of onset of symptoms, past medical interventions, and current medications. The exact dosages

CLINICAL RATING SCALE

Name _____ Date _____ Time _____ AM/PM

Last dose: amount: _____ Time _____ AM/PM

1. Facial expression: Poker face / sl. abnorm. / moderate / severe
   1   2   3   4

2. Seborrhea: Oily / mild erythema and scaling / moderate / severe
   1   2   3   4

3. Salivation: excess in pharynx / min. drooling / moderate / marked
   1   2   3   4

4. Speech: Slight loss of volume / monotone and slurred / marked / unintelligible
   1   2   3   4

5–9. Tremors:

	RUE	LUE		RLE	LLE		Face, Lips, etc.
Slight and infrequent (1)							
Moderate and intermitt. (2)							
Mod. and most of time (3)							
Marked and most of time (4)							

10–14. Rigidity:

	RUE	LUE		RLE	LLE		Neck
Slight or activated (1)							
Mild to moderate (2)							
Marked (3)							
Limited range of motion (4)							

15–20. Dexterity:

	Finger tapping			Succession movement			Foot tapping	
	RUE	LUE		RUE	LUE	(Grip)	RLE	LLE
Slightly slow (1)								
Slow (2)								
Markedly slow (3)								
Unable (4)								

21. Arising from chair: Slow / push with arms / falls back (>1 try) / unable
    1   2   3   4

22. Standing: Slight stoop / mod. flexed / marked and kyphosis / extreme flexion
    1   2   3   4

23. Stability: Retropulsion / would fall / fall spontan. on Romberg / unable
    1   2   3   4

24. Gait: Slow-shuffle / festinate-freeze-pulsion / requires assistance / unable
    1   2   3   4

25. Bradykinesia: Minimal slowness and deliberate / mild slow and poverty /
    1   2

    mod. slow and occasional hesitancy or freeze / marked slow and frequent hesitancy
    3   4

26. Action/Postural: Slight-action / mod.-action / mod-posture / marked—interferes with feeding
    Tremor   1   2   3   4
         RUE:
         LUE:

27. Pronation/supination: Mild slow- ↓ amplit. / mod. fatigue—occasional arrest /
    (simultaneously)   1   2

    marked-hesitation / barely able
    and arrests
    3   4

28. Leg agility: Mild slow- ↓ amplit. / mod. fatigue—occasional arrest /
    1   2

    marked-hesitation / barely able
    and arrests
    3   4

29.   RLE:
         LLE:

FIGURE 14–2. Clinical rating system for parkinsonism patients.

and time schedules are obtained. The time required for the patient to experience a decrease in symptoms after taking the medications is recorded. Physical limitations experienced by the patient, as well as adaptive and coping mechanisms, are identified. The patient's general medical history includes hospitalizations, surgeries, allergies, any coexisting health problems, and current medications.

Neurologic Examination

The patient's preoperative neurologic status must be accurately assessed and documented. Baseline data are used postoperatively to assess any changes in the patient's status. Some research protocols include videotaping the patient's neurologic examination in order to supplement written observations.

The patient's level of consciousness (LOC) is assessed by ascertaining orientation to person, place, and time and ability to follow simple directions. Patients with PD may require a longer time to answer questions or follow directions because of difficulty with articulation and with initiating movement. Failure to complete a task immediately should not be interpreted as an inappropriate response, although any delay should be carefully documented.

Level of consciousness provides the basis for assessing the patient's cognitive function. Areas to be evaluated include attention span, concentration, memory, sequencing of activities, logical reasoning, and perception. A PD patient can experience confusion and memory disorders secondary to pharmacologic agents. Alterations in cortical neurons and cholinergic projections that occur in PD can cause dementia (Moses, 1986).

Pupillary observations, including size, shape, and reactivity to light and accommodation, provide valuable information for postoperative comparison. The patient's blink reflex is assessed. Patients can have a decrease in the normal blink rate of ten or more times a minute, leaving them at risk for corneal damage. Supplemental lubrication or eye patching may be indicated.

An orderly assessment of the patient's motor function will reveal the extent to which PD has affected the patient's neurologic status. Bradykinesia is slow, deliberate movement, which may be misinterpreted as akinesia because of delayed response time in initiating movement. Akinesia is a disturbed state in which a patient cannot initiate or execute simple voluntary acts or motor activities. To assess bradykinesia ask the patient to perform a series of rapid movements, such as opening and closing of the hand, tapping the thumb and index finger, or tapping the foot.

Involuntary movements in the form of tremors are commonly observed. The classic parkinsonian tremors will decrease with movement and are usually absent during sleep. The severity of the tremors and the effect they have on the patient's ability to perform activities of daily living are assessed.

Rigidity in PD results from increased muscle tone, primarily in the striated muscles. To assess rigidity the patient's extremities, head, and trunk are moved passively to detect resistance. Rigidity exists when the patient exhibits resistance to both flexion and extension of the joint.

Abnormalities in postural reflexes and gait are noted. Postural reflexes are diminished in PD, causing the patient difficulty in righting when suddenly jarred. Assessment of postural instability is performed by having the patient stand in front of the examiner with eyes open and feet slightly apart. The patient is then pulled toward the examiner with a tug on the shoulder. The normal response is to take one step backward, throw arms forward, and regain balance. Patients with PD take several small steps backward before regaining balance or lose balance completely. Precautions must be taken to prevent injury to the patient during this test.

Neuromuscular changes cause difficulty in coordinating movements of the arms and legs, leading to abnormalities in gait and posture. A patient with PD has a distinct, flexed, dystonic posture and walks with a shuffling gait. The muscles used in speaking and swallowing are also affected. The patients will experience difficulty with articulation related to the lack of coordination and decreased movement of muscles that aid in speech. The rate, rhythm, and intonation of the patient's speech are documented.

Dysphagia results from impaired swallowing movements and excessive salivation secondary to lack of spontaneous swallowing. The patient's ability to handle oral secretions is closely assessed and monitored. One potential problem that can occur is ineffective airway clearance, leading to aspiration pneumonia or respiratory arrest if the airway becomes occluded. Suction equipment may be necessary at the bedside if a severe swallowing disorder exists. Dietary and speech consultations will assist in problem solving for these complications.

Cardiovascular Assessment

A complete assessment of the patient's cardiovascular system will provide baseline data for postoperative comparison. Electrocardiography is performed. PD patients may develop cardiac arrhythmias secondary to anticholinergic and carbidopa-levodopa therapy (Moses, 1986). Arrhythmias usually occur only if the patient also exhibits orthostatic hypotension. Orthostatic hypotension can result from Sinemet or bromocriptine (Parlodel) therapy and as a result of autonomic dysfunction. Supine, sitting, and standing blood pressures and pulse rate are measured. The patient needs to be cautioned to sit before standing, to change positions slowly, and to wear support stockings.

Respiratory Assessment

Rigidity affects the expansion of the PD patient's chest wall. The patient may experience a decrease in tidal volume. The flexed posture of the PD patient also leads to changes in the patient's respiratory pattern. Lung sounds are evaluated as well as the rate, rhythm, and depth of breathing. A preoperative evaluation by a respiratory therapist will assist in developing a pulmonary toilet regimen before surgery.

Patient Preparation

The results from the initial assessment provide information necessary to classify the patient into one of five stages used to document the degree of disease progression (Table 14–4). Classification is based on the degree of involvement of the disease process and the resulting gdisability (Hickey, 1986). The progression of PD will provide valuable information to incorporate to pre- and postoperative care planning.

The nurse carefully assesses the patient's and family's understanding that autotransplantation is an experimental procedure developed to ameliorate the signs and symptoms of PD. In addition, the effect of the procedure on the progression of PD will be evaluated. The patient and family must be cautioned not to view the procedure as a cure for PD. Possible risks and benefits must be explained. A teaching plan is developed to enhance the patient's and family's realistic expectations of the autotransplant and to explain preoperative, operative, and postoperative regimens. The preoperative nursing care for the adrenal-caudate autotransplant patient is summarized in Tables 14–5 and 14–6.

Operative Period

The autotransplantation of the adrenal medulla to the caudate nucleus involves two simultaneous procedures. A team of general surgeons

TABLE 14–4. CLASSIFICATION OF PARKINSON'S DISEASE

Stage I:	Unilateral involvement
Stage II:	Bilateral involvement only
Stage III:	Diminished postural reflexes; mild to moderate disability
Stage IV:	Severe disease; marked disability
Stage V:	Confinement to bed or wheelchair

will perform a right adrenalectomy while the neurosurgical team performs a microsurgical stereotaxic craniotomy. The procedure takes approximately four to six hours.

On the day of surgery the patient is taken to a minor surgery suite where her head is shaved and a stereotaxic frame is applied. During this procedure the patient is awake and will experience some discomfort. The frame is secured to the skull using four carbon pins. Pin sites are identified, and a local anesthetic is injected into the scalp and periosteum. A drill is used to penetrate the scalp, periosteum, and the outer table of the skull. The bits are removed and carbon pins are inserted to secure the frame. This procedure is similar to the placement of a halo brace. The patient is then taken to the radiology department for a CT scan. The stereotaxic scan provides the basis for a three-dimensional approach to an anatomically defined point (the caudate nucleus) in relation to a second set of fixed external points (Marinari, 1984). After the scan the patient is returned to the operating room for the autotransplantation.

Removal of the right adrenal gland is performed by the general surgeon because it is more easily accessible than the left. A flank incision is made and the adrenal gland is identified and dissected. The surgeon waits until the neurosurgical team is ready for the gland before it is clipped and removed. There is a possibility that the 12th rib may be removed to better visualize and remove the gland.

The neurosurgical team, using a twist drill, passes a catheter through the nondominant hemisphere into the right frontal horn of the lateral ventricle near the caudate nucleus. This area is determined using the coordinates from the stereotaxic scan. An Ommaya reservoir is placed on the opposite side. The catheter from the reservoir extends into the left frontal horn of the lateral ventricle on the side opposite the transplant. The Ommaya reservoir is located under the scalp for easy access for CSF sampling postoperatively. After the completion of these two procedures the stereotaxic frame is removed.

A frontal craniotomy is turned using the catheter as a guide. After the adrenal gland is removed the neurosurgeon dissects the adrenal medulla into tiny pieces and rinses the pieces in saline solution. The tissue is placed on a wire spiral holder and inserted into the area of the caudated nucleus. The craniotomy is closed and anesthesia is reversed.

POSTOPERATIVE RECOVERY

Before returning to the neuroscience intensive care unit the auto-transplant patient has an initial postoperative head CT scan to detect the presence of intracranial air, the degree of swelling present, and the location of the transplanted tissue and Ommaya reservoir. Computed

Text continued on page 338

TABLE 14–5. PREOPERATIVE TEACHING PLAN FOR THE ADRENAL-CAUDATE AUTOTRANSPLANT PATIENT

Behavioral Objectives	Content	Teaching Strategies	Evaluation
The patient and family will verbalize an understanding and acceptance of the autotransplantation procedure as an investigational procedure designed to help decrease the signs and symptoms of PD.	History of the procedure Theories behind development Investigational nature Research protocol Current results	Meet with the patient and family members at a convenient time for them, keep teaching sessions brief, do not provide too much information at any one time, give written information whenever possible, allow time for the patient and family members to review information and ask questions. Clarify the physician's explanation of the procedure and its possible risks and benefits. Allow time for the patient and family members to express concerns and feelings.	The patient and family members will participate in all teaching sessions and verbalize an understanding and acceptance of the procedure.
The patient will demonstrate the proper method to splint flank incision for postoperative coughing and deep breathing, and the use of the incentive spirometer for pulmonary toilet.	Rationale for the importance of vigorous pulmonary toilet postoperatively	Explain the importance of postoperative coughing, deep breathing, and the use of the incentive spirometer in the postoperative recovery phase. Demonstrate the proper use of pillows to splint the flank incision for coughing and deep breathing. Ask for a return demonstration.	The patient will correctly demonstrate the proper method.

Goal	Intervention	Expected Outcome
The patient will explain the purpose of each preoperative test and procedure and what is to be expected during each.	Preoperative testing and rationale for each. Include the following tests: abdominal and head CT, MRI, PETT scan, lumbar puncture, blood work, 24-hour urine and videotaping. Review preoperative testing procedures with the patient and family. Review the purpose of each, where it will be done, preparation required, and what can be expected before, during, and after the procedure. Provide patient information material for each test and procedure to reinforce teaching.	The patient will explain the purposes and rationale for each test. Repeat teaching when patient cannot state rationale and purpose.
The patient will state the sequence of events on the day of surgery.	Procedures and routines the patient can expect on the day of surgery, including after midnight, preoperative medications and the effect they will have, transport to the minor surgery suite for the application of the stereotaxic frame and what to expect during the application, transport to the CT scan, return to the suite for the surgery, transport to the neuro intensive care unit. Review the sequence of events on the day of surgery. Inform the family where they can wait during the surgery.	The patient will verbalize an understanding of the sequence of events on the day of surgery.
The patient will be able to state the rationale for the initiation of Dilantin therapy preoperatively.	Information about Dilantin, the drug's use and importance, wide effects, and dosage schedule. Review with the patient the rationale for Dilantin therapy. Provide a written drug information sheet to the patient that describes the purpose of the drug, the drug's actions, possible side effects, and scheduling. Review the time scheduling with the patient, telling her that she may be receiving the drug more often until a therapeutic level is achieved.	Patient will state rationale and time scheduling of Dilantin therapy.

TABLE 14–6. PREOPERATIVE CARE PLAN FOR ADRENAL-CAUDATE AUTOTRANSPLANT PATIENT

Nursing Diagnosis	Expected Patient Outcomes	Nursing Interventions
Impaired physical mobility related to rigidity, tremors, and bradykinesia, possibly manifested by inability to walk with a steady gait, complete ADLs, difficulty initiating movement, shuffling gait, dystonic posture, and loss of balance	Patient will not suffer from complications of decreased mobility as evidenced by clear breath sounds, no skin breakdown, and no signs of phlebitis. Patient will maintain or improve joint mobility. Patient will participate in ADLs.	Discuss with the patient the importance of physical activity and physical therapy in maintaining physical mobility. Obtain physical therapy and occupational therapy consults. Place a foam mattress on the bed; consider the use of an air flotation bed. Instruct the patient on the use of antiembolism stockings. Remove the stockings every 8 h and examine for signs of phlebitis, including pain with dorsiflexion, warmth, redness, and swelling. Auscultate breath sounds and note presence of rales. Assist patient with turning every 2 h. Perform range of motion to all extremities every 4 h. Examine skin, especially over pressure points for redness and swelling; massage area gently with lotion. Encourage participation in ADLs.

| Alteration in nutrition related to dysphagia, possibly manifested by difficulty chewing and swallowing and by inadequate secretion clearance | Patient's nutritional status will be maintained as evidenced by maintaining or achieving optimal body weight.
Patient will be able to clear oral secretions. | Consult the dietitian and speech therapist to evaluate the patient's swallowing.
Help the patient select foods that she likes that meet nutritional requirements. Help choose a soft diet and small feedings.
Encourage the patient to take small bites and swallow frequently.
Massage neck and throat muscles before eating.
Have the patient sit in a chair or at a 90-degree angle when eating.
Maintain a caloric count and daily weights. |
| Ineffective breathing pattern related to rigidity of chest wall and dystonic posture, possibly manifested by rapid, shallow respirations and decreased tidal volume | Patient will develop an effective respiratory pattern as evidenced by respiratory rate of 12–24 breaths per minute, clear breath sounds all lobes, pO_2 80–100 mmHg: pH 7.35-7.45; and $pCO_2 < 45$ mmHg | Consult respiratory therapy.
Evaluate effectiveness of patient's respiratory pattern.
Encourage deep breathing and use of the incentive spirometer.
Turn patient every 2 h.
Instruct patient on the importance of deep breathing, coughing, and the use of the incentive spirometer postoperatively. |

tomography scans are routinely performed every two to three days postoperatively until the swelling and air are resolved. Changes in the patient's condition are assessed and compared with the information obtained in the preoperative assessment.

An initial and ongoing assessment of the patient's neurologic status is performed to detect changes that are indicative of increasing intracranial pressure. Hourly assessment of the patient's LOC, pupillary reactions, and body movement provides early clues to changes in intracranial pressure. Nursing activities are directed toward maximizing the patient's neurologic status. Elevating the head of the bed, maintaining the patient's head in a neutral position, and providing a quiet environment minimize the effects of transient increases in intracranial pressure. Changes in the patient's neurologic status need to be reported immediately.

The patient may return to the unit intubated, depending on her LOC and pulmonary status. Assessment of rate, depth, and pattern of respirations is performed. The quality of breath sounds is also assessed. A pneumothorax can occur because the operative manipulation to remove the adrenal gland may nick the pleural cavity. The symmetry of chest wall expansion, the position of the trachea, and the quality of breath sounds will help in assessing the presence of a pneumothorax. A postoperative chest x-ray will confirm the diagnosis. The placement of a chest tube is necessary to reexpand the collapsed area of the lung. Emergency equipment should be ready if the patient's respiratory status deteriorates and necessitates reintubation.

Deep breathing is difficult for the autotransplant patient because of the high flank incision. Respirations tend to be shallow. Deep breathing and the use of an incentive spirometer are encouraged immediately to prevent atelectasis. If the patient is intubated, endotracheal suctioning is performed every one to two hours. The nurse needs to hyperoxygenate and hyperventilate the patient during the suctioning procedure to prevent increases in intracranial pressure. Arterial blood gases are measured. Hypercarbia causes cerebral arteries to dilate. This action could lead to increased intracranial pressure secondary to increased blood flow to the area. Thus, a partial pressure of carbon dioxide between 25 and 35 mm Hg is desired. Repositioning the patient every one to two hours will help to prevent the pooling of secretions in the dependent lobes of the lungs.

Monitoring the patient's cardiovascular status provides information about the patient's circulating volume. The patient's heart rate and rhythm, blood pressure, and central venous pressure (CVP) are assessed hourly. Postoperative bleeding is uncommon but can occur. Serial packed cell volumes are measured.

The removal of the adrenal gland can lead to an acute adrenal insufficiency crisis. The likelihood that a crisis will occur is slight, but the possibility does exist. Petechial hemorrhages, hypovolemia as evidenced by increased heart rate, low blood pressure and CVP, hyperkalemia, and hypoglycemia are signs of an acute adrenal crisis. Accurate hourly intake and output with determination of urine specific gravity is performed. Close monitoring of serum and urine electrolyte levels is necessary in order to detect early signs of a crisis. Electrocardiogram changes, including tall peaked narrow T waves and a shortened QT interval, are indicative of hyperkalemia. Therapy is directed toward maintaining an adequate circulating volume and replacing levels of circulating cortisol. The patient may be started on vasoactive drugs to maintain adequate perfusion to the brain and other vital organs. Overzealous fluid resuscitation can lead to pulmonary edema. The presence of rales in the lungs, a heart gallop, and jugular venous distention needs to be assessed.

Because of immobility secondary to pain or altered LOC, the autotransplant patient is at risk for deep vein thrombosis. Passive range of motion to the extremities every four hours will help to prevent this complication. Range of motion also helps to keep the muscles from becoming more rigid until more aggressive physical therapy can be initiated.

Postoperative pain is managed with a transcutaneous electrical nerve stimulation (TENS) unit. The TENS unit allows for pain control without the use of narcotic analgesics, which can alter the patient's LOC and depress deep breathing. Electrodes from the TENS unit are placed along the flank incision to control pain. This temporarily decreases pain by electrically stimulating peripheral nerves through the electrodes. Patients report a decrease in their incision pain, leading to increased mobility and depth of respiration.

Sinemet and other chemical antiparkinsonian therapies are initiated postoperatively, based on the neurologist's evaluation. The dosage and scheduling of the drugs change frequently until the desired effect is achieved. A delay in receiving a dose may cause an exacerbation in the patient's condition and should be avoided. The nursing care of the adrenal-caudate autotransplant patient during the first four to five days postoperatively is summarized in Table 14–7.

The patient is transferred to the neuroscience general care unit approximately four to five days postoperatively. Neurologic assessment continues, as does vigorous pulmonary toilet. The patient's medications continue to be adjusted until the desired effect is achieved. The Ommaya reservoir is tapped for CSF sampling, and the results are compared with preoperative results.

During this period occupational and physical therapy teams work with the patient to increase mobility and independence. Progressive ambulation begins after neurologic and cardiovascular stability have been

TABLE 14–7. POSTOPERATIVE CARE PLAN FOR ADRENAL-CAUDATE AUTOTRANSPLANT PATIENT

Nursing Diagnosis	Expected Patient Outcomes	Nursing Interventions
Potential alteration in tissue perfusion (cerebral) related to craniotomy, possibly manifested by altered LOC, unequal pupils, lack of spontaneous movement, decreased strength of spontaneous movement	Patient will not experience any alteration in cerebral tissue perfusion as evidenced by absence of neurologic deterioration from baseline, equal reactive pupils, spontaneous movement	Elevate head of bed 30 degrees. Maintain head in neutral position; avoid hyperextension and hyperflexion. Provide a quiet environment. Do not cluster nursing activities. Neurologic checks every hour, noting LOC, pupillary reaction, and strength and character of spontaneous movement. Monitor arterial blood gases and maintain P_{CO_2} less than 45 mm Hg.
Alterations in breathing patterns related to surgical incision and alterations in LOC possibly manifested by shallow, rapid respirations, absence of breath sounds, presence of rales, asymmetrical chest expansion, abnormal arterial blood gases	Patient will maintain an effective breathing pattern as evidenced by unlabored, deep respirations, respiratory rate of 12–24 breaths per minute, clear, equal breath sounds, $P_{O_2} > 100$ mm Hg pH 7.35 to 7.45; and $P_{CO_2} < 45$ mm Hg, symmetrical chest expansion	Auscultate lungs every 2 h, noting quality of breath sounds. Incentive spirometer every 2 h. Teach patient to splint flank incision with pillows for coughing. Cough, deep breathe, and turn every 2 h. Monitor arterial blood gases. Assess symmetry of chest expansion. Administer oxygen as ordered.
Alteration in comfort related to flank and cranial incision possibly manifested by verbalized complaints, restlessness, elevated heart rate and blood pressure, facial grimacing	Patient will achieve maximum level of comfort as evidenced by verbalization of relief, heart rate and blood pressure returning to baseline, absence of grimacing	Noninvasive pain measures as needed: backrub, repositioning, quiet environment. Ensure proper functioning of TENS unit. Medicate with nonnarcotic analgesics as ordered before activity. Assess effectiveness of pain measures.
Potential alteration in fluid volume (deficit) related to postoperative bleeding and an acute adrenal insufficiency crisis possibly manifested by increased heart rate, low blood pressure, falling hematocrit, low CVP, decreased or increased urine output, petechial hemorrhages, hyperkalemia, hypoglycemia, abnormal urine specific gravity	Patient will maintain an adequate circulating volume as evidenced by heart rate of 60–100 bpm, SBP greater than 90 mm Hg, CVP between 8 and 12 mm Hg, hematocrit between 40% and 50%, urinary output > 40 ml but < 200 ml/h, urine specific gravity 1.005 to 1.010, serum potassium level between 3.5 and 5 mEq/liter, serum glucose level between 70 and 110 mg	Circulatory assessment every hour. CVP every 2 h. Hematocrits as ordered. Strict intake and output hourly. Urine specific gravity every 2 h. Serum and urine electrolyte levels as ordered. Serum cortisol level as ordered. Examine character and amount of drainage on dressings.

achieved. Patients may continue to experience postural hypotension, and precautions should be taken to prevent injury.

Discharge planning is begun when the neurosurgeon and neurologist state that the patient's condition is stable. Evaluation of the patient's level of independence will provide information concerning the need for home health referrals and home aides (e.g., walker, lift chairs). A multidisciplinary discharge conference, which includes the patient and family members, is held. The autotransplant patient and family members have lived with PD before the procedure and usually have adapted their lives to it. Adaptive mechanisms identified in the patient's admission history are evaluated for their appropriateness for discharge. After discharge the patient will need to return to the medical center for further testing as determined by the team. This visit will include videotaping and CSF testing.

SUMMARY

The autotransplant of the adrenal medulla to the caudate nucleus in the treatment of PD offers a new alternative for patients suffering from this progressive, disabling disease. It is too early to predict the role of autotransplantation as a definitive treatment of PD, but preliminary evidence shows it to be a promising one. Cooperation among research centers is vital to help evaluate the effectiveness of the autotransplant. The usage of standardized rating scales and evaluation techniques at all of the autotransplant centers is necessary. As research protocols are expanded to include more patients in a variety of medical centers, nurses need to continually increase their knowledge of PD and the autotransplant procedure in order to provide consistent quality care for the patient. The procedure provides a unique experience for neuroscience nurses to combine their knowledge of a neurologic disease process with their expertise in caring for a neurosurgical patient. The ggnursing process provides a vehicle for coordinating a multidisciplinary team to meet the challenge of caring for the adrenal-caudate autotransplant patient.

ADDENDUM

In April 1988 an adrenal-caudate autotransplant was performed on a 41-year-old man who suffered from Huntington's chorea. The rationale for performing this procedure at Vanderbilt University Medical Center was based on evidence from research obtained at Vanderbilt using a model for Huntington's chorea in rats. This was the first time the autotransplant was performed to treat this disease, whose symptoms include uncontrollable movements, slow mental and physical deterioration, extreme depression, and emotional disturbances. Huntington's chorea is caused by degeneration of nerve cell bodies within the caudate nucleus. The mechanism of degeneration is not known. Researchers believe that the autotransplant will not cause any improvement in the clinical symptoms, but will hopefully slow down or stop the progression of the disease. This autotransplant was the first in a series of 24 patients whose range in age is from 24 to 50 years, and who are at varying degrees of disease severity.

The role of fetal transplantation is also currently being explored in animal models throughout the country as a possible treatment for PD. This, if it becomes a reality, opens a new frontier for neuroscience nursing. Ethical, moral, and legal issues will have to be addressed.

References

Backlund, E.O., Granberg, P.O., Hamberger, B., Knutsson, E., Martensson, A., Seduall, G., Seiger, A., & Olson, L. (1985). Transplantation of adrenal medullary tissue to the striatum in parkinsonism: First clinical trials. *Journal of Neurosurgery, 62*(2), 169–173.

Garrett, E. (1982). Parkinsonism: Forgotten considerations in medical treatment and nursing care. *Journal of Neurosurgical Nursing, 14*(1), 12–17.

Goetz, C.G., Olanow, C.W., Koller, V.C., Penn, R. D., Cahill, D., Morantz, R., Stebbins, G., Tanner, C.M., Klawans, H.L., Shannon, K.M., Commella, C.L., Witt, T., Cox, C., Waxman, W., & Gauger, L. (1989). Multicenter study of autologous adrenal medullary transplantation to the corpus striatum in patients with advanced Parkinson's disease. *New England Journal of Medicine, 320*(6), 337–341.

Guyton, A.C. (1986). *Textbook of Medical Physiology* (7th ed.), Philadelphia: W.B. Saunders.

Hickey, I.V. (1986). *The Clinical Practice of Neurological and Neurosurgical Nursing* (2nd ed.), Philadelphia: J.B. Lippincott.

Illson, T., Bressman, S., & Fahn, S. (1983). Current concepts in Parkinson's disease. *Hospital Medicine, 19*(11), 33–56.

Madrazo, I., Drucker-Colin, R., Diaz, R., Martinez-Mata, J., Torres, C., & Becerril, J. (1987). Open microsurgical autograft of adrenal medulla to the right caudate nucleus in two patients with intractable Parkinson's disease. *New England Journal of Medicine, 316*(14), 831–834.

Marinari, B. (1984). Stereotaxis. *Journal of Neuroscience Nursing, 16*(3), 140–143.

Moses, H. (1986). Parkinson's disease. In R.T. Johnson (Ed.). *Current Therapy in Neurologic Disease,* (pp. 236–243). Philadelphia: B.C. Decker Co.

Penn, R.D., Goetz, C.G., Tanner, C., Klawans, H.L., Shannon, K.M., Commella, C.L., & Witt, T.R. (1988). The adrenal medullary transplant operation for Parkinson's disease: Clinical observations in five patients. *New England Journal of Medicine, 319*(22), 999–1005.

15

Patient Education: Theory and Strategies

Katherine M. Sigardson-Poor and Lois Bartell

Patient education is an integral component of successful transplantation. A comprehensive, multidisciplinary plan needs to be developed in order to meet the clients' and their families' goals; however, it is primarily the nurse who is responsible for patient teaching. This chapter focuses on the theoretical components of education as well as practical methods to assist in patient education throughout the transplant process. Specific teaching and learning barriers and suggested means to overcome them are also discussed.

THEORETICAL FRAMEWORK

Dorothea Orem's theory of nursing is based on four broad concepts: (1) self-care, (2) self-care agency, (3) therapeutic self-care demand, and (4) nursing agency. Self-care refers to the activities of daily living that a person performs every day for herself. Self-care agency is a person's ability to perform the activities of daily living. Any activity that a person cannot carry out is a self-care deficit. Therapeutic self-care demand describes what is required to maintain a particular person's health and well-being. Some requirements may be imposed because of health-deviation demands. The concept of nursing agency refers to people who, because of education and experience, are able to care for those who are unable to meet their self-care demands.

Human beings are viewed as a whole by Orem with three functions: (1) biological, (2) behavioral, and (3) social. These would appear to be self-explanatory.

Nursing uses five methods of assisting a person to health: (1) acting for, (2) guiding, (3) supporting, (4) providing a developmental environment, and (5) teaching.

343

"Acting for" should be replaced as soon as possible with another method of assisting. The goal is to return the patient to a state in which she is able to meet her own self-care demands. This is accomplished by designing a system of assistance. Orem (1985) speaks of three systems. These are wholly compensatory, partially compensatory, and educative-developmental. Patients who are critically ill are wholly compensatory; they are unable to perform self-care activities. The nurse also makes all of the decisions regarding care.

Partially compensatory refers to a patient who is able to perform some or most self-care activities. Decision making is shared between the patient and nurse. The nurse must compensate for any self-care demands that the patient cannot meet.

The patient is able to meet her own self-care demands in the educative-developmental system; however, the patient may still need support and education to accomplish the self-care demands. The patient makes all of the decisions in this system, but the nurse may be able to influence these decisions through the teaching-learning process.

Orem's theory can be applied to the nursing process and is illustrated with clients undergoing organ and tissue transplantation. This, combined with a holistic view of the patient and family, will assist in individualizing patient education.

PRETRANSPLANT EVALUATION PHASE

Most transplant recipients are active, enthusiastic participants in the teaching-learning process. Many have been chronically ill and have received some information before consideration for transplant. This information may have come from relatives, the media (i.e., television, newspapers, pamphlets), or, more commonly, other patients (who may or may not have had a transplant) and nurses or other health professionals. Prior knowledge of the transplant process may have left the patient with some preconceived ideas (all of which may not be accurate) of what to expect. Before their first visit, some centers provide prospective patients with written or audio information consisting of basic facts regarding transplantation, which may dispel some previous misinformation.

Assessment

Assessment is the most important step of the nursing process because all other care is developed from this first step. It occurs during each patient encounter. In preparing to meet a patient and family for the first time it is important to set the "right" atmosphere. Comfortable chairs, plants, and refreshments may help to set the stage. It is important for the practitioner to be relaxed and warm, but not too familiar.

The nurse should be honest in answering the patient's questions and do this before asking questions herself. This will provide the nurse with information she needs to complete her assessment and will help to relax the patient.

After answering the patient's questions the nurse needs to take a health, social, and education history. Questions included in the health history relate to who currently assists the patient in meeting self-care demands, previous experiences with health care systems, and how therapeutic self-care demands are currently being met.

It is important to identify who the client is during the interview. This refers to the patient, family, significant others, or even the community in which the patient lives and works and how they react with each other. These people will be assisting the patient to meet her therapeutic self-care demands after transplant, and it is vital to assess their abilities before the planning stage. The nurse's relation to these people is shown in Figure 15–1.

A social history assessment question might be, "How do you spend

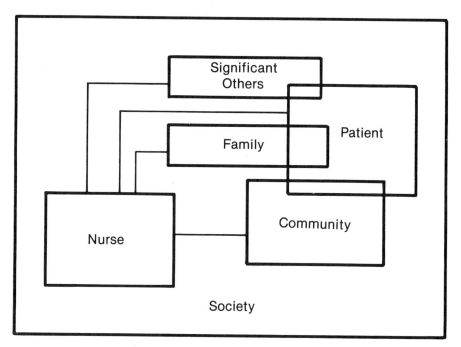

FIGURE 15–1. Nurse's relationship to clients.

your day?" A forward-looking follow-up would be, "How would you like to spend your day?"

It would be expedient to review with the patient how she has learned best in the past. Is it by reading, watching video, listening to audio cassettes, role playing, or playing games? Assess formal educational experiences, whether positive or negative. Finding out the highest level of formal education attained is not sufficient. During this part of the assessment the interviewer will need to determine the literacy status of the patient, if this has not already been noted by the referral source. It is not enough to judge whether the patient is able to read and write, but to what degree this is currently operating. Some people are able to read word by word, but their level of comprehension is low. This can be tested. A suggested method is to present the patient with a short (four to six sentences) information paragraph including some facts about transplantation, followed immediately by a multiple-choice question-and-answer test designed to ascertain understanding of what was just read. If the patient does not do well having read it to herself, it should be read aloud. A judgment can then be made as to whether the patient is having trouble with reading per se or with understanding what was read. It is important to document the findings so that this can be taken into consideration when planning the patient's educational program. It is also vital that this information be posted in confidentiality but so that all other care givers are aware of this factor. In this way inaccurate assumptions and expectations will not be made of the patient during her hospital stay.

Another question in the assessment phase should be, "What are your life goals?" This question may cause reflection on the part of the patient, but it may help to focus on realistic expectations of transplant. A summary of information to be garnered during the assessment is shown in Figure 15–2. It may be prudent to contact the source of the patient referral to verify information and impressions regarding the patient.

Analysis and Diagnosis

The second step is to analyze the data gathered during the assessment and identify deficits in the patient's ability to perform self-care. This includes demands foreseen owing to progressive illness requiring transplantation. Some nursing diagnoses may require the involvement of other members of the health care team, such as the dietitian. Current ability to meet self-care demands should be analyzed. The client may have some misconceptions regarding her current illness and any concurrent chronic illness.

THESE GOVERN NEED AND READINESS TO LEARN

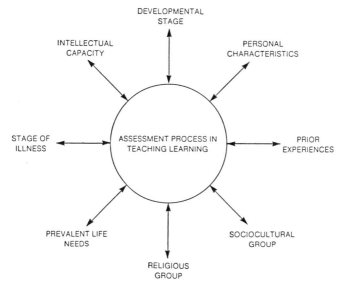

FIGURE 15–2. Areas for assessment. (Reprinted with permission from Stanton, M.P. [1985]. *Nursing Management, 16,* 59.)

Plan

At this stage the nurse and patient determine ways of meeting specified goals. It is important to differentiate what the patient wants and needs to know and what the nurse would like the patient to know. The identified goals need to be stated in such a manner as to be measurable. Goals can be divided into three types of objectives using the following categories: knowledge, comprehension, and application (Stanton, 1985). Dividing a goal into measurable stages can help the patient understand why it is important. To illustrate this, a patient may be asked to take serial blood pressure readings at home before transplant.

> Goal: The patient will take her blood pressure, record the measurements, and understand how this relates to her health status.
> Objectives:
> *Knowledge:* The patient defines blood pressure.
> *Comprehension:* The patient is able to discuss why it is important to take blood pressure measurement pretransplant.
> *Application:* The patient measures blood pressure and records the results.

In this way there are three means of evaluating whether or not the teaching-learning process accomplished the goal. Both the teacher and the learner will be able to identify where the process failed if the goal is not met. This method can be used whether the goal involves knowledge or psychomotor or attitudinal changes (Stanton, 1985).

Implementation

In the pretransplant phase the goals generally revolve around completing the evaluation. Patients need to know what tests are to be performed, why they are necessary, and how to complete the evaluation. Methods of assisting the patient to meet therapeutic self-care demands include possibly providing a checklist of patient responsibilities and encouraging the patient to make her own appointments for testing. Meeting another patient or participating in a support group may also be helpful. See Table 15–1 for specific steps to be completed pretransplant.

A group class is an effective and cost-efficient way to provide information regarding organ transplantation for prospective patients and family members. The use of overhead transparencies and clinical examples in informal presentation allows for learning, even though a two-hour class is necessary to cover all the material. If the system provides written information before the first clinic visit, the class and clinic visit will be shorter and provide reinforcement, rather than new information. After class a brief one-on-one encounter with each patient and family can clear up their immediate questions and concerns. Videotape programs may also be used. The colors need to be bright so as not to wash out when shown on television on a closed-circuit system.

At the conclusion of each teaching session the points covered should be summarized. Then the patient should be asked to state in her own words what she learned. By way of reinforcement, it is good strategy to

TABLE 15–1. PRETRANSPLANT EDUCATIONAL NEEDS

Physical evaluation tests	Quality of life after transplant
How to arrange for testing	Success rates, surgical risks
Where testing will occur	Adverse effects of medications
Why testing is necessary	Short-term complications
What patient will experience	Rejection
during test	Infection
Surgery	Ability to work
Posttransplant hospital care	Activity guidelines
Family involvement	Sexual functioning
Discharge criteria (expectations)	Long-term complications
Patient education and learning	Cancer
required	Eye and bone disease
Therapeutic self-care demands	Infection
Medications	Rejection
Dietary guidelines	Recurrent disease (if appropriate)
Physical self-assessment	Financial obligations

begin each teaching session with a review of the previous session. Verbal feedback from the patient can help the instructor to decide whether to proceed with the planned program or reteach the previous lesson. If the latter is decided, it is wise to use a different approach.

Evaluation and Documentation

Pretransplant goals need to be evaluated and documented. Many of the goals will be fairly easy to evaluate (e.g., were the physical evaluation tests completed?). Written or oral goals, quizzes, and discussion also assist in evaluation. Patients may also be able to state probable quality of life, therapeutic self-care demands, and financial obligations. Whether this information was internalized often cannot be evaluated until long after transplantation.

Documentation should include an evaluation of the patient's learning style. Posttransplant care may be assigned to a staff nurse whose teaching style best fits with a particular learning style. It is also important to document patient attitudes exhibited during this phase. If a patient calls frequently to question the outcome of each test, this pattern needs to be known to the staff who will be caring for the patient postoperatively. Documentation provides for continuity of care.

POSTTRANSPLANT MANAGEMENT

Assessment

Assessment of the patient's level of anxiety is central when beginning posttransplant education (see Chapter 16). Anxiety can be reduced by assuring the patient that she is safe and being properly cared for. Clear, concise explanations should be provided regarding all procedures and activities. Patient care should be coordinated in order to provide for rest periods. An atmosphere that is calm and reassuring can relax a patient so that she can identify reasons for anxiety.

In assisting patients to prepare for a teaching experience it is important to care for their physical needs. Acute symptoms such as pain, nausea, and vertigo should be alleviated.

One way of assessing readiness to learn is to place a medication wall chart in the patient's room soon after transplant (Fig. 15–3). Most patients will begin asking questions regarding information on the chart within one to two days post transplant. This practice has been useful in teaching not only the patients, but also their families. The chart should be fairly

MEDICATION	DOSAGE/ TIME	ACTION	ADVERSE EFFECTS
Cyclosporine	3.5 ml/ 8 AM and 8 PM	Prevents rejection	Nausea, hirsutism, tremors
Prednisone	25 mg/ breakfast	Prevents rejection	Increase blood pressure, water and salt retention, sun sensitivity, acne
Mycelex (Clotrimazole)	1 troche/ after meals or at bedtime	Prevents *Candida*	Bad taste
Zantac (Ranitidine)	150 mg/ breakfast and dinner	Prevents ulcers	
Lasix (Furosemide)	breakfast	Gets rid of excess water	Decreased potassium level

FIGURE 15–3. Medication wall chart.

large, about two by three feet. The large size enables it to be read across the room. Patients can take the chart home with them and refer to it until they are more comfortable with their medication routine.

Research has shown that anxiety is high and learning significantly decreased at two different times. These are just after transfer from the intensive care unit and just before discharge (Griesbach, 1985). Therefore, it may be best to plan teaching activities between these times.

Once it has been determined that the patient is ready to begin learning, it is important to implement the nursing process once again. An assessment should be made of what the patient already knows, what she would like to know, and what she needs to know.

A study was conducted in 1984 to determine which areas of patient teaching were most important for patients. The nurse responders identified the following as most important: (a) signs and symptoms of rejection, (b) signs and symptoms of infection, and (c) medication side effects (Sigardson, 1985). These and other areas are listed in Table 15–2.

One way of determining the patient's existing level of knowledge is to administer a pretest consisting of various types of questions (i.e., true-false, matching, fill in the blanks). The questions should cover content that the health care team thinks is vital for the patient to know in order to meet therapeutic self-care demands. Not all patients will be able to take a test, possibly because of illiteracy or other learning barriers. Discussion may be a means of determining what these patients already know.

Patients will be taking certain medications for the rest of their lives after a transplant, so the nurse needs to assess past medication compliance. Ask open-ended questions such as, "Do you have a hard time remembering to take your medications?" or, "Is there anything that could be done to make this task easier?"

The nurse needs to present questions and respond in a nonjudgmental manner. Many patients have a different life-style than that of the

TABLE 15–2. POSTTRANSPLANT EDUCATIONAL NEEDS

Rejection
    Prevention
    Signs and symptoms
    Treatment
    Possible outcomes
Infection
    Prevention (include safe sex, pets, gardening, travel)
    Signs and symptoms
    Treatment
Medications
    Name
    How much to take
    When to take
    How to take
    Why taking
    Adverse effects of medication and how to alleviate these
How and when to contact transplant personnel
    Routine
    Emergency
Activity restrictions
    Lifting
    Sexual
Exercise recommendations
Dietary recommendations
Follow-up clinic
    Laboratory
    Yearly Pap smear, chest x-ray, physical exam, cancer screening
General health care
    Dental
    Vaccinations

nurse. Patient responses may be geared to cause a reaction on the part of the nurse. If the nurse can remain calm and relaxed, this may go a long way toward developing a positive nurse-patient relationship. Some questions may be uncomfortable to ask, especially those dealing with sexual practices, but these may be vital in determining the posttransplant education plan.

Analysis and Nursing Diagnosis

Just as during the pretransplant phase, the data gathered need to be analyzed. Information obtained during the pretransplant interview and the evaluation phase needs to be included in the analysis. If a particular teaching-learning method was not effective before, it probably will not be now. The appropriate goals that need to be met before discharge should be determined.

The analysis may reveal that the patient is not able to meet therapeutic self-care demands without assistance. Sources of assistance (i.e., family, friends, visiting nurse) may need to be brought into the teaching-learning process at this time.

Plan

The patient should be presented with options on how to learn the specific teaching facts that need to be mastered before discharge. Priority is given to the learning deficits that the patient has identified. Goals should be realistic and able to be met before discharge. Goals that involve knowledge of specific anatomy and physiology may need to be met after hospital discharge.

When deciding which tools would best meet the learning style of the patient, it is important to keep in mind that people remember 15 per cent of what they read, 20 per cent of what they see, 30 per cent of what they hear, 50 per cent of what they see and hear, 70 per cent of what they see, hear, and personally experience, and 90 per cent of what they see, hear, personally experience and practice (Ojule, 1983). Consequently the more senses used in learning, the greater the degree of learning. Figure 15–4 shows various teaching techniques used in transplant programs and the percentage of use.

The advantages of videotapes are obvious: patients can view the tapes when they're feeling receptive or late in the day, when their family is interested, rather than when their nurses have time to teach. Patients can repeatedly view a tape to reinforce their knowledge. Before a patient views the tape, a nurse on the unit outlines the intended objectives and

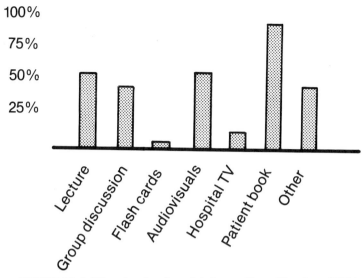

FIGURE 15–4. Educational tools and their use. (From Sigardson, 1985.)

mentions concepts that the patient should look for in the program (Banks-Gould & Hufschmidt, 1982).

Microcomputers with computer-assisted instruction will probably be as commonplace in the future as videotapes are today for patient education. The microcomputer, in conjunction with high-quality educational software, can present learning objectives to the user, maintain records of educational activities completed, and evaluate learner performance. Computer-assisted instruction provides an opportunity for patients to be actively involved in learning basic information about their conditions in a nonthreatening environment. Several hundred patient education software packages are being marketed on such topics as allergy, cancer, cardiology, diabetes, environmental health, family planning, human physiology, pregnancy, rheumatology, nutrition, ophthalmology, physical fitness, stress, substance abuse, medications, neurology, surgery, and weight control. Once a patient completes a lesson, the health care professional's time may be more efficiently used to answer the patient's specific questions. Computer-assisted instruction can be available in waiting rooms and patient education rooms, at the bedside on portable carts, at organization health fairs, or even at home with borrowed diskettes from a clinic with transmission of their answers by way of modems. The cost of computer-assisted instruction can be recovered in many ways, including savings in staff time, increased patient satisfaction, increased referrals, fees for educational services, and, under some circumstances, direct third-party reimbursement. The cost of microcomputer hardware and software is falling rapidly as technology improves and the market becomes glutted.

Because transplantation is complicated and difficult to understand, written and audio materials are often inadequate for those who are illiterate and those with cultural or language barriers. Special materials need to be developed. Refer to the section on special needs at the end of this chapter.

Implementation

Initial teaching sessions should focus on what the patient wants to know. At the beginning of each teaching session the patient is told what information will be presented, then the information is presented, and finally, either the nurse or the patient summarizes what was presented.

Because new medications represent a concrete change in the patient's life, this topic is frequently taught first. A chart similar to that shown in Figure 15–3 may already be in the patient's room. Additionally, the nurses have been bringing the patient medications and answering questions. The nurse should begin by sitting down with the patient and developing a medication schedule, taking into account the patient's daily routine. The schedule should be arranged for the patient's convenience. Scheduling doses around mealtimes and bedtime may help the patient to remember when to take the medications.

A container large enough to hold all of the patient's medication bottles should be provided. Individual bottles of medication similar to what the patient would obtain from her regular pharmacy can be supplied by the hospital pharmacy. Each bottle should be labeled with the name and strength of the medication. Each time a medication is scheduled, the patient should obtain the correct medication from the bin, set aside the indicated dose, and call the nurse. The nurse can then check for patient accuracy, answer any questions, and quiz the patient about the medication. This system provides the nurse with the necessary information for medication charting. Later on, as the patient becomes more familiar with the medication routine, information regarding possible adverse effects can be presented, followed by a discussion of how to cope with these effects.

It is important to observe patients writing changes on their medication record. Frequently dosages are changed over the telephone after discharge, and the staff needs to be reassured that the patient is able to do this accurately. Patients who participate in self-medication programs feel a sense of control over some aspect of their posttransplant hospital care. It also makes them responsible and accountable for their own self-care. The self-confidence developed by this program can also spur the patient to learn other aspects of self-care before discharge.

Many transplant programs also place medication responsibility with their pediatric patients. Generally, a child between four and six years of age who has mastered the alphabet can match the medicine names on the bottle with the name on the medication card or list. The child can then count out the number of pills needed, as indicated on the list. Parents do need to check to make sure the correct dose is taken, especially if elixirs are involved.

Middle school–age children like to be more independent. Ideally, the parent should observe the medication routine. Realistically, parents may need to look for signs of skipping doses. Counting how many pills are left is one method. A child who becomes angry and belligerent when discussing medications may also be missing doses.

Sometimes dealing with the adolescent patient can be the most difficult. Conflict over control is common, and adherence to the medication regimen may be part of the conflict. Adolescent noncompliance may also be due to the effects of medication on body image. A peer support group may be helpful so that the teenager does not feel alone in her situation. Peers may also convince the patient that the consequences of not taking medication as prescribed are serious.

In some programs it is important for patients to obtain their own laboratory values. The names of the tests and what they indicate should be reviewed (Sophie & Bartell, 1981). The nurse can look over several days' worth of values with the patient and then discuss the trends, the reasons they occurred, and their implications. The fact that values are looked at each day in relation to the previous day's values, not necessarily in comparison to a chart of normal values, should be emphasized to the patient and family. This information may need to be repeated many times before they begin to understand, but it doesn't mean that they should assume any responsibility for whether the test value requires treatment. In future teaching sessions the nurse can outline parameters of normal results, if the patient and family indicate an interest. The patient should be shown where to record values in her handbook (described later). The nurse can record the first set of values or dictate the numbers and guide the patient in where to write them. With each set of numbers the nurse should assist less and less until the patient is recording all the values without any assistance. Then the patient should be given responsibility to ask for and record her values each day.

Almost all transplant programs provide their patients with a handbook. The handbook contains information regarding medications and laboratory tests, self-care recommendations, and charts for keeping track of data. Patients are encouraged to read the information, highlight or underline as they wish, and write down their questions. Patients can use the handbook after discharge as a reference and to reinforce information presented during hospitalization.

Before discharge it may be helpful for the patient to imagine being at home and meeting her own therapeutic self-care demands (e.g., self-medication, vital sign monitoring, trips to the laboratory, and clinic visits). Questions may arise from this experience as the patient begins to plan for discharge.

Evaluation and Documentation

After each teaching-learning session the nurse needs to document what material was presented, by whom and when, and the results (see Fig. 15–5).

Evaluation of cognitive learning can be done through written or oral quizzes or, for example, by checking the patient's dietary choices. The nurse needs to decide which method is best for a particular patient.

Psychomotor skills can be evaluated by using the return demonstration technique. The patient may be asked to lay out all of the medications she needs to take at a specified time; or she may be asked to take her own blood pressure with the nurse verifying the results using a stethoscope with two sets of earpieces.

Affective or attitudinal learning may only be evaluated months or years after initial teaching occurs. Teaching in this area may require repeated reinforcement from both the patient's support group and the nurse in the clinic after discharge.

Evaluation is an ongoing process during teaching-learning sessions. If one teaching tool has not been effective, another should be tried. Some patients need more time to learn, or a variety of tools with which to learn. A comprehensive catalog of existing tools is available through the North American Transplant Coordinators Organization and the American Council on Transplantation.

Documentation of patient teaching and learning is vital in providing continuity of care, especially in large transplant centers. Pretransplant evaluation and posttransplant coordination may be divided among several staff members. Nurses on the posttransplant care unit are involved in patient care too, as well as outpatient clinic nurses.

Referral

Because of pre-set reimbursement rates for transplant, patients may be discharged home before meeting their learning needs completely. Referral may be necessary to arrange for nursing support of these needs.

The nurse making the referral needs to assess the capabilities of the referral agency. Many have had little experience working with transplant patients and may need an education program before working with the patient.

Special Teaching-Learning Situations

Special consideration must be given to patients who are unable to learn the necessary self-care activities because of sensory deficits and illiteracy. Another group of patients, those who are labeled "noncompliant," also have special needs.

Sensory deficits

Patients frequently have sensory deficits because of their original disease that necessitated transplantation in the first place (i.e., diabetes, Alport's syndrome, brachio-oto-renal syndrome). Each deficit can be effectively dealt with, enabling a patient to achieve self-care.

Blind or partially sighted patients can provide much of their own care after transplantation. Many devices have recently been developed to measure temperature, blood pressure, and blood glucose and deliver a verbal response. If these are not available, a significant other or public health nurse can be of assistance.

Medication bottles with raised letters or braille labels can be provided for the patient. When these bottles need to be refilled it should be done by a pharmacist or two sighted persons to lessen the chances for mistakes. Medication cards with raised letters or braille can also be provided for these patients. The cards should have a hole punched in them and be bound together on a ring so that one is not accidentally lost. This way the cards can easily be changed to reflect medication dose changes. Also, consider referring blind patients to specialized agencies or schools when needed. Plastic syringe cards to assist such patients in drawing up their own insulin are available commercially. Audio teaching materials may be best for these patients.

Hearing-impaired patients can also present a teaching challenge. Some patients with a hearing loss may refuse to use a hearing aid for cosmetic reasons, because of discomfort from the device, or because of the increased background noise that they hear when they wear it. It is important to remember that a hearing aid amplifies all noise, not just the voice of an individual, and the background noise is more difficult to "filter out" for a hearing-impaired person. When speaking with a person who uses a hearing aid eliminate extraneous noise, look at her, talk slowly, and enunciate clearly. Low-pitched voices are easier to hear. Patients with a hearing loss frequently become frustrated with their

UNIVERSITY OF MINNESOTA HOSPITALS & CLINICS
PATIENT TEACHING FLOW SHEET
ORGAN TRANSPLANTATION

INSTRUCTIONS:
1. Complete INITIAL ASSESSMENT; DATE and INITIAL.
2. Identify Patient Teaching Outcomes (skills or knowledge that the patient needs to demonstrate).
3. Identify all methods and patient teaching materials used. Include classes attended by patient.
4. Note DATE/INITIALS each time the patient/family is taught; along with comments regarding patient's progress when indicated.

PATIENT IDENTIFICATION PLATE

5. Note DATE/INITIAL when outcome is met (when learning has occurred).

INITIAL ASSESSMENT		
(DATE)	PATIENT READINESS TO LEARN (E.G., ASKING QUESTIONS, INTEREST IN DISCHARGE) BARRIERS (HANDICAPS, ACUITY OF ILLNESS) MOTIVATION	
	I am willing to participate in learning how to take care of myself at home (patient/parent/guardian signature):	
(INITIALS)	LEARNING NEEDS IDENTIFIED BY PATIENT	

	PATIENT TEACHING OUTCOMES	METHODS MATERIALS (DATE/INITIAL)	TAUGHT (DATE/INITIAL)	PROGRESS & COMMENTS	PATIENT OUTCOME MET — PATIENT (DATE/INITIAL)	FAMILY (DATE/INITIAL)
DIET	1. States rationale for diet plan	Handbook				
	2. Describes ways of adjusting diet plan/fluid restriction	Dietician's Instruction				
DIABETES CARE	GLUCOSE MANAGEMENT:					
	1. Demonstrates ability to use glucose monitoring devices— state method(s) used:	Handbook				
	2. States plan to manage glucose at home with L.M.D.	Diabetes Care Class				
	3. States effects of Prednisone on glucose/insulin					
	4. Describes appropriate treatment for hypoglycemia					
	5. Demonstrates ability to record glucoses/insulin in Handbook	Nurse's Instruction				
	FOOT CARE:					
	6. States significance of Daily DFC					
	7. Report any foot trauma as an emergency					
A.D.L.	1. Describes actions to maintain health and hygiene regarding:	Handbook				
	—exercise	Home Care Class				
	—incisional care					
	—bath/shower					
	—skin care/acne treatment					
	—hair care/permanent/coloring	Nurse's Instruction				
	—oral care					
	—returning to work/school					
	—bowel function					
	—CONTINUED—					

SIGNATURE & CLASSIFICATION		

28068, MAY 84

FLOW SHEET

PATIENT TEACHING

FIGURE 15–5. Teaching checklist.

PATIENT TEACHING OUTCOMES	METHODS MATERIALS (DATE · INITIAL)	TAUGHT (DATE · INITIAL)	PROGRESS & COMMENTS	PATIENT OUTCOME MET	
				PATIENT (DATE · INITIAL)	FAMILY (DATE / INITIAL)

HOME MANAGEMENT

1. Demonstrates ability to monitor and record:
   - temperature (BID)
   - pulse (before certain meds)
   - blood pressure (3 times/week and prn) lying and standing if orthostatic
   - weight (daily in a.m.)
   - height (monthly under 18 yr)
   - intake and output (oxalosis only)
   - lab values (3 times/week)

   Handbook

2. States rationale for and significance of:
   - no ASA or ASA containing meds
   - sunscreen daily to prevent skin cancer
   - wearing or carrying emergency medical identification
   - no pet bird
   - antibiotic coverage before dental work (no routine dental work for 6 months)
   - no corrective eye lens change for 6 months
   - no smoking
   - use of alcohol

   Home Care Class

SEXUALITY:

3. Identifies that there are no restrictions on sexual activity

4. States method of birth control to be used after surgery

5. States rationale for yearly pap and breast exam

   Nurse's Instruction

6. States potential change in male sexuality

7. States procedure for communicating with transplant office/answering service regarding:
   - routine lab values/follow-up care
   - current L.M.D. name/phone
   - L.M.D. treatment
   - mailing cyclosporine levels
   - illness/exposure to infectious disease (temp greater than 100°F, rapid weight gain or other unusual changes)
   - return to clinic

MISC.

LIST OTHER TEACHING FLOW SHEETS USED (i.e., R. Atrial Catheter, Ostomy, IV Therapy)

1. Operative Checklist

2. Medications (Organ Transplant)

Clinic Follow-Up

CLINIC NURSE RESPONSIBILITIES:

1. Monthly breast exam instruction

SIGNATURE & CLASSIFICATION				

FIGURE 15–5 *Continued.* **Teaching checklist.**

inability to hear and may nod as if they understand. It is vital for the teacher to validate what the learner has heard and understands. Lip reading has been shown to be fairly inaccurate. Visual teaching materials may be best for these patients.

Illiteracy

Determining whether someone is illiterate may be difficult because many people go to elaborate lengths to hide the fact that they cannot read or write. Some camouflage the problem by surrounding themselves with newspapers, books, and magazines. Some circumvent the problem by asking hospital visitors to read things to them. Others claim to have forgotten their glasses or may be anxious or hostile toward any "book work." It is possible to discover this situation early in the pretransplant period, and it is highly recommended that it be done then. (Refer to Pretransplant Evaluation Phase above.) One way of assessing the patient is simply to ask her to read the paper cover of a disposable tongue blade or other such item readily available. This will enable the nurse to assess whether the patient can read words, but not whether she can understand what she reads. A suggested method of determining comprehension has been previously discussed. Refer the patient to the social worker to arrange for an adult education course in her area if the patient appears receptive to this course of action.

Some points to be aware of regarding the illiterate patient: Adults who have struggled for years with this handicap often have a low sense of self-esteem and need more bolstering than do others who take this attained skill for granted. They have a tendency to measure their self-worth in terms of this one factor only. These patients may display defiance and defensiveness when the subject comes up or their handicap becomes known, depending on how sensitive they are about it. Others are more open and forthcoming about it and appear to have come to some kind of terms of acceptance regarding this lack in their lives. In either instance, it is well to watch and listen for remarks of self-denigration (e.g., "I'm so stupid" or "I guess I'm just too dumb"). Each time one hears these or similar statements, firmly and dispassionately disavow the statement. Focus on what they can do as evidenced by their life experiences. Often this is a revelation to them, a new way of looking at themselves. Emphasize to the patient that she is no less a worthy person because she is not able to read and write. Assure her that you will help her learn what it is she needs to know regarding her health and self-care, and that it can be done whether or not she can read. Together you will find a way.

It is important to keep lines of communication free and open. Watch for and be aware of body language and facial expressions that might be indicative of a lack of understanding (e.g., frowning, shaking of the head) and respond immediately. Verbal repetition may be necessary. If so, make sure that the same terminology is used each time in explaining some item of use or care. If you think that it is necessary that the patient know more than one word for an item (e.g., catheter, tube), be certain that the patient understands that these words are being used interchangebly.

Some patients may feel intimidated by hospital or professional personnel; they may feel that the nurse, doctor, technician, or clinician has all sorts of knowledge that they do not and can never have. They may be sensitive about their lack of formal education and very much aware of the hospital staff's. This can also be true of patients who are not illiterate. These kinds of barriers to learning can be broken down by a genuine show of concern, caring, and constant reassurance that they, too, can take control of their situation just as the hospital staff is now doing for them. Avoid scientific terminology when possible and explain it when it must be used. Also, avoid "in-house" abbreviations such as EKG, BP, BUN, and MCV, particularly when talking about laboratory values. These abbreviations are confusing to those who are not familiar with hospital jargon. If you do decide or prefer to use abbreviations in conversation with patients, be prepared to explain not only what they stand for, but their meanings as well.

Illiterate clients do not have to be viewed as a teaching problem; in fact, it may be better to think of illiteracy as a factor in considering teaching strategies rather than as a problem. It can be viewed as a challenge that requires alternative and innovative teaching techniques, such as story typing, a strategy used in beginning reading. Often, out of necessity, illiterate people have highly developed compensatory observational skills. Take advantage of this skill if it is demonstrated and use it as part of the teaching strategy. If a client cannot tell time, an alternative is to draw clocks, or the sun or moon in the sky as a time indicator (Dunn, Buckwalter, Weinstein, & Palti, 1985). For the foreign patient who is unable to read English, one can use a medication flip card, 4 by 8 inches, bound in plastic. Cards can easily be added or subtracted as dictated by the patient's medication regimen. For an activity prescription, draw pictures or use magazine pictures and photographs to construct pages of both allowed and not allowed activities. Draw a large red X across disallowed activities (Dunn et al., 1985).

Nonadherence

Noncompliance, or nonadherence, describes the behavior of a category of patients who are not taking medications properly, not coming for clinic visits or laboratory appointments, not calling the transplant center as previously instructed for problems, not staying on prescribed diets, and not following health advice in general. As a group, they are difficult to deal with and can provide a constant source of frustration to their caregivers. Patients who are unable to adhere to their medical regimen have many reasons for their behavior. The nurse is in a unique position to seek out these reasons, especially if she has a good rapport with the patient.

Many concerns can occupy the patient's attention while the nurse is attempting to teach new and complicated information. These concerns need to be alleviated to some degree before the patient can learn even the most basic self-care post transplant. The patient is unable to "hear" or be attentive to what is being taught because of these other concerns.

Medications and abnormal blood chemistries can diminish the patient's ability to concentrate and remember information. One category of medication commonly implicated is steroids, along with pain-relieving medication the patient may also be taking. The use of diuretics may shorten the time a patient has to sit before she has to urinate. If attention and concentration are diminished by elevated blood urea nitrogen and creatinine levels, then higher intellectual functions of abstraction, generalization, and language skills cannot be effectively executed. There is some support of the notion that every dialysis patient is experiencing at least mild organic brain dysfunction that affects learning (Redman, 1984).

Once it has been determined that the patient understands what has been taught, it is important to determine why she is not complying with the prescribed regimen. Consider these questions:

- Is the prescribed regimen too restrictive (e.g., diet)?
- Are there too many, too often (e.g., medications, laboratory tests)?
- How does it taste (e.g., medication, diet)?
- What does it cost (e.g., medications, laboratory tests, time)?

Decreasing complexity should improve compliance by reducing medications to the minimum number necessary to produce the desired result and by minimizing the frequency of pill taking. Also, those monitoring practices that don't really matter and that interfere with quality of life, such as measuring intake and output at home, wearing a mask, and avoiding crowds, can be eliminated. Cost should be considered, and reduced when possible. It is less expensive and more convenient to take a single pill that contains more milligrams once a day than a pill that contains fewer milligrams twice a day. By tailoring the prescribed regimen to their specific characteristics, patients feel as though they are being treated as individuals, and this should improve their compliance.

Consider this example: A patient who is experiencing a decreasing white blood cell count, presumably caused by azathioprine, is instructed to decrease her azathioprine dose and start a low dose of cyclosporine. The last time she was on cyclosporine she experienced severe gastrointestinal symptoms that made her quality of life unbearable. Her highest motive is wanting to please the health care professionals responsible for her care. Fear of diminishing her quality of life hindered her from taking even one dose of cyclosporine. This shows how a patient can be noncompliant, without the health care team's knowing, because of fear—fear of reprisal for not following instructions.

Promoting patient autonomy can also improve adherence to the prescribed regimen. Logical decision-making practices should be taught when possible. Of concern are patients who use logic but end up with the wrong decision. One patient knew that excessive vitamin C would negate the effect of her prophylactic sulfa antibiotic. However, she believed that high doses of vitamin C made her diabetic neuropathy better, so she chose to take the vitamin C and not take the prescribed co-trimoxazole, since it wouldn't be effective anyway. She didn't report her choice for several weeks.

After discovering the causes of nonadherence, it is important to reach a mutually agreed on course of action and document the plan. Both the nurse and patient should sign this documentation, thereby giving the patient responsibility for following through with the plan.

CONCLUSION

Education of the organ transplant recipient is complex, involves all aspects of health and wellness, and is supremely rewarding when the patient's well-being is improved because of the nurse's knowledge.

It is important not to assume that the person is managing a chronic illness well just because it was diagnosed many years ago and a treatment regimen was established.

The goal of teaching is to help the patient feel comfortable and confident managing self-care at home. If the environment and equipment in the hospital are different from what the patient will experience at home, a difficult learning situation is created for the patient. Patients frequently voice their concern at "not being able to remember to do everything right" once they are at home. When they feel comfortable performing a procedure at home because they did exactly the same thing when they were in the hospital, going home becomes more comfortable and safer.

Points to remember:

- The number of drugs and administration times should be kept to an essential minimum.

- Drug regimens should be worked out to fit in with the patient's daily routine.

- The patient should have a suitable drug container that she can handle. Large bottles should be used so that labeling can be adequate. Palm-sized, brown plastic containers with screw or snap tops are the most satisfactory, especially for patients with neuropathy.

- Labels should be clearly printed using large letters, preferably typed.

- A clear, handy medicine card or list that names all prescription and nonprescription medications is necessary to enhance communication to all health care providers of the patient's medication program.

- Instruction sheets should be supplied as necessary.

- All those concerned with the patient's care should be aware of what one another are doing and what instructions have been issued.

- Specially designed pill containers and dispensers with times and days improve adherence.

- Concern should be shown and the patient confronted if noncompliance is demonstrated.

References

Banks-Gould, M. & Hufschmidt, A.P. (1982, July/August). When you're the teacher—turn on the television. Nursing Life, 20, 54.

Dunn, M.M., Buckwalter, K.C., Weinstein, L.B., & Palti, H. (1985). Innovations in family and community health. Family and Community Health, 8(3), 76–80.

Griesbach, E.H. (1985, Summer). Anxiety and the timing of diabetes teaching in the hospital: A literature review. The Diabetes Educator, 20, 43.

Miller, A. (1985, July). When is the time ripe for teaching? American Journal of Nursing, 20, 801.

Ojule, C. (1983, March). Workshop in intercultural training sponsored by Washington

Association of Professional Anthropologists. Annual meeting of the Society for Applied Anthropology, San Diego, Calif.

Orem, D.E. (1985). *Nursing: Concepts of Practice* (3rd ed.). New York: McGraw-Hill.

Redman, B.K. (1984). *The Process of Patient Teaching in Nursing* (5th ed.). St. Louis: C.V. Mosby.

Sigardson, K.M. (1985). Renal Transplant Center Survey. Paper presented at a meeting of the North American Transplant Coordinators Organization, San Diego.

Sophie, L.R. & Bartell, L. (1981). Patient education: The patient as partner. *Dialysis and Transplantation, 10*(5), 444.

Stanton, M.P. (1985, October). Teaching patients: Some basic lessons for nurse educators. *Nursing Management, 16,* 59.

16

Managing the Psychosocial Responses of the Transplant Patient

Virginia H. Carr

Jake was 12 years old when he was diagnosed as having Wilson's disease, a rare liver disease that, if untreated, results in liver failure and death. His parents had no warning of this catastrophic news, except for Jake's vague complaints of intermittent "stomach aches" over the past few weeks.

When their family doctor offered them no hope for Jake's recovery, they began an intense search for information relating to their son's condition. In the process they found an article in a lay publication describing liver transplantation as an option for treating end-stage liver disease. This discovery changed their lives. They moved from a position of helplessness and grief to one of hope through transplantation.

With support from their family doctor, Jake's parents contacted the nearest transplant center. Their hope began to wane as they were informed that not only must Jake be evaluated and meet the criteria necessary for transplantation but also, if he were chosen, there would be a chance that a matched organ would not be donated in time to keep him alive.

During their first interview with the transplant team Jake and his family discovered that the waiting period was unpredictable. They realized that they would need to secure financial support not only for the surgery, but also for the secondary expenses of out-of-town lodging, loss of work time, and provisions for the care of their three younger children. In addition, they must manage Jake's potentially deteriorating condition and be available to come to the transplant center with only a few hours' notice.

Spared a long wait, they were notified that an organ was available the week after Jake's evaluation. The wheels began to turn before the family had an opportunity to sort through their needs. They were launched into a state in which their hope, joy, and fear were felt simultaneously.

Jake's surgery was successful and his recovery smooth, but his world would never be the same. What would accompany Jake for the remainder of his life would be a regimen of life-sustaining medications and the perpetual threat of rejection of his new organ. Jake and his family would come to view his every physical discomfort as a potential threat to life and would have to relinquish the view of their world as secure. The limits imposed by this view would be countered, however, by the gradual awareness that Jake had been given a second chance at life.

Jake's case presents, in part, a concept known by transplant recipients and their families as the "emotional roller coaster" of organ transplantation. The same concept has been described in the literature as a distinct psychological process, marked by specific stages and experienced by both recipients and their families. These stages coincide with specific time periods during transplant therapy and are characterized by common stressors and emotional responses (Allender, Shisslak, Kaszniak, & Copeland, 1983; Christopherson, 1987; O'Brien, 1985).

Nurses are often present at every stage of the transplant process. They are always touched, and sometimes overwhelmed, by the emotional needs and responses of this group of patients and their families. This chapter focuses on these issues and the nurse's role in their management.

A model based on the stages of transplantation is presented in this chapter, and the common stressors of both patient and family are identified. Nursing diagnoses are used to categorize the characteristic psychosocial responses, and assessment and intervention strategies are offered.

It is important when using this mode to individualize treatment and recognize that many factors affect the transition through these stages, including patient age, cause of illness, patient and family knowledge level regarding the illness, treatment available, degree of pain and disability, rehabilitation potential, changes in family role, state of growth and development in the life cycle, and premorbid personality traits (Gulledge, Buszta, & Montague, 1983).

This chapter is limited to the normal responses that occur in relation to the transplant process. Although premorbid personality style and psychopathology brought on by the situational crisis of a life-threatening disease may be apparent in some individuals and will create special treatment problems, others have addressed the special needs of these individuals in more depth (Castelnuovo-Tedesco, 1971; Watts, Freeman, McGiffin, Kirklin, McVay, & Karp, 1984).

STAGES OF TRANSPLANTATION

Transplant Proposed

The first stage begins when a transplant is initially offered to a patient as a treatment option and ends when a decision to be evaluated is made. Patients enter this period in various states of health. Whereas one may be at the end stage of a chronic illness, another may be experiencing her disease for the first time after a sudden and severe onset. There are times, especially with acute disease, when family members must make the transplant decision for the patient. In many cases the transplant proposal accompanies the devastating news that this treatment is the patient's only hope for survival.

One of the greatest stressors for the transplant patient and family during the proposal stage is the fear of death (Christopherson, 1987; O'Brien, 1985). Patients are faced with the reality that without treatment, they will die. Although this fear may be the focus, a more unspoken fear is that of the dying process. One patient shared her experience: "It is not death that frightens me, but a vision of myself lying in the hospital bed dying alone while my pain and fear become invisible to those around me."

During this stage overwhelming anxiety may occur as the patient and family struggle with the myths and unknowns of transplantation. The combination of fear and anxiety, along with the multiple stressors that have accompanied their particular illness, can leave both the patient and family at risk for ineffective coping.

The anger, depression, and sadness associated with the grieving process may be apparent as the recipients and their families attempt to cope with the many real and potential losses. In addition to the most obvious loss of physical well-being, both the family and the patient may be dealing with the loss of roles, financial security, self-esteem, and their view of the world as predictable and safe.

Evaluation

The evaluation stage begins when the patient first undergoes assessment for transplant candidacy and continues until she is put on the list to await a suitable organ. In addition to the stresses of their illness during this period, patients and families must deal with the disruption that a period of hospitalization brings. There is additional stress for those who reside out of town and are separated from their major support systems.

The stage of evaluation is a time of much uncertainty as patients await the verdict of whether they will qualify for an organ. If they do not, it will guarantee them a shortened life.

Even as they are being evaluated, it is not uncommon for patients to express doubt about their decision. They may perceive that their family members are pressuring them to be evaluated, and sometimes these perceptions are accurate. Stresses over finances become an issue as the hospital assesses the patient's ability to pay for the procedure. Some patients are confronted with the fact that their insurance will not cover expenses and that they must raise the funds themselves in order to survive.

Awaiting a Donor

The third stage begins when a patient is placed on the waiting list and ends when the call is received that an organ is available. Despite the fact that they have been informed of the realities of receiving an organ, pretransplant patients and their families hope for immediate results and may fantasize that they will be called the day they are listed. It is not unusual for patients and families to report experiencing a physical response when the telephone rings in expectation that an organ is available. It is common, especially in the early stage, for patients and their families to experience a change in life-style requiring that all family members be on alert and put all their plans on hold. Although a family must be prepared and available for the time an organ does become available, an intense vigilance can be unnecessarily stressful for the family. The logistics about waiting and notification must be thoroughly explained. Patients and families need to be reassured that every effort will be made to locate and contact them.

As the waiting period continues, fears of dying reemerge (Christopherson, 1987; O'Brien, 1985). Patients and families begin to question whether an organ will become available in time. They may even begin to doubt that their names were placed on the list. They may have met other candidates who were evaluated after them, yet have already received their organs. Their trust in the team and the transplant process may wane as stresses build and coping diminishes.

Another prevalent response seen during the waiting stage is guilt (Christopherson, 1987; O'Brien, 1985). The source of guilt may be based in the patient's feeling that she is using too much of the family's resources, or she may realize that another human being must die for her to live. Another less verbalized source emerges from the patient's or family's hope that someone's death will occur soon and admit to tracking local accidents in the hope that an organ will become available to them.

Another response often felt during the waiting period is powerlessness (Christopherson, 1987). Potential recipients are confronted with certain death if they do not receive a transplant, but the process of obtaining this treatment is out of their control. They must depend entirely on a family donor or another's death to remain alive. Patients and families are expected to wait an indefinite period, wondering whether the patients will live long enough to benefit from this treatment. It is a difficult period for all as they attempt to live normal lives, feeling little power to move toward recovery.

Perioperative Period

The perioperative stage begins when an organ is matched and ends when the transplant surgery is complete. The predominant responses seen at this time are fear and anxiety mixed with excitement and relief (O'Brien, 1985).

The fear, again, relates to survival as the patient and family wonder whether they will see each other again. It is at this point that the anxiety level of the family increases. Although relieved perhaps of a long period of waiting for an organ, they must now endure a second wait as they focus on the outcome of surgery. Their concerns continue to be the survival of their family member and whether they will be competent to care for the patient after surgery.

Postoperative Period

The postoperative period begins when the patient arrives in the recovery room or intensive care unit (ICU) and is complete at the time of discharge. This time can be divided into two distinct stages: the early postoperative period (the time spent in the ICU) and the late postoperative period (the time spent on the transplant unit).

The ICU experience is marked by increased anxiety and powerlessness for both the patient and the family. The patient's physical appearance may be dramatically changed because of the long surgery, and she may be unable to communicate. Despite the fact that the family may have been prepared, intense anxiety may reemerge on seeing their family member for the first time. Because the ICU environment can be intimidating, and they are entering after a long and tiring wait, the family may easily lose confidence in its role as caregiver.

After making the transition from the ICU to the transplant unit, patients experience a "honeymoon stage" (Christopherson, 1987; O'Brien, 1985). During this time they feel all the joys and hopes of a rebirth. Families share this experience, as it serves as a much deserved respite for all. During this time, however, families' anxieties continue to increase. They wonder what their responsibilities will be now that the surgery is over. They may begin to question their abilities to manage the patient's care at home. Many struggle with the unspoken fear of losing their roles as caregivers now that the patient is moving toward recovery.

Complications and Death

The honeymoon stage can end abruptly for patients who face complications, such as the first rejection episode. Their fantasies about "being cured" must be abandoned as they realize that they have replaced their pretransplant symptoms with threats of rejection, infection, and other complications of transplant surgery.

Many patients have minor complications that are resolved during a short hospital stay, whereas others experience more serious problems (e.g., life-threatening infection and total rejection of the graft) and must endure a long and frustrating period of recovery in the hospital. The resolution of these complications may take from weeks to months. The fear of death and dying and the anxiety of the unknown underlie this period of complications. The patient and family often struggle with decreasing amounts of energy to cope.

Guilt emerges as the patient and family begin to question their decision to have a transplant. This is a difficult time for the transplant patient, family, and health care team. The crescendo of hope and joy experienced initially gives way to discomfort and loss of confidence in the transplantation process. It can be a time of great discouragement as the injustices of life are deeply felt by all.

In addition to managing the fear of death that returns when complications arise, the patient and family must continue to deal with the loss of control over their lives brought on by a long hospitalization. The patient, family, and transplant team may suffer with their perceived inability to control the situation.

There are times when, after a long period of suffering, the transplant treatment ends with the death of a recipient. Under these circumstances the family can be expected to manifest intense feelings of relief, sadness, depression, and anger (Christopherson, 1987). Depending on the stage of grieving, these feelings will emerge with varying intensities and with different targets. Most families will allow the staff to mourn with them as they all deal with feelings of loss, whereas other families will direct their anger toward the staff, blaming them for not having saved their family member's life.

Discharge

The discharge stage extends from the time patients are told that they are going home until they leave the hospital. It is marked by continued anxiety for both the patient and the family (Allender et al., 1983; O'Brien, 1985). The anxiety at this point is primarily related to the issues of physical separation from the hospital and transplant team.

A common cause for concern at this time is organ rejection. Patients may express such fears as doing themselves harm by eating certain foods or dislodging the organ through too much activity. Recipients who live out of town worry about their ability to make it back to the hospital in time for treatment. Families worry that they will be unable to manage the patient at home and take on the responsibility for any problems that may occur. Some patients may become so anxious about leaving that physical symptoms of anxiety may occur that prevent them from being discharged (e.g., increased blood pressure or stomach pains).

Postdischarge

The postdischarge stage begins when the patient leaves the hospital and extends indefinitely. The most predominant responses seen initially are anxiety, the depressive stage of the grieving process, disturbance in self-image, and alteration in family process (Allender et al., 1983; Christopherson, 1987). As they adjust to the separation from the hospital, the concerns experienced by patients and families at discharge are replaced by anxiety surrounding long-term issues (e.g., returning to work, stabilizing their finances, and attempting to return to the mainstream of life).

Once at home, the depressive stage of the grieving process may become apparent for both patients and their families. By this time they may have experienced multiple losses related to physical changes, finances, self-concept, and roles. It is only now that their sadness is felt so completely. Those recipients and families who have experienced acute and sudden onset of the disease are at greater risk for depression, since these individuals may have had little opportunity to incorporate lifestyle changes.

Postdischarge marks a new period of life for the transplant family as they attempt to reintegrate as a family and cope with role changes. Patients are anxious to start living again, feel added strength and energy from the effects of steroid therapy or emotional mood swings secondary to steroids. Both the patients and their families may have high expectations. Instead of a smooth path forward, however, this time may be fraught with conflicts between the expectations and realities of recovery. Whereas some patients may be reluctant to give up their dependent roles for fear they will not survive, others have forgotten how to be a "healthy person" after years of chronic illness. This situation can be made worse by family members who hesitate or refuse to relinquish their roles as caregivers. Many patients describe a period immediately after discharge when they felt that their families' overprotectiveness interfered with their own needs to pursue independent lives.

Carol was 19 years old and preparing for her first year of college when she was struck with acute liver disease. After a six-month illness and a two-month hospitalization after transplant surgery she returned home to continue her life. Her need on discharge was to get back into the mainstream of life with her peers, which included late-night parties and what appeared to her parents as overindulgent behavior. Her developmental needs conflicted with the needs of her parents, who believed that they must continue to closely monitor her life, as they had in the past seven months, and to continue to make decisions that were best for her well-being. Role transitions create changes in the family and are a paramount task at this time (Allender et al., 1983; Christopherson, 1987).

By the time of discharge, transplant patients have experienced much assault on both their bodies and body images. In addition to the changes brought on by major scarring from the surgery itself, patients must continue to go through the adjustment of incorporating another human being's body part as part of their own. This process takes energy as they unravel their concerns about whether the organ will reject or whether it will change the way they look and feel. During this time the patient must also deal specifically with the physical changes that may accompany the immunosuppressive therapy (e.g., weight gain and abnormal hair growth). Some patients' appearances will change dramatically over time, causing great distress, especially to adolescents and young adults, whose appearance is paramount in their developmental tasks.

The stages of transplant and corresponding diagnoses are summarized in Table 16–1.

TABLE 16–1. STAGES OF TRANSPLANT AND POTENTIAL NURSING DIAGNOSES

STAGE	NURSING DIAGNOSIS
Transplant proposed	Fear and anxiety, potential for ineffective coping, anticipatory grieving
Evaluation	Anxiety
Awaiting a donor	Anxiety, guilt, powerlessness
Preoperative	Fear and anxiety
Postoperative	Anxiety, powerlessness, grieving
Discharge	Anxiety
Post discharge	Anxiety, grieving, disturbances in body image, alteration in family process

NURSING DIAGNOSIS

Fear and Anxiety

Fear is a feeling of dread related to an identifiable source that the person validates (McFarland & Wasli, 1986). Anxiety, on the other hand, is an uncomfortable warning of varying intensity of an impending subjective danger for which the source of the danger is unknown (McFarland & Wasli, 1986).

Both anxiety and fear can be manifested with different intensities, depending on how the individual perceives the danger or threat. A patient or family member may experience feelings on a continuum from slight discomfort, sleeplessness, and irritability to a "panic" stage manifested by extreme discomfort, unrealistic perceptions of the situation, and immobility (McFarland & Wasli, 1986). There are also differences in the way people express this response.

A 56-year-old recipient waited for six months after evaluation before she received her new organ. During that time she attended a support group. She was able to articulate with little effort her anxiety and the coping strategies she used to manage it. She shared that it has always helped her to talk openly about her problems.

Another patient denied his anxiety. He offered his view that one must have total trust in the world and that he saw no cause for concern. This same patient suffered with physical symptoms of anxiety that were causing serious delays in the evaluation process.

It is a nursing responsibility to assess the presence and level of fear and anxiety in both the patient and the family. Many times they are obvious as the person becomes jittery and irritable and verbalizes her anxiety. But it is the hidden response couched in aggressive, demanding, or other destructive behavior that challenges nurses to understand and intervene.

In setting the stage for intervention it is important to establish with the patient and family that fear and anxiety are normal responses. Presenting an attitude that the management of these responses is important to their recovery will give patients and families permission to share more openly, and thus receive appropriate comfort more readily. It is important to assess the patient's and family's coping abilities and supports and their current stress levels as well as evaluate their resources.

The first step in assessing and managing a patient's anxiety and fear is the establishment of a therapeutic relationship. Offering a sense of availability, openness, and consistent presence will create a trusting environment for the patient and family to share their anxieties and sort through their feelings. Use active listening, especially silence, to encourage the patient and family to express what they are feeling. Keeping silent can be a challenging intervention, as it requires us to resist giving helpful reassurances and to allow the person to feel and express her pain. If this expression is allowed, a natural break will occur that will provide an opportunity to offer reassurance and support. It is only after validation of their feelings that many patients and families will be able to internalize the hope that transplantation offers.

It is important at every stage of the transplant process to offer both the patient and family a consistent and updated flow of information about what is occurring and what to expect. They should be instructed on the routes of communication and how and to whom they should direct their questions and concerns. Clear and accurate information not only reduces anxiety, but also offers the patient and family control. Because selective hearing may accompany anxiety, expect that information may need to be repeated several times throughout the process before it can be internalized by patients and their families. It is always important when giving information to balance the hope of transplant with the possibility of complications and failure.

Another critical intervention to reduce anxiety is continuous reassurance to the patients and families that they will not have to go through the process alone. If a support group is available for transplant patients and their families, it would be helpful to encourage them to attend. This intervention is well supported in the literature and, when designed and facilitated by skilled health professionals, can serve a multitude of patient and family needs throughout the transplant process (Hyler, Corley & McMahon, 1985; McAleer, Copeland, Fuller, & Copeland, 1985; Mann, 1985).

The purpose of a support group is to provide patients and families with the opportunity to gather important information from other recipients and transplant team members about what to expect during the transplant process. In addition, patients and families can share their feelings and concerns with other recipients who have successfully come through this difficult process and can suggest helpful coping strategies. An added benefit to the staff is that the support group serves as an avenue for assessment of psychosocial needs, since much is revealed about patients' resources and coping as they describe their situations in the group.

The support offered in a group has the potential to extend outside the group and become, for the patient, an extended family where continued sharing and support can take place. This is particularly helpful if the family does not reside locally. Some of the patients will return to the group after discharge to give support to other patients and families. Their successes with transplants and restored lives give other recipients a hope, one that can never be instilled through the words of the staff. If a support group is not available, a nurse can introduce transplant patients and families to each other informally or through an educational program.

Anxiety can be managed cognitively by helping the patient to problem-solve around specific issues. For example, during the waiting period a nurse can offer ideas about how the patient and family can manage their need to be vigilant. A list of telephone numbers where they can normally be reached can be kept by the transplant team, and a beeper can be made available to them, allowing for more freedom and decreased anxiety. One family awaiting an organ for their six-year-old daughter was helped by designing a plan delineating each member's responsibility. This plan was to take effect as soon as the "call" was received. This plan not only served to decrease their anxiety through preparation, but also gave each member a sense of control and purpose once an organ was matched.

Although information, reassurance, and problem-solving can relieve a significant amount of patient and family anxiety, there is a certain level of anxiety that can be relieved only through a successful transplant. Management at this point includes the use of distraction as well as instruction on the use of relaxation therapy and other stress management techniques.

When anxiety is expressed as doubt about the adequacy of care, as may occur during the waiting period and when complications occur, it is important not to respond defensively. It is more effective to listen, validate their feelings, and provide information, reassuring them that they are being cared for. Encourage them to discuss their feelings with other patients and families who have gone through similar processes.

People manage their anxiety uniquely. The use of defense mechanisms (e.g., denial, repression, and rationalization) is normal and productive to the extent that it serves to encapsulate the immobilizing forces of anxiety and allows the person to manage everyday life. Problems occur when these defenses become destructive and interfere with the patient's well-being.

Mr. L. showed little emotional response throughout the transplant process. Although he experienced a rejection episode during the postoperative period, his ending emotional response continued to be one of stoic indifference. After discharge, Mr. L. was readmitted to the hospital several times in the first month for treatment of rejection. He finally experienced total rejection of his organ and a second transplant was performed. After the second transplant the patient again experienced a series of readmissions, not only for rejection, but also for treatment of injuries associated with auto accidents in which he was charged with drunken driving. On close investigation Mr. L.'s problems became clear. Throughout his recovery Mr. L. was not complying with his medication regimen and was exposing himself to other situations, such as alcohol abuse, that were self-destructive to his well-being.

After a psychiatric evaluation it was determined that Mr. L.'s non-compliant, self-destructive behavior was based on fear that resulted in massive denial of both his illness and the anxiety that is expected when a person is confronted with a life-threatening disease. This patient had endured multiple separations and crises throughout his life with little support and had learned to cope with the painful feelings by ignoring their presence.

A less dramatic example was Mr. N., a wealthy, high-level executive, who was diagnosed as having severe heart disease. When he was offered a transplant he handled his anxiety by "bulldozing" the transplant team. Before being evaluated Mr. N. demanded that he be made top priority and be given immediate consideration. His behavior not only alienated the health care team but also increased his anxiety level as his caregivers responded to him with anger and withdrawal.

Such patients present nurses with the greatest challenge. The first step in their care is to recognize that fear and anxiety are the sources of their destructive behavior. Interventions aimed at reducing anxiety are paramount. There is never a more important or difficult time to maintain a consistent and caring relationship. Within this relationship the nurse can provide the support and feedback a patient needs to understand how her behavior is affecting herself and others. Sometimes simple feedback within a caring relationship will enable a patient to change behavior and share anxieties. If the behavior does not improve, firm limits must be set.

Sometimes nurses feel "uncaring" when it is suggested that they set limits with patients and families. They feel that the patients are already stressed and fear that they will make the situation worse. It is important to understand that patients have a need for limits at this time. Limits give them boundaries when they feel out of control. Setting limits in a caring manner can help to reduce a patient's anxiety. If feedback and limit-setting are unsuccessful in controlling patient behavior, a referral should be made for further psychiatric evaluation and treatment.

With difficult patients it is important for nurses to be aware of their own feelings and responses and not let them interfere with care. It is understandable that over time this situation can become overwhelming as the team's energy diminishes. The goal is to remain in control and help patients to deal with their anxieties so that they do not continue to be destructive. Utilizing resources is crucial. It is important to arrange a regular care conference with other team members, including those who specialize in behavior management and psychosocial issues. The purpose of the conference is to discuss ways to best manage the patient's care.

When dealing with anxiety or any other emotional response it is important to document the behavioral characteristics of the problem as well as the effects of the interventions. Not only is this necessary for consistency in treatment, but it may also serve as a useful record if future psychiatric intervention becomes necessary.

Potential for Ineffective Coping

Ineffective coping occurs when the amount of stress experienced overrides a person's ability to cope (McFarland & Wasli, 1986). This state becomes apparent when the patient's and family's behavior becomes dysfunctional and disorganized. They may be unable to perform activities of daily living and manifest extreme anxious or depressed behavior.

Mary and Janet, the two adult children of Jason, were found in a panic state. Their father, who was undergoing a kidney transplant, was not expected to survive. The clinical transplant coordinator was called to intervene. As soon as she arrived she gently guided the two daughters to a corner of the waiting room and asked them to sit down. She told them that she understood that they had received difficult news and wondered if they had any other family or friends that she might call for support. With their permission she notified the rest of the family. She waited with the daughters until other family members arrived, allowing them to ventilate their feelings and reassuring them that they did have the strength to handle this situation. Before she left she told them that she would keep in touch with them about their father's condition and that they could expect a call from her regularly.

This family was in crisis. The transplant coordinator used crisis intervention to help them gain control of the situation. The family needed a caring person who was in control to give them specific direction and help them take action. She both supported their defenses and reminded them of their strengths. She provided them with a system that they could rely on to get the information they needed to keep in control.

After the initial intervention many families are able to resolve their crisis and stabilize with standard support. Others may require additional support and can be referred for counseling.

Grieving and Anticipatory Grieving

Grieving is a normal process by which a person adaptively adjusts to a significant loss (McFarland & Wasli, 1986). Anticipatory grieving takes place before and in preparation for an actual significant loss. This process is seen throughout the transplant process and can be assessed by observing for the behavioral characteristics that define the common stages of grief, including denial, anger, bargaining, depression, and acceptance (McFarland & Wasli, 1986).

Patients and families can be helped through this process by being encouraged to express their feelings openly and by having their experiences validated as being normal and expected as part of the grieving process. It is important to respect the differences in the way people move through this process and allow them adequate time to incorporate the reality of their losses.

In many cases the realities of loss do not present until the patient and family are home and in their own safe environment. The depression that is commonly seen in the postdischarge period is related to this process. It is also this response that may be responsible for the noncompliant behavior sometimes seen after discharge. Patients can be assessed for depression during return visits to the clinic by noting the common signs and symptoms, including sleeping or eating disturbances, social withdrawal, verbalization of worthlessness, hopelessness, and helplessness, and a general loss of interest in life (McFarland & Wasli, 1986).

If depression is diagnosed, it is important to encourage patients to share their feelings about losses and reassure them that these feelings are normal. It is also helpful to encourage and assist the patients to make a plan of action for their lives. For example, if withdrawal is the symptom, encourage them to make contact with a friend one time during the next week and to increase the contact little by little until they are back in the mainstream of their support system. For those people who suffer from lengthy depression without resolution, a referral should be made for counseling and for medication management.

Guilt

Guilt is a method of interacting, manifested by extremely poor self-concept and feelings of having done something wrong and fear of punishment (McFarland & Wasli, 1986). It is manifested most clearly in those who express self-worthlessness, bitterness, and failure. For example, the family of one patient suffering from severe complications shared the following thoughts: "I shouldn't have talked him into a transplant. I should not have trusted those other recipients and staff who praised the treatment. I should have thought it out more clearly. It's all my fault."

Sometimes the guilt is so pervasive that it affects other recipients and their families as well. Ben was in the support group when Louise, the mother of a recipient who was suffering from a severe infection, shared her anger about the transplant process. Afterward Ben shared with the staff his feelings of guilt at having encouraged this patient to have a transplant. The nurse's role is to encourage patients to express this guilt, validate their feelings, and reassure them that they are normal.

Powerlessness

Powerlessness is the perceived lack of control over one's current situation or immediate happening (McFarland & Wasli, 1986). As with anxiety, there are levels of powerlessness and behavioral characteristics that mark each level (McFarland & Wasli, 1986). With low levels, passivity and self-concern about fluctuating energy levels are experienced by the patient and family. A moderate level is commonly manifested by the patient's participation in self-care and expression of doubt regarding role performance by the family. Severe levels are marked by depression over physical deterioration that occurs despite patients' compliance with the medical regimen, apathy, and verbalization of a lack of control over life (McFarland & Wasli, 1986).

The nurse's first task is to assess the level of powerlessness and provide the patient and family with feedback about the behaviors. They should be encouraged to discuss their feelings and identify areas of their lives in which they do have control, and assisted to make a plan and take action in those areas. Although stress management techniques are often effective in helping patients to resolve their feelings of helplessness, some cases that involve severe powerlessness necessitate further intervention.

Jack, 43 years old, and his wife, Julie, came to the Midwest from their home in south Florida to undergo a transplant procedure. Jack developed a serious infection and was returned to the ICU one week postoperatively. He was hospitalized for five months, in and out of the ICU. Jack's and Julie's behavior changed dramatically during the course of hospitalization. They went from being trusting and cooperative to being hostile and noncompliant. They blamed the team for being incompetent and insensitive to their needs. Jack became demanding and aggressive toward the nursing staff as they attempted daily care. The nurses felt helpless as Jack refused to accept their care. The staff began to withdraw from Jack and avoid both him and his wife. They felt guilty about not providing adequate care and did not know how to respond to this couple. Their powerlessness turned into anger, and they accused Jack of not trying to help himself. Julie complained that the transplant team was avoiding them and giving up hope for Jack's recovery.

Powerlessness can create multiple problems in communication among the patient, family, and staff. Anger and guilt may emerge as self-esteem decreases. This helplessness is contagious and can be one of the greatest detriments to the patient's health and well-being. It has potential to lead to serious depression and, in some cases, death.

During pervasive powerlessness it is important for the nurse to step back and obtain a perspective from those outside the system who are not so intensely involved. Support is needed for the health team, as well as for patients and families. A series of conferences that include psychological consultants are helpful at this point to assist in sorting through the issues and developing an effective care plan.

Although patients and families may require additional emotional support during these times, a support group does not seem to be the intervention of choice. Many times these people are dealing with their own doubts about the decision to have a transplant and may be struggling with the anger they feel about their loss. Families have commented that they do not believe that they can be helpful at this time. What they are also saying is that they cannot give hope when they do not feel it. It is best to allow them space, respect their needs, and recommend individual counseling instead.

Disturbances in Body Image

Problems in body image can be described simply as a disruption in the way one perceives one's body (McFarland & Wasli, 1986). The major signs of this disturbance include preoccupation with and repetitive negative comments about their affected body part as well as refusal to look at or touch it. This response can become a major problem when it interferes with the patient's needs.

Jean was an avid member of a support group throughout her transplant but stopped coming approximately two months post discharge. When asked about this she admitted that she was embarrassed about the weight she had gained and couldn't bear to have anybody see her out of control. This patient benefited from the support group throughout her transplant experience, but because she viewed herself as overweight and repulsive, she risked the isolation that would come from not being part of the group.

Patients can be helped with body image problems by both support for their feelings and encouragement in making a plan to help them adjust. For example, those patients who suffer from weight gain can be helped by meeting with a nutritionist to assist them in making a plan for weight control. A patient who has difficulty looking at her body could be helped with a behavior modification plan in which, with support, she could be helped to slowly view her body. If problems continue, it is appropriate for the nurse to suggest counseling for the patient, as this could be an indication that more serious psychological problems exist.

Alteration in Family Process

Problems in family process occur when a family experiences disruption in the structure and function of its system (McFarland & Wasli, 1986). In the case of the transplant family, role transitions are the main source of this disruption. Many times these issues emerge during the postdischarge period and the adjustment to home. They are commonly manifested in marital conflict and conflict in general among family members. Patients complain that their families are overprotecting them, while families lose patience with the perceived careless behavior of patients. Communication problems emerge and family tension builds.

The problems associated with alteration in family process can be assessed during clinic visits by listening closely to the patient's and family's descriptions of life at home. Sometimes such problems surface in the verbal and nonverbal interaction between family members during the visits.

It is helpful to intervene in these role transitions before discharge by offering anticipatory guidance. Patients and families should be instructed about the changes they may face as the patient moves toward recovery. They should also be taught the importance of communicating their needs to one another openly and reminded that these adjustments are to be expected. If problems in family process continue for more than a month or two with no signs of resolution, the family should obtain professional counseling to assist them in sorting out their issues and improving family communication.

THE CAREGIVERS

Transplant nursing challenges nurses to draw heavily not only on their knowledge base in psychosocial nursing, but also on their own personal strengths. The joy that comes from sharing in the process of transplantation is balanced only by the challenge that is faced in helping patients, families, and themselves manage the fears and disappointments surrounding it.

Although the needs of the transplant patient and family seem complex at times, they are simple. First, they need to be heard and understood; second, to be given consistent information about their progress; and third, to know that support is there if they need it. To meet these needs nurses must have a clear understanding of the psychological process inherent in the experience of transplantation. Active listening on the part of the caregiver allows patients and families an opportunity to express their emotional pain. It is through this process that they can be relieved of their loneliness and fear. It is important for nurses to understand their impact on this process.

It is also important to understand the impact that working with the transplant patient and family has on nurses as caregivers. There is a great deal of psychological work involved in the care of this group of patients. As nurses listen to their fears and feelings of powerlessness, they must struggle to keep their own anxieties and helplessness intact. It is difficult to respond to a patient or family when, in their grief, they ask, "Why did this have to happen to me?" One is reminded of one's own vulnerability with each difficulty that these patients encounter.

To balance the psychological work, nurses must take action to get replenished. It is crucial to create and maintain the boundaries necessary to experience a personal life in which support from others and an active leisure life can renew energy. In addition, it is important to be involved in a professional network in which others in the same role can provide support through the sharing of problems, ideas, and feelings.

References

Allender, J., Shisslak, C., Kasniak, A., & Copeland, J. (1983). Stages of psychological adjustment associated with heart transplantation. *Heart Transplantation, 2,* 228–231.

Castelnuovo-Tedesco, P. (1971). *Psychiatric Aspects of Organ Transplant.* New York: Grune & Stratton.

Christopherson, L.K. (1987). Cardiac transplantations: A psychological perspective. *Circulation, 75*(1), 57–62.

Gulledge, A.D., Buszta, C., & Montague, D.K. (1983). Psychosocial aspects of renal transplantation. *Urologic Clinics of North America, 10*(2), 327–335.

Hyler, B.J., Corley, M.C., & McMahon, D. (1985). The role of nursing in a support group for heart transplantation recipients and their families. *Heart Transplantation, 4,* 453.

McAleer, M.J., Copeland, J., Fuller, J., & Copeland, J.G. (1985). Psychological aspects of heart transplantation. *Heart Transplantation, 4,* 132.

McFarland, G.K. & Wasli, E.L. (1986). Nursing *Diagnosis and Process in Psychiatric Mental Health Nursing.* Philadelphia: J.B. Lippincott.

Mann, L.M. (1985). A group approach to teaching and support in a renal transplant unit. *American Nephrology Nurses Association Journal, 12*(2), 102–106.

O'Brien, V. (1985). Psychological and social aspects of heart transplantation. *Heart Transplantation, 4,* 229.

Watts, D., Freeman, A.M., McGiffin, D.G, Kirklin, J.K., McVay, R., & Karp, R.B. (1984). Psychiatric aspects of cardiac transplantation. *Heart Transplantation, 3*(3), 243–247.

17

Extended Role of the Nurse

Linda M. Haggerty and Becky A. Harris

The role of the clinical transplant coordinator (CTC) is broad, complex, challenging, and rewarding. The CTC functions in a variety of settings in order to promote successful organ and tissue transplantation. CTCs come from a variety of backgrounds, from staff nurses to nurse clinicians to clinical specialists. Certain aspects of the role reflect the differences in training, expertise, and program needs. In any case, the CTC has unique opportunities to directly and indirectly influence the transplant recipient and the transplant process. The CTC has significant influence on the health care milieu, providing essential communication links, providing and assuring quality of care, and promoting continuity of care. This is done by way of systematic assessment of problems, nursing intervention, and evaluation.

DEVELOPMENT OF THE CTC ROLE

The nursing process is useful in defining the role, in terms of personal, professional, and institutional needs. As a newly hired CTC in a recently developed position or as a CTC in an established program, the nursing process allows the CTC to assess and define these needs and evolve a role that fits in with the transplant program's goals and objectives.

Assessment and Planning

During the process of assessing the CTC's professional needs and planning role activities, it is necessary to evaluate and identify the CTC's professional and personal needs and to assess the flexibility available to the CTC to incorporate these needs into the role. It is important for the CTC to keep in mind role perceptions and ideas and to incorporate these as much as possible. The resulting role, then, will be one in which the CTC can satisfactorily and effectively work.

Initially the job description should be reviewed. It will probably outline the following major areas of responsibility:

- Evaluating transplant candidates and potential living donors
- Coordinating the pretransplant testing and evaluating results
- Maintaining the cadaver transplant waiting list
- Coordinating the transplant admission and preoperative preparation
- Assessing and educating the posttransplant patient in collaboration with the nursing staff and other members of the multidisciplinary transplant team
- Providing short- and long-term outpatient management
- Educating professional and lay personnel
- Providing consultation
- Designing and participating in research projects.

Any combination of the activities above may be associated with the CTC role or may be shared by two or more CTCs working together. By assessing the CTC's own expectations, as well as those of other people and departments with whom the CTC will interact, activities can be prioritized. Frequent evaluation of the evolving role may assist in redefining priorities in order that personal and professional needs are being met and the transplant process is effectively coordinated.

Developing a solid and broad base of knowledge regarding transplantation and the transplant process is crucial. This can be accomplished through research, literature review, and attendance at professional conferences. Self-motivation to maintain current knowledge is essential in order to facilitate effective team collaboration and patient care.

Another critical step is the development of professional relations with other members of the multidisciplinary transplant team. Such team members include the nursing staff involved in direct patient care, nursing management personnel, discharge planners, social workers, dietitians, physicians, laboratory managers and personnel, pharmacists, operating room personnel and administrative personnel from other departments. A mutual needs assessment can be performed and an understanding gained of each team member's contribution to the transplant process. Subsequently coordination of activities is achieved.

Networking and communicating with other CTCs may assist in role definition. Such collegial relations will also be helpful in gaining information regarding other transplant programs, including methods of data collection, policies and procedures, protocols that may be shared or revised, educational materials, and identification of other available resources. Interaction with other CTCs may also provide a future sounding board when new or difficult patient situations arise with which the CTC has had limited experience.

Additionally, there are a number of regional and statewide organizations that merit investigation. The purpose of each and the CTC's role in collaboration should be identified. Examples of such agencies include regional organ procurement organizations (OPOs), organ-specific registries for data collection, the United Network for Organ Sharing, and the American Council on Transplantation. A major function of several of these organizations, with which the CTC is involved, is data collection. Specific data are required for research purposes and documentation to the federal government. The regional OPOs are an extension of the transplant process, and it is important to identify the relationship between the transplant center and the OPO.

Other professional organizations include the North American Transplant Coordinators Organization, the American Nephrology Nurses Association, and the American Association of Critical Care Nurses. These can provide valuable professional growth and networking opportunities.

During the assessment process a great deal of information is gathered from which a job description and plan for implementation can be devised. Evaluation of quarterly, yearly, or biannual objectives will also help the CTC function effectively within the job description.

THE CTC ROLE IN THE TRANSPLANT PROCESS

Implementation

As stated in preceding chapters, the goal of organ and tissue transplantation is physical and psychosocial rehabilitation for the transplant recipient. The CTC is necessarily and intimately involved in all aspects of the complex transplant process in order to help the recipients meet their goals. The CTC is involved in direct and indirect patient care, and in formal and informal patient, family, professional, and public education, as a multidisciplinary team member and as a patient and family advocate. The nursing process is used for effective interaction and outcome in each phase.

Initial Evaluation

The first phase of the transplant process involves providing information to the potential organ recipient and family members. The CTC participates in the initial meeting between the patient, family, and transplant surgeon. Such a meeting can be conducted on an individual or family basis or in groups. At this time a significant amount of education is provided regarding the risks, benefits, procedures, and responsibilities associated with the transplant process. Transplantation as a therapeutic option is discussed. Patients and their families are made aware that transplantation is not a panacea, but a generally successful form of treatment for many forms of end-stage organ or tissue disease. Patient and family responsibilities throughout each phase of the transplant process are made clear. Assessment of basic knowledge, readiness to learn, and understanding will help to tailor the interview to the appropriate level as well as guide areas of future needs and interactions. Similar data may be obtained from the referral source.

During the initial visit, a complete history is taken and a physical examination is performed. Medical records and referral summaries are reviewed. A careful assessment helps to direct the evaluation process, identifying potential problem areas that necessitate additional review. Physical problems are identified and evaluated. Similarly, psychosocial factors are assessed, and appropriate interventions and referrals are applied.

The tests required to evaluate transplant candidacy, the procedures and their rationale, are reviewed with the patient. Histocompatibility testing, blood tests, x-rays, and the required consultations are explained. Information regarding the surgical procedure, hospitalization, and outpatient management is given in order to achieve the goal of informed consent.

At this time the CTC assesses the recipient's level of understanding, interest, and anxiety. An opportunity for the patient and family to ask questions is essential. Also, the rapport that is established in this initial phase is vital and will influence subsequent phases.

The CTC may also be involved in the assessment and education of a potential living-related donor. As with the recipient, the CTC helps to ensure that all aspects of the donor evaluation, surgical procedures, risks, hospitalization, and long-term implications are explained. An assessment of family relations is made. The importance of the decision to donate is appreciated, and confidentiality is assured.

Recipient Evaluation

The CTC assures that all aspects of the recipient evaluation are completed. The CTC reviews all reports and identifies any abnormal results that may necessitate further evaluation. Communication is maintained with the patient in order that each step and the associated requirements are understood. Throughout the evaluation phase repeated opportunities for assessment of patient understanding and concerns, as well as for patient education, are created and used.

After the evaluation the CTC should again review what the process has been and explain the waiting period until a suitable organ is found. Frequent communication is important while patients are awaiting transplantation in order to assess and evaluate anxieties, maintain rapport, obtain the patient's current medical status, and reassure the patient and family that they are not forgotten. See Chapter 16 for a discussion on the anxieties frequently associated with this waiting period. Communication with other health care providers involved in the patient's care is maintained in order to promote continuity of care.

Immediate Preoperative Period

The CTC may be involved in informing the patient and primary care physician of the availability of an organ. An assessment is made to rule out any current contraindications to transplant, such as active infection. The patient is reminded of what to expect during admission and the preoperative period. The CTC may assist in coordinating the patient's admission and immediate preoperative education, although in many cases this may be done by the transplant nursing staff. Reinforcement of previous teaching will help to decrease the patient's level of anxiety. A similar review is given to the donor in the case of living-related donation.

Immediate Postoperative Period

During the immediate postoperative period the CTC coordinates the recipient's care with the primary nurse. The recipient and family may be anxious about the patient's status as well as the function of the newly transplanted organ or tissue. An explanation of the patient's medical status and expected procedures may help to allay some anxieties. The CTC interacts with members of the multidisciplinary team. It is important to take advantage of opportunities for informal education about such matters as medication administration, rationale for planned procedures, and an explanation about the individual patient's history while interacting with the health care team. Similarly, members of the health care team should communicate with the CTC about the patient's current status. Often the CTC is the person most available to other health care providers and the patient, and can most effectively maintain communication and promote continuity of care.

Postoperative Period

Again, assessment of the patient's organ function and medical status is made in cooperation with the primary nurse and members of the health care team. Ideally the CTC interfaces with the primary nurse to identify the recipient's specific needs. The CTC assists in preparing the transplant care plan that is appropriate for the individual patient. A list of potential and actual problems is prepared and evaluated daily and as needed. Specific nursing care during this phase has been described in earlier chapters.

During the postoperative phase patient education is intensified. With an appreciation for the patient's responsibilities at the time of discharge, thorough education is provided. It is essential to individualize patient education, based on the patient's ability and readiness to learn. An appreciation of the patient's own environment, culture, and life-style will influence the CTC's teaching strategies, with the understanding that such factors play a significant role in the patient's acceptability of health care (Dever, 1975; Fuchs, 1974; Somers, 1971; see Chapter 15). The CTC should, in collaboration with the primary nurse, assess the recipient's needs, strengths, stressors, and skills. The rapport developed and assessments made during prior phases of the transplant process will help the CTC to assess these factors and direct an effective teaching program. Certainly there is a minimal amount of knowledge that the patient must gain in order to perform self-care after discharge. Some patients will desire additional details. The content and methods of teaching, as well as the methods of evaluation, should reflect information gathered in the assessment regarding patient needs and abilities. The goals of care are then identified and a nursing care plan is devised and implemented (see Chapter 15, Table 15–2). The patient may be evaluated by means of verbal feedback, repeat demonstration, or written examination. Areas of additional need are readdressed as appropriate, the teaching plan may be modified, and, if appropriate, the goals may also be modified. Recipients should not be discharged unless the CTC has evaluated their learning and is confident that they have mastered the necessary skills to provide effective self-care. Larger transplant programs may promote group teaching, which, when applied appropriately, may be as effective as one-on-one teaching. Evaluation, however, of individuals in the group is essential in order to ascertain that each recipient is gaining the necessary knowledge.

Family attitudes and support can strongly influence the commitment and ability of patients to manage their conditions, particularly for long-term treatment plans that require continuous patient participation. Families can enhance supervision and assist and encourage patient compliance (Becker, 1985; Eraker, Kirscht, & Becker, 1984). It is important to develop rapport with the recipient's family, assess family relations and concerns, and provide education to family members as well as to the recipient.

Outpatient Management

Outpatient management is a critical aspect of the CTC's role with significant potential to influence the transplant recipient's state of health and well-being. The CTC is often the main link between the patient and other members of the health care team.

Consistent care provided by a familiar person can increase compliance and patient satisfaction. In many settings the CTC can provide that consistency and build on the rapport that was established during prior interactions. Lipkin (1976) reported that a patient who trusted a physician was far more likely to freely discuss symptoms, feelings, and problems. The trust that is established between the CTC and the patient can be seen in the same way, particularly since it is the CTC with whom the patient spends the greatest amount of time during the outpatient phase.

A systematic approach to patient assessment is required. The CTC assesses the recipient's current medical status, with emphasis on function and evidence of a rejection episode, signs and symptoms of infection, and the development of other complications. Astute physical assessment is of paramount importance. An abnormal finding requires further evaluation by an appropriate member of the transplant team. Referrals to other departments, such as dermatology, radiology, cardiology, and internal medicine, are made as necessary. Two-way communication with members of these departments is required.

During outpatient visits, the CTC can evaluate the recipient's degree of adjustment and rehabilitation. Such visits provide an opportunity for reinforcement of patient education and the addressing of other patient issues. It is critical for the CTC to maintain rapport with the patient without promoting dependence.

Communication with the recipient's primary care physician is essential. In many centers the transplant surgeon or transplant nephrologist will remain involved in all aspects of immunosuppression, but promote collaboration regarding the patient's general health care. Visits to the transplant clinic may become less frequent over time as the patient reports more often to another primary health care giver. However, with an appreciation of the transplant and specific issues such as the development of complications and drug interactions, frequent communication is essential. The CTC may set up a regularly scheduled means of communicating such as summary letters, telephone calls, or meetings. Similarly, the patient should understand the need to inform the CTC of such changes as new medications, procedures, and hospitalizations. A systematic approach will help to promote the continuity of care that is essential for long-term, uncomplicated success.

EDUCATOR

Education is a key responsibility of the CTC. She can create an educational approach and program that best uses her established expertise and personal capabilities to uniquely contribute to quality patient care.

In addition to patient education, the CTC is often formally and informally involved in professional and public education in a variety of settings. She may be asked to lecture at medical, nursing, and other professional meetings on various aspects of the clinical care of the transplant recipient. Depending on the needs of the group, and the group members' roles in the transplant process, any number of issues can be discussed. The kidney transplant CTC may, for example, address the staff of dialysis units. Because a dialysis patient may first seek information from the staff, accurate information is essential. The staff should have a basic understanding of the transplant process as well as know where to refer the patients for further information. Other CTCs may organize seminars for professional referral sources.

The CTC must assess the needs of the team and staff members directly involved in the delivery of patient care. Each group will have different educational needs based on their involvement. For example, nursing staff education should consist of patient care issues, protocols, nursing diagnoses, and patient education. Consistent information must be provided by all team members in order to avoid patient confusion or misunderstanding. The CTC should be involved in the writing and editing of written materials for both patients and staff, as well as in designing educational programs for staff orientation. An in-service program can also be developed that involves other members of the transplant team. In this way multiple needs can be met and multidisciplinary team relations can be reinforced. As a CTC, it is important to become established as a resource person to all team members.

The transplant coordinator may also be involved in the education of students, providing direct and indirect clinical instruction to undergraduate and graduate nursing students. The CTC is also frequently asked to lecture for a variety of student groups on various aspects of the transplant process.

The CTC may also be involved in education of the lay public. Through the hospital's public relations department, the OPO, or community resources, the CTC may be asked to present a program to a group of interested public. Information regarding organ donation, as well as the clinical aspects of transplantation, may be discussed. The public often possesses a significant amount of misinformation, and any opportunity to provide a realistic picture of transplantation is important.

CONSULTANT

A major role of the CTC is to provide consultation services to patient care groups. For example, the CTC may act as a consultant to other nursing groups regarding such issues as the writing of care plans, outpatient clinic management, independent nursing practice, physical assessment, immunology, pathophysiology, administrative issues in transplantation, and any other areas in which the CTC has established expertise and credibility. Requests for consultation may originate from inside one's hospital or from other hospitals and transplant centers.

It is important to establish oneself as having expertise and offer consulting services. Marketing of the role and one's abilities is important for role development. In addition, by providing such services, the CTC will contribute to quality patient care. It is important to assess areas of need, develop a plan of addressing those needs, and offer interventions on a consultative basis. Such marketing activity can begin at the coordinator's institution and later expand to include professional organizations and the community. The goal is to simultaneously create opportunities for exposure and provide information. Involvement in nursing education, participation in opportunities to educate the public, involvement in professional organizations, and seeking opportunities to provide both informal and formal learning will help to market both the role of the CTC and the realities of transplantation. It will also encourage understanding, commitment, and involvement on the part of those who work directly and indirectly in the field of transplantation.

RESEARCHER

Transplantation offers innumerable research possibilities for the CTC. Bowie (1980) has delineated eight roles of the nurse researcher. These roles are as consumer, participant, supporter, technician, consultant, investigator, collaborator, and interpreter. The CTC can become involved in research at any or all of these levels. There may be opportunities for collaborative research with other health care providers, and certainly any effort contributed to a research study should be credited. Familiarity with the research process, including subject selection, data analysis, and conclusions, in order to accurately interpret results, is critical. Research, however, should not be limited to collaboration. Ideally the CTC should design and initiate research studies and publish the results as often as possible.

EVALUATION

An evaluation process is critical for role development, both for self-growth and to determine one's impact on patient care. As defined by Veney and Kaluzny (1984), evaluation constitutes analysis of the relevance, progress, efficiency, effectiveness, and impact of activities. Once an assessment of institutional, patient care, and personal needs has been made, objectives should be written. Such objectives should be prioritized and organized into short- and long-term goals. They should be frequently reviewed in terms of the criteria above. The CTC role is dynamic. Reassessment of needs and goals is expected and should be performed when appropriate. Because the CTC role includes such a variety of areas of responsibility, realistic prioritization of activities is important in order to promote effectiveness in the role and minimize invaluable time expenditure.

As described, the role of the CTC involves many important nursing activities. The rewards are many:

- independence in practice,
- high degree of responsibility,
- feelings of professional competency,
- feelings of accomplishment,
- intimate, long-term involvement with patients and families and opportunities to participate in their rehabilitation, and
- opportunities for self-growth.

These provide the CTC with self-satisfaction, pride, and professional growth. It is important to make use of every opportunity to learn from one's peers, from others in the medical community, and from one's patients. Thus the uniqueness of one's role and patient-care activities can be strengthened and appreciated.

The CTC role, however, is not without difficulty. The CTC must learn to effectively balance the many patient and role demands with personal needs and abilities. The role is often emotionally demanding and time-consuming. The CTC must recognize the limitations of the role and the ability to intervene. One must balance the emotional rewards of successes with the difficulties associated with complications. One must recognize the rewards of the intense patient involvement while discouraging inappropriate patient dependency. With such recognition the CTC can provide effective, therapeutic interventions to transplant patients and benefit from a multidimensional, challenging, and rewarding nursing role.

References

Becker, M.H. (1985). Patient adherence to prescribed therapies. *Medical Care, 23*(5), 539–559

Bowie, R.B. (1980). The nurse researcher's roles and responsibilities. *AORN Journal, 31*(4), 609–611.

Dever, G.E.A. (1975). *An Epidemiological Model for Health Policy Analysis.* Atlanta: Georgia Department of Human Resources.

Eraker, S.A., Kirscht, J.P., & Becker, M.H. (1984). Understanding and improving patient compliance. *Annals of Internal Medicine, 100*(2), 258–268.

Fuchs, V.R. (1974). *Who Shall Live? Health, Economics, and Social Choice.* New York: Basic Books.

Lipkin, M. (1976). Quality of care assessment in light of the relation between doctor and patient. *Bulletin of the New York Academy of Medicine, 52,*9–15.

Somers, A.R. (1971). *Health Care in Transition: Direction for the Future.* Chicago: Hospital Research and Education Trust.

Veney, J. & Kaluzny, A. (1984). *Evaluation and Decision Making for Health Services Programs.* Englewood Cliffs, N.J.: Prentice-Hall.

18

Legal and Ethical Issues

Susan Neely and Nancy S. Davis

The dynamic evolution of transplant technology has forced society to face a myriad of legal and ethical issues. All of these issues stem from disparities in supply and demand. This chapter provides an account of what has transpired and what is yet to be done.

Improved technology, immunosuppressive therapy, and the availability of non-Medicare funding have led to a proliferation of transplant centers. Easier geographic access and greatly improved survival rates have made transplantation a viable option to patients with end-stage organ or tissue failure. The resulting escalation of recipient candidate referrals has placed additional stress on a procurement system that is already struggling to meet the demand for donor organs. Efforts have been made to increase the number of organs available, but the supply still cannot keep pace with the demand.

Transplantation is an expensive technology. Many who could benefit do not have adequate personal funds or insurance. Although the general opinion is that health care is a basic human right, who will pay for those who cannot? If adequate funds and donor organs cannot be supplied, decisions will have to be made as to who does and who does not benefit from available resources.

ORGAN AND TISSUE DONATION

Living Donation

Before the development of immunosuppressive drugs, the only successful organ transplants were those performed between identical twins. According to Starzl (1985), the use of azathioprine and prednisone led to the first successful transplant between nonidentical twins in 1959. The potential donor pool was expanded shortly thereafter to allow for the use of cadaver donors when there were no acceptable family donors. Despite the limited resource, living-related donors were preferred because of a 30 per cent higher success rate. The increased advantage to the recipient was considered to far outweigh any risk to the living donor. During this period, however, there were also frequent requests from emotionally attached, but unrelated, people (e.g., spouses) that they be considered for donation. Because no better result could be expected than that achieved with cadaver donors, it was considered unacceptable to put these people at risk. The requests were seldom given consideration.

Assessing candidates for living-related donation is a three-part pro-cess aimed at ensuring (1) the histocompatibility of the donor and recipient tissues; (2) that the donor is free of any underlying disease process, is a good surgical candidate, and is not likely to experience disability as a result of the donation; and (3) that the donor's motivation is genuine.

The first two determinations are based on objective criteria easily obtained through a thorough medical evaluation. The third, however, is subjective, and warrants close scrutiny. It is important to confirm that the decision to donate is one of free choice, not a result of coercion from family members or the health care community. Potential donors may be acting out of guilt; they are well while a loved one is sick. It is not uncommon for such candidates to feel forced by family obligation, be it real or perceived. When coercion is a possibility the transplant team must provide an escape hatch through which the donor may withdraw without fear of reproach. When the live-donor candidate is a minor or deemed mentally incapable of agreeing to donation, the practice in most states has been to obtain court approval. This approach avoids any uncertainty regarding the motives of the parent or guardian (Brant, 1984).

In 1979 a new immunosuppressive drug, cyclosporin A, was made available for clinical use. The specificity and steroid-sparing character-istics of this drug dramatically improved the one- and five-year transplant survival rates. The results with unrelated cadaver grafts moved to a more acceptable plateau. As the margin between results with cadaver versus living-related donors narrowed, a reassessment of donor resources and their use occurred. Two strongly opposing views emerged.

One faction, concerned with short- and long-term risks to the donor, believes that the substantially improved results with cadaver donors has invalidated the once-accepted risk-benefit ratio associated with living-related donations. Thus living donors should no longer be accepted. A second viewpoint focuses on the increasing shortage of transplantable organs and supports the continued use of living-related donors. Addi-tionally, it is considered that these current improved results warrant accepting the living-unrelated donor candidates that once were rejected. This practice is not opposed by the American Society of Transplant

Surgeons, but they insist that its application be limited and hope that it will be discontinued when and if the supply of cadaver kidneys becomes adequate (Morris, 1987).

The decision to use emotionally related donors brought two additional challenges to the transplant team. The first was to ensure that the consent to donate is truly informed. Although the concept of informed consent is not new, its application in this situation involves some unique issues. It is critical that any live donor understands that (a) there are short-term surgical risks associated with the donor nephrectomy, (b) a potential for long-term harm related to having only one kidney exists, and (c) there is another donor source available (cadaveric) that offers their loved one an almost equal chance for success. It is true that selecting a cadaver donor over a live donor most often means that the recipient will have to wait longer for a transplant. Although this is a consideration, particularly with uremic children, it is seldom justified as a primary motive. The second challenge—confirming the appropriateness of the unrelated donor's motive—requires additional vigilance (Levey, Hou & Bush, 1986).

An unfortunate aside to permitting unrelated donation has been the emergence of commercialism. According to Morris (1987), "this has proved to be a quite common practice in the developing world, especially in the Indian subcontinent" (p. 17). The danger of allowing payment for organs and tissues has become evident. In Tokyo, according to Schneider and Flaherty (1985), a loan shark persuades his debtors to repay him in kidneys. In a typical deal the recipient of the kidney pays $85,000; of this, $80,000 is retained by the loan shark to cover the administration fee and the donor's debt. The remaining $5,000 is given to the donor. In another case cited by Schneider and Flaherty (1985) a warehouse worker from New Delhi was coerced into donating a kidney to his employer's wife. His payment for donating under the guise of being a distant cousin was a free trip to London for the surgery and being allowed to keep his job.

In the communities in which such scenarios take place the availability of donor organs is almost nonexistent. Insufficient medical technology, conflicting religious and cultural views toward donation, an absent or undeveloped system for procurement, and widely disseminated poverty may contribute to commercialism. Tolerance for the buying and selling of organs varies greatly around the world. Many perceive it as an application of pure economics and think that it is acceptable as long as there is no coercion or intended harm to the buyer or seller: the principle of nonmaleficence (Irwin, 1986).

The United States, however, has taken another view. In 1983, when faced with two similar attempts to develop systems for brokering kidneys, albeit of a less coercive nature, this country's response was firm and swift. Discovery of these activities spawned a series of congressional hearings that resulted in the passage of the National Organ Transplant Act in October of 1984. Adoption of this U.S. law made it illegal to buy, sell, or otherwise profit from the commerce of human organs. Violation is a felony with a maximum penalty of a $5000 fine or up to five years in prison, or both (Schneider & Flaherty, 1985).

Disallowing the commercialization of organ donation in the United States was not a denial of the shortage, but an effort to preserve the foundation on which organ transplantation has developed: altruism. This law also protects those who might be exploited through coercion or their own desperation. Traffic in tissues would probably have been from the indigent, depressed, and mentally handicapped to the wealthy, but seldom in the other direction (Morris, 1987). "If we are to make organ donation a financial transaction, then we demean the relationship between the donor and recipient and, indeed, begin to dismantle the fabric on which our society is built" (Morris, 1987, p. 18).

Cadaveric Donation

The question of when death occurs has perplexed societies throughout history. In 1740 *The Uncertainty of the Signs of Death and the Danger of Precipitate Interments and Dissections* prompted the first attempt to categorically define when death occurs (Slemenda, 1983). The fear of being buried alive and the possibility of premature diagnosis led to the creation of "waiting mortuaries" (Martin, 1983). Here, burial was delayed until observable signs of putrefaction occurred or when a full glass of water was placed on the chest of a corpse and no evidence of respiratory effort was present. These fears and precautions were precipitated by numerous reported cases of suspected premature burial.

In 1875 a medical journal published 25 major signs of death. By the mid-1900s the medical community began to agree that irreversible cardiorespiratory cessation constituted death. In 1959 two French neurologists referred to a condition of "coma dépassé." They described a state beyond coma in which the patient failed to recover from severe neurologic insult and was apneic with negative mesencephalic reflexes resulting in circulatory collapse (Slemenda, 1983).

In the 1960s thousands of lives were saved with the advent of external artificial circulatory and respiratory devices. Patients with severe head injuries were maintained beyond acute trauma, providing the ability to differentiate levels of neurologic deficit. Some survived while others remained comatose for years with minimal response. Others failed to recover, were totally unresponsive, and, despite aggressive medical management, suffered cardiac arrest.

The historic view that death occurred with the loss of heart and lung function no longer applied. Cardiorespiratory integrity could be maintained by mechanical ventilation and other medical interventions, despite loss of total brain function. The disparity between accepted biomedical practice and the common law definition of death became apparent, leading to the development of the landmark "Harvard Criteria." In 1968 an ad hoc committee of the Harvard Medical School examined the characteristics and symptoms of death based on cessation of neurologic function. The resulting criteria included 24-hour persistence of deep coma, total areflexia and apnea, normothermia, and absence of central nervous system depressants. It further recommended electroencephalography as a confirmatory test. These were the first standardized guidelines for the diagnosis of cerebral death and recognized such a state as being equivalent to cardiorespiratory death.

Between 1970 and 1980, 25 states enacted legislation permitting determination of death based on neurologic criteria. The first statute was passed in Kansas in 1970 (Stuart, Veith, & Cranford, 1981). In 1972 Dr. Leon Kass and Professor Alexander Capron developed a "Statutory Definition of the Standards in Determining Human Death: An Appraisal and a Proposal" (Capron & Kass, 1972, 1973). In 1975 the Law and Medicine Committee of the American Bar Association drafted a Model Definition of Death Act. In 1978 the National Conference of Commissioners on Uniform State Laws completed the Uniform Brain Death Act. In 1979 the American Medical Association developed its own Model Determination of Death Statute.

In May of 1980, owing to a lack of uniformity and standardization of statutes, the members of the President's Commission for the Study of Ethical Problems in Medicine and Biomedical and Behavioral Research developed a uniform model law referred to as the Uniform Determination of Death Act (Stuart, 1984). It was drafted in conjunction with the National Conference of Commissioners on Uniform State Laws and provided a comprehensive basis for determining death in all situations. Although this law was not required in order to make a determination of death based on neurologic criteria, it provided a legal cushion for an already accepted medical diagnosis. All 50 states, including the District of Columbia, have either adopted a form of the Uniform Determination of Death Act or had precedent set in appellate court decisions.

Initially the President's Commission was reluctant to endorse a recommendation on standards for criteria and tests required to establish a diagnosis of brain death. However, a consensus was reached after testimony from 60 professionals in the fields of neurology, neurophysiology, neurosurgery, and electroencephalography. The resulting published report, "Guidelines for the Determination of Death," in 1981, became the standard clinical criteria for the determination of death based on neurologic criteria (Stuart, 1984). The primary contrast between the Commission's report and the previously established Harvard criteria was the acknowledgment of spinal reflexes and motor activity as being of spinal origin.

Although brain death was established both medically and legally, it was still a difficult concept for society to grasp. A mechanically ventilated cadaver, warm and retaining healthy color, offers the illusion of life. This can present a paradox for the family members if the diagnosis of brain death is not explained thoroughly and methodically in direct, simple lay terms. For families who are traumatized by a tragedy, commonly clinging to every ounce of hope that their loved one will survive, additional time and effort are required to assist them as they attempt to understand that death has occurred and all efforts to sustain life are futile. In order to relay the information adequately and support them through this process, medical professionals must thoroughly understand brain death. They must also be willing to accept the loss of a patient, accept the fact that, medically, nothing more can be done and acknowledge that the only way to accomplish this is full acceptance of one's own mortality. This task can be painstaking, but denial of this professional responsibility will lead to a multitude of tragic and complex dilemmas.

First, the physician may become reluctant to make an expeditious declaration of brain death. Although this can offer the element of time and perhaps temper the discomfort and grief that the family may be experiencing, some believe that it is cruel and unnecessarily extends their vigil. Some families, for a variety of reasons, never accept that death has occurred until the point of cardiac cessation. It is not uncommon for health care providers to assume that the family is unable to cope. They must use caution and carefully scrutinize who is deciding that the family is unable to accept the diagnosis. This has the potential of becoming a method of avoiding an extremely difficult situation. The family is being denied the opportunity to consider the option of organ donation. Although this is not something that every family will choose to do, it can provide a precious opportunity to salvage something positive from an otherwise tragic and seemingly senseless situation. Additionally, maintaining a patient beyond death not only places a needless financial burden on the family and society, but can also be demoralizing to the nurse and preclude availability of beds to other patients (Stuart, 1984). Finally, there is the responsibility to those potential recipients awaiting transplantation. Organs that are healthy at the time of brain death generally deteriorate and are not viable for transplantation if the patient is maintained on a ventilator for days or weeks.

The second dilemma often experienced in the face of brain death is that a declaration will be made and then explained very coarsely to the family, compounding their confusion and grief. At this point the family may become unwilling to discuss the next step—termination of treatment (ventilator) or organ donation. The result is a cadaver being maintained in the unit, a confused family, a frustrated medical staff, and no resolve.

Several forces were in opposition during the developmental phase of brain death statutes. Although there was widespread acceptance of the concept of brain death among the theological, ethical, and medical communities, some minority groups within the major religions opposed the concept in principle. Most have neglected to publish their view (Stuart et al., 1981). The literature does reveal that most major religions do support the concept of organ donation and recognize it as the person's choice. There was also fear that if brain death was recognized medically and legally, there was potential for it to lead to support of active or passive euthanasia and the so-called right-to-die or death-with-dignity laws. Members of the pro-life movement have now begun to realize the difference between brain death laws and euthanasia or right-to-die advocacy (Stuart et al., 1981).

Anencephalic Donation

According to the Centers for Disease Control, 3000 babies are born every year with fatal anencephalopathy (Capron, 1987). With the developing success of pediatric organ transplantation, there has been a drastic increase in the demand for transplantable infant organs. Yet there are limited resources for supplying the estimated 400 to 500 infant hearts and kidneys and the 500 to 1000 infant livers needed in the United States annually (Capron, 1987). Although most donors are victims of suicide or automobile or motorcycle accidents, relatively few newborns die under such circumstances. On a national scale, efforts continue to refine the organ procurement system in hopes of drawing us closer to meeting the need. There have been proposals to allow organs to be recovered from anencephalic newborns. These proposals not only have significant support from the transplant community, but there has also been a strong utilitarian initiative from the parents of these babies.

Under current law, organs cannot be recovered from a patient who does not meet the criteria for whole brain death (i.e., irreversible cessation of all function of the brain, including the brain stem). The anencephalic infant is often born with some lower brain stem function despite an incomplete cranial vault and absent cerebral cortex. The brain stem can maintain vital functions for hours or even days.

Because of the prognosis of 0 per cent survivability for these infants, the usual method of care is to withhold supportive measures and allow multisystem failure and cardiorespiratory arrest to ensue. Seldom do they fulfill the criteria for brain death before cardiac arrest. The appeal from the parents is to interrupt this process long enough to recover viable organs. Brain death, under these circumstances, has been viewed as a legal technicality that, if followed under current guidelines, will result in not only the inevitable fetal death, but also the loss of viable organs and potentially the death of the waiting recipient. This frustration is compounded by the currently legal and acceptable practice of allowing abortion of anencephalic pregnancies up to 24 weeks or induction of labor at any point during gestation. The question of how to deal with these issues remains the focus of intense debate.

Two forms of legislation have been proposed, neither of which has passed. The first, by the California Senate, was to amend the Uniform Determination of Death Act to include anencephalic infants. Capron (1987) points out that if this were to occur, the standards for determining death must also be expanded to include standards for determining anencephaly, sparing any risk of misdiagnosis of other neurologic defects (e.g., hydrocephalus, microcephaly). He further stresses that the anencephalic is a dying infant, not a dead infant. To include this category in a death statute lends itself to the potential for expanding the law to include the permanently comatose, dying, incompetent, and unconsenting patient. If this is indeed what society is prepared to do, the question has been raised regarding the appropriateness of setting such a precedent with the weakest member of our species.

The second proposal was to amend the Uniform Anatomical Gift Act (UAGA). The New Jersey Assembly Bill No. 3367 permitted the donation of organs from an anencephalic infant despite the requirement that organs be removed only after a physician not involved with the transplant procedure determined death had occurred (Capron, 1987). If death has not occurred, we are allowing organs to be recovered on the basis of imminent death or nonviability. Are we not opening the door to encompass a much broader category of patients? If so, do all patients with a terminal prognosis become candidates for donation . . . before death?

Clearly, the whole-brain interpretation of death was created to protect the severely brain injured patient who has the potential for recovery. This precaution, according to Harrison (1986), is not applicable to the anencephalic infant who will never have higher brain or cognitive function. His recommendation is to create an entirely new category of "brain absence," limited to the anencephalic and excluding all other neurologic defects. This would avoid amending any law, parallel current medicolegal implications of brain death, and allow for termination of treatment and for organ recovery. As the cadaveric donor depends on external mechanical support for maintenance of organ function, the anencephalic fetus depends on maternal support for its very existence. Yet birth is inevitable, and birth for these infants begins the dying process.

There are three deliberate distinctions that must be made as we strive to resolve these concerns: (1) the pregnant female, (2) the waiting potential recipients, and (3) the anencephalic fetus. We must work within a framework that ultimately realizes the moral, ethical, and medical responsibilities to each. For the woman, the decision of whether or not to carry the pregnancy to term should be a result of free and informed consent and independent of any decision about organ recovery. Prolonging gestation to term carries risks, and to assume these risks simply for the purpose of organ donation is inappropriate. If the mother chooses to donate, it must be done safely and with the hope that she gain consolation from offering the humanitarian gift of life to another child. To the waiting recipients, we owe dedication to perfecting the organ procurement system, ensuring that viable organs are recovered in a moral and equitable manner without trivializing human life. For the anencephalic infant, we must permit fetal demise without discomfort and maintain dignity throughout the dying process.

Fetal Tissue Transplants

Worldwide research has led to impressive advances in the field of neuroscience in the past decade. We now have the potential for brain cell transplants, stimulation of nerve fiber production, regeneration of nerve pathways, and neuron replacement. It is now within the vision of neurobiologists to treat chronic illness (e.g., Parkinson's disease, epilepsy, and Alzheimer's disease) and neural tube defects (e.g., spina bifida and spinal cord injury) and, possibly, reverse brain damage. Experimental treatment has proved successful in the transplantation of neural tissue from fetal primates into adults. Whether the same results can be obtained in humans remains to be seen. Science is moving in that direction. Yet the primary source for neural tissue is aborted human fetuses. The current legal system does not allow for access to tissue obtained from nonviable fetuses. Elective abortion is considered an acceptable practice, medicolegally, but remains an area of ongoing debate. This issue becomes even more complex when related controversies are introduced. Although thousands could potentially benefit from this tissue, there are some who are concerned lest we create an older generation that depends on the sacrifice of the young for its survival.

UNIFORM ANATOMICAL GIFT ACT

During the 1960s, as transplants were occurring with increasing frequency, one of the most pressing issues faced by medical professionals was the question of liabilities associated with donation and removal of organs and tissues. Improved survival rates with the use of cadaveric tissue led to the need for legal and moral guidance. In 1965 the National Conference of Commissioners on Uniform State Laws and the American Bar Association began efforts to modify public policy in order to encourage cadaveric donation. The resulting Uniform Anatomical Gift Act (UAGA) was drafted in 1968. By 1973 all 50 states and the District of Columbia had adopted some form of the model law.

Those directly involved with cadaveric organ recovery must adhere to the UAGA guidelines to ensure legally valid donation. Although failure to act in accordance with the terms of this statute does not necessarily establish criminal or civil liability, it could result in the loss of good faith (UAGA Sect. 7[C]) and immunity from civil or criminal action (Overcast, Merriken, & Evans, 1985). Under the guidelines set forth, any living person, 18 years or older, has the legal authority to make a gift of organs or tissues, effective at the time of death. This may be done in a will, on a driver's license (in those states that include this designation on driver's licenses), or by donor card. Even in the presence of documentation of intent to donate, the most crucial step in the entire donor process is obtaining secondary consent from the next of kin. Although this is not required by law, proponents of this practice believe that it is consistent with the altruistic philosophy of donation and avoids the possibility of alienating the next of kin, which, in the long run, could lead to litigation. The lack of emphasis on a donor card or driver's license is understandable when one imagines the futility of facilitating the donor process based solely on a donor card when family members strongly object.

Organ donation must take place immediately after death in order to ensure organ viability. Wills and donor cards are often difficult to locate and are frequently not examined for days or weeks after death has occurred. When finally discovered it is too late to carry out the wishes of the deceased. It is best if those who did sign a donor card also relay their feelings to family members so that the family members may assume responsibility for carrying out their loved one's wishes. In situations in which the next of kin cannot be located, even after diligent attempts have been made (which must be well documented), it is permissible to proceed with the donor process in the presence of a signed license or donor card. Again, this is a clear deviation from the Act. No states routinely recognize these provisions of the UAGA. The practice of not retrieving organs based solely on a donor card or driver's license has been the focus of widespread debate. The person's rights were being denied and the original intent of the UAGA was not being realized.

Subsequently, in 1987, the National Conference of Commissioners on Uniform State Laws (NCCOUSL) amended the UAGA, which, among other things, added more credence to the "document of gift" (i.e., donor cards), requiring that the intentions of the donor be followed. The amended section 2(h) reads: "An anatomical gift that is not revoked by the donor before death is irrevocable and does not require the consent or concurrence of any person after the donor's death" (UAGA, 1987, drafted by the NCCOUSL at its annual conference meeting in its 96th year, July 31–Aug. 7, 1987). As of January 1988, no state had adopted the amended version of the UAGA.

Medical Examiner's Cases

Under the UAGA, cases that fall under the jurisdiction of the medical examiner (ME) take precedence over organ donation. Section 7(d) stipulates that the provisions of the UAGA are subject to the state laws with respect to autopsies. Though content varies most states have adopted some form of an ME's or coroner's law. In some states the law contains a clause delegating priority to organ donation. However, prior notification and release from the ME is required before organ recovery can take place.

Many donors die under circumstances that require investigation by the ME, and in most cases the ME's office and the organ procurement organization cooperate with each other. For example, if an abdominal examination is required by the ME, he will observe the organ donation procedure and inspect the organs as they are recovered. Seldom will an autopsy or ME's investigation preclude organ recovery from taking place.

CONSENT

In obtaining consent for organ donation it is important that the medical professional be cognizant of several issues. A 1985 Gallup poll reported that 93 per cent of Americans surveyed had heard of organ transplantation. Of these, 75 per cent approved of the concept, 27 per cent indicated that they were likely to donate their own organs and a mere 17 per cent have completed donor cards. Of those likely to donate, nearly half had not indicated their desires to family members (National Conference of Commissioners on Uniform State Laws, 1987). An earlier study by Overcast and co-workers (1984) revealed that 45 states have a designated area on the driver's license to indicate desire to donate (all states excluding Delaware, Florida, Hawaii, Nebraska, and Pennsylvania, as well as the District of Columbia). Although there is no method of obtaining exact figures on the number that sign driver's licenses, the literature suggests that it is less than 20 per cent. And, as discussed earlier, family consent is still required by the vast majority of states, regardless of the donor card. The likelihood of discovering or relying on a donor card or driver's license at the time that organ donation is a viable option is minimal. Therefore, it is left up to the physician, nurse, and organ procurement coordinator to explore this option with the next of kin.

Although the goal of public policy is to obtain informed consent, there are those who argue whether anyone can fulfill this responsibility in light of the circumstances. The family is usually in a state of shock, in an alien and confusing environment, grief-stricken, and psychologically devastated. Even with the best intentions it is thought to be presumptuous to profess that informed and free choices are made within these constraints. Furthermore, sometimes it is difficult to differentiate between encouragement and coercion. As Caplan (1983) points out, specialists in the field are well educated in the consent process and aware of the issues. It is up to these medical professionals to remain fully focused on the individual family and to do all within their power to meet the family's particular needs.

The Centers for Disease Control have found that more than 27,000 patients who fulfill criteria for vascular organ donation die annually in hospitals across the United States (Bart, Macon, Whittier, Baldwin, & Blount, 1981). Of these, only 10 per cent to 15 per cent ever become donors (Stuart, 1984). A variety of factors have been cited as being responsible for the disparity between potential supply and actual utilization. Ongoing proposals are being considered in an effort to bridge this gap.

One recommendation has been to move from the current volunteeristic approach of organ donation to a more mandatory "presumed or implied consent" philosophy. In other words, everyone is "presumed" to be an organ or tissue donor unless they declare otherwise. Presumed consent policies have been adopted in 13 countries (Stuart et al., 1981). In six of these countries (Norway, Greece, Finland, Spain, Sweden, and Italy) the physician still obtains secondary consent from the next of kin. In the remaining seven (Austria, Czechosloviakia, Denmark, France, Israel, Poland, and Switzerland) organs are recovered unless there is known prior objection (Moskop, 1987). Those who oppose this approach argue that it is in direct conflict with the freedom of choice philosophy on which the United States is founded. Some believe that changing to this type of system would do little to solve all of the existing problems and would probably create others. A survey conducted by Manninen and Evans (1985) revealed that only 7.4 per cent of those surveyed favored the presumed consent concept. Proponents believe the presumed consent system would bring us closer to recognizing cadaveric organs as a social and national resource. Some speculate that our current approach places an unjust and cruel burden on family members, by requiring that they make a difficult decision at an emotional time. Rather, presumed consent would become routine and expected at the time of death, and medical personnel would be more willing to broach the subject (Caplan, 1983).

Interestingly, the precedent may have already been set regarding how a presumed consent statute might be viewed in the United States. In April 1968 the Virginia General Assembly passed a law allowing the ME to remove body parts in cases in which a patient was in immediate need of an organ transplant. It was further stipulated that the ME need not obtain consent from the next of kin if the time lost would prohibit the use of the organ, or if there was no known objection made by the decedent. Virginia was the first state to develop such a law, and its original version actually preceded the UAGA (Lombardo, 1981).

In 1980 an amendment was proposed to include routine pituitary gland removal. The impetus behind this amendment was the wish to make desperately needed pituitary hormone available to a Virginia community of dwarves. Because of the unavailability of the gland, those who suffered from hypopituitary dwarfism were rationed only enough hormone to reach five feet. The idea was to obtain free access to these glands so that all dwarves could have unrestricted access to the therapy needed (i.e., extract from one pituitary gland per week) to realize their full growth potential (Lombardo, 1981). With this goal in mind, the amended version excluded the three qualifiers contained in the original law; the "immediate need" clause was changed to "need," the viability clause was changed to require no contact with the next of kin, and the objection clause was deleted. This proposal allowed an organ procurement agency or a physician to request organs and tissues from all unclaimed bodies and the ME was given the right to fulfill this request without ever attempting to notify or locate the next of kin.

The debate began. Negative reaction was based on religious principles. The American Civil Liberties Union protested on the basis of the First Amendment; others argued that it threatened the "right to property" clause of the Fourteenth Amendment. On the opposing side the medical community lobbied for the dwarves and the potential benefit to society. One year later compromise was achieved. The resulting law had forfeited all impact originally intended. The final version included a "good faith, nonobjection" clause, required next-of-kin consent, and allowed for religious beliefs that might prohibit organ removal.

EQUITABLE ACCESS AND ALLOCATION
OF A LIMITED RESOURCE

In 1972, the Social Security Act was amended to extend benefits to all patients who had chronic renal disease that required dialysis or kidney transplantation. This piece of legislation, titled the End Stage Renal Disease (ESRD) Program, removed most financial obstacles to kidney transplantation in the United States. This, combined with the rising success rates of transplants, led to increased public demand for access to these new techniques.

Research led to a broader understanding of tissue compatibility and histologic matching proved critical to the ultimate success of kidney transplantation. It became clear that in order to maximize the use of cadaveric kidneys, it was necessary to have a large pool of potential donors and recipients. In 1969 one of the first attempts to regionalize organ-sharing was the establishment of the South-Eastern Organ Procurement Foundation (SEOPF). This decreased the organ wastage rate by providing a system of kidney-sharing through a computerized network and offering a program for serum exchange. This system created a mechanism for identifying the best-matched recipient for the kidney being offered. The federation also had responsibility for quality control and assurance of appropriate organ removal and preservation methods. In order to provide this service on a national scale, SEOPF incorporated the United Network for Organ Sharing (UNOS) in 1976.

By the late 1970s the increased availability and added demand for kidneys and other solid organs accelerated. In 1982 SEOPF created the Organ Center in Richmond, Virginia, to house UNOS and provide administrative, technical, and organizational support. The Organ Center became the mainstay for national kidney placement and was funded by Medicare. Extrarenal organs were also being recovered during this period. UNOS incorporated a separate system for nonrenal organs. Medicare funding for this was not available, as extrarenal organs do not qualify for reimbursement under the ESRD program.

In September 1982 the North American Transplant Coordinator's Organization developed a phone-accessed extrarenal organ-sharing system coined 24-ALERT. This system complemented UNOS in that it was for nonrenal organ and tissue sharing. It matched donors and recipients by body size and ABO group rather than by histology. Recipient selection was based on proximity of donor organ to the transplant center and priority of medical need.

Legislation and Policymaking

In the formative years the organizational framework of the organ procurement process was known to few outside the field. A limited supply of organs was available for thousands of people suffering from end-stage organ failure. The only hope for their survival was a lifesaving transplant. Many, however, died while waiting. In a desperate plea for help many recipients and their families turned to their congressmen. The investigation began. It was discovered that there were approximately 110 organ procurement organizations (OPOs) in the United States, some hospital-based and some independent. The OPOs' role included interacting with physicians, nurses, families, other OPOs, tissue-typing laboratories, and transplant teams. They were responsible for facilitating the organ donor process, providing viable organs for transplantation, and ensuring equitable organ distribution. Coordinators were employed to carry out these functions, and as a means of encouraging organ donation, informal hospital educational programs were instituted. Education focused on identification of potential donors and initiation of the donor process. Once a potential donor was identified and the process under way, the coordinator was responsible for organ placement. Local recipients were usually considered first. If no local recipient was identified, UNOS and 24-ALERT were consulted.

There were no standard guidelines for recipient selection. Quality assurance was informal and varied greatly from site to site. No process existed for certifying coordinators, OPOs, or transplant programs, and monitoring of their activities was minimal. This entire system was funded by Medicare through kidney acquisition fees as part of the ESRD program.

Meanwhile public outcry grew. The critical shortage of organs was evident, but it was difficult to ascertain why. It was obvious that a remarkable job was being done because the number of transplants performed and success rates were on the rise. However, until each phase of the process became more clearly understood, it was difficult to define those areas in need of improvement.

In April 1983 the Subcommittee on Investigation and Oversight of the Committee on Science and Technology (U.S. House of Representatives), chaired by Albert Gore, Jr., held hearings on the "Procurement and Distribution of Organs for Transplantation." In June of that year the Surgeon General convened a workshop on organ transplantation. Experts in the field were brought together to find a way to increase the donor supply. One of the outgrowths of this workshop was the formation of the American Council on Transplantation. The aim of this organization was to increase the supply through public awareness and professional education and to ensure equitable access and distribution.

Congressional hearings scrutinized every aspect of the system. Finally, after months of debate, the Democrats and Republicans together unveiled the nation's first organ transplant policy. In October 1984 the National Organ Transplant Act was signed into law.

The National Organ Transplant Act addressed three primary issues:

1. *The establishment of a task force on organ transplantation.* During the developmental phase of this law it was quickly realized that

although a great understanding of the system had been realized, the surface had barely been tapped. The 25-member team conducted a comprehensive examination of the legal, ethical, medical, economic, and social issues presented by organ procurement and transplantation. In April 1986 the Final Report to Congress was published. The recommendations in the area of procurement were as follows:

a. That uniform determination of death be enacted in all states and that each state medical association develop and adopt model policy and procedure for the determination of death based on irreversible cessation of brain function and make those protocols available to hospitals.

b. That states enact legislation requiring that the medical examiners offer the option of organ and tissue donation to families unless the surgical procedure would compromise medicolegal evidence.

c. That all health professionals voluntarily accept the responsibility for identifying and referring all potential donor candidates.

d. That all hospitals adopt a required request/routine inquiry policy for identifying potential donors and for providing the next of kin with appropriate opportunity for donation.

e. That the Joint Commission on the Accreditation of Hospitals and the Commission for the Uniform State Laws develop model legislation and standards that require all acute-care hospitals to have agreements with local OPOs and policies and procedures for the identification of potential organ and tissue donation candidates and provisions for offering the option to the next of kin.

f. That the Health Care Financing Administration incorporate into Medicare conditions of participation, requiring that hospitals have a required request/routine inquiry policy.

g. That all states adopt required request/routine inquiry statutes.

The report also provided detailed recommendations on methods of:

h. improving public and professional education;

i. certifying OPOs and organ procurement coordinators;

j. developing a cohesive, standardized organ-sharing system and a scientific registry for procurement and transplantation data maintenance;

k. providing equitable access to organs, ensuring nondiscriminatory standardization of recipient selection based on medical criteria and probability of outcome; and

l. regulating the diffusion of transplant technology by certifying designated transplant centers.

2. *Authorization of financial assistance for the establishment, initial operation, and expansion of qualified organ procurement agencies.* Allocation of grants was pending any task force recommendations and

was to first consider any geographical areas not adequately served. It further outlined criteria for certification of all OPOs.

3. *Provision of funding for the establishment of an organ procurement and transplantation network (OPTN)*. The OPTN was to refine and consolidate the efforts of UNOS and 24-ALERT into a single, cohesive 24-hour network that handled all organs. It was to be a nonprofit entity (as was every aspect of organ procurement), governed by a board of directors representing organ procurement, transplant centers, voluntary health organizations, and the general public. The OPTN was also to develop and maintain a scientific registry of data on all organ procurement and transplant activity.

The Secretary of the Department of Health and Human Services was mandated responsibility for these provisions. Subsequently the Office of Organ Transplantation was developed to oversee the implementation of the Transplant Act, a process that is still under way.

REQUIRED REQUEST/ROUTINE INQUIRY

Before the passing of the National Organ Transplant Act and the task force report that followed, there were ongoing debates and proposals as to how to increase supply. Ideas of presumed consent, mandatory consent, opting in and opting out, commercialism, and organ marketing systems were balanced against the current informed voluntary system. Each carried its own set of moral, ethical, and social consequences. Public opinion polls suggested that most Americans would donate if asked, and it was estimated that the current system was actually recovering 10 per cent to 15 per cent of all transplantable organs nationwide (Stuart et al., 1981). In light of these statistics, the concept of the altruistic volunteer approach was reexamined. There was predominant unwillingness among medical professionals to assume responsibility for initiating the process. The potential donors were there, but the families were not being asked.

The consensus was to develop a paternalistic approach consistent with the benevolent and humanitarian ideal: required request. It was simple; every hospital would be required by state or federal statute to ensure that the option of organ donation was presented to the family of every potential donor. It was a policy of free choice. It encouraged the use of donor cards. It made discussion of organ donation routine and respected a person's right to make a decision.

Oregon was the first state to mandate required request, in 1985, followed by California and New York. Most states have followed suit. The content of the laws differ slightly from state to state regarding whose responsibility it is to offer the option (hospital or OPO) and noncompliance penalties. In the fall of 1986 the UAGA was amended to include a required request/routine inquiry provision, and the Joint Commission of Accredited Health Care Organizations adopted new policies for required request in their 1988 standards.

In 1986, to further enhance the impact of the state laws, Congress moved to amend the Social Security Act. This led to the passage of the Federal Omnibus Reconciliation Act of 1986. Selected sessions addressed "Hospital Protocols for Organ Procurement and Standards for Organ Procurement Agencies."

Hospital protocols for organ procurement require the following:

- Written policy and procedure for the identification of all potential donors that ensure that their families are provided the option of organ donation (and their option to decline);

- Consideration of circumstances and beliefs of such families;

- A certified OPO be notified of all potential donor candidates; and

- Hospitals that perform transplants must affiliate with and abide by the rules and regulations of the OPTN.

Certification and performance standards for OPOs fall under the jurisdiction of the Department of Health and Human Services. Requirements include that the OPO is a member of and abides by the rules and regulations of the OPTN and that only one OPO be designated per service area. Noncompliance with mandates of the Reconciliation Act will result in revocation of all Medicare funding.

As the field of organ procurement and transplantation grows and becomes more regulated, potential liability increases. For example, some think that physicians should be held accountable for failure to refer patients to transplant centers for evaluation. Further questions address failure to offer the option of donation to families of potential donor candidates. The health care professional may not believe in, or be aware of, the efficacy of transplantation, or she may have an ethical and moral conflict with organ donation. Does that negate the responsibility to inform, or justify breach of duty? As laws increase so will the potential for civil liability. Acquaintance with state and federal regulations, basic knowledge of the process, and how to seek assistance when necessary are paramount during this regulatory era.

ORGAN SHARING AND DISTRIBUTION

Two weeks ago, my office received urgent calls from the governor's office in South Carolina and the Children's Defense Fund. They were told that a child whose parents resided in South Carolina would die soon unless a liver donor could be found.

How could they help? If only they could get the child onto the national networks. Did they mean UNOS and NATCO? No, they meant ABC, CBS and NBC.

—Senator Albert Gore, Jr. (November, 1986).

There is little doubt that media attention heightens awareness about the need for organs. Few stories are as tender and heart-rending as that of a dying child whose only hope of survival is through a transplant. Many were convinced that the system could be manipulated. This strategy by no means constitutes a long-term resolution of the problems in organ placement, not to mention the inequity to those less fortunate.

After transplant candidates are placed on the waiting list a new set of selection criteria must be met. These include length of time waiting, ABO matching, degree of tissue match, presensitization levels, medical need, organ size, and geographic proximity. Although this seems fairly straightforward, the scarcity of organs makes rationing necessary. There is usually direct competition for an organ. Quite often, when one organ becomes available, someone must be denied.

One allocation issue is that of nonimmigrant aliens pursuing transplantation in other countries. Since the late 1970s, foreign nationals have been coming to the United States to receive kidney transplants. Although some have a living-related donor (or living-unrelated donor), the majority receive cadaveric kidneys. It appeared that nonimmigrant aliens were being given preference based on their financial status. In 1985 an estimated 300 foreign nationals received cadaveric kidney transplants in the United States (5.2% of all kidney transplants performed). In that same year approximately 250 kidneys were exported to other countries (Office of Inspector General, 1986).

This issue was first brought to light during the congressional hearings that preceded the development of the National Organ Transplant Act. There have been defensible arguments on both sides. Unanimous agreement was that Medicare not fund this practice. Beyond that there has been little accord, and consensus has been difficult to attain.

Organs are considered a community resource, but there has never been a clear definition of "community." In the case of organ-sharing, community has been defined on local, regional, national, and international levels—in that order. Should citizenship—better yet, residency—play a role in allocation? Worldwide research is responsible for the strides in technological accomplishment. Most nonimmigrant aliens come from developing countries that do not offer the same technological expertise as is available in the United States. Likewise, few had access to dialysis. For most, the only alternative to transplantation in the United States was death.

Yet the organ procurement system is supported by public money. The United States has committed resources for education, research, and public awareness, and as a result has developed the most sophisticated system in the world. If precedent was to allow nonimmigrant aliens equal access to transplants in this country, would that not diminish the inducement for other countries to establish programs? Is it realistic to expect one country to share a precious, lifesaving resource at a sacrifice to its local community?

The 1986 task force addressed this issue. Recommendations were to allow kidney transplants of nonimmigrant aliens, but not to exceed 10 per cent of total transplants performed at any single center. Nonrenal organs should not be offered unless no other suitable recipients were found. It was recommended that these guidelines be followed until more accurate data could be gathered through the OPTN.

The Office of the Inspector General of the Department of Health and Human Services performed a study that same year. It recommended that exclusive access to all kidneys be given to U.S. citizens. If no U.S. citizen match was identified, then alien foreign nationals could be considered. Additionally, kidneys should be exported only when they could not be used within the United States. If kidneys are exported, Medicare should prohibit reimbursement of acquisition fees to the donor center. The standards adopted by UNOS were to have one, unified list, providing equal access to United States citizens and foreign nationals. Ten per cent of each transplant center's patients may be foreign nationals. Any transplant center serving a greater percentage of foreign nationals having transplants will undergo investigation.

PROLIFERATION OF TRANSPLANT CENTERS

Equitable allocation of donor organs became an even greater challenge as the number of transplant candidates burgeoned. Many factors precipitated this rapid growth in demand. Aside from major improvements in immunosuppression in the early 1980s, some credit is due to the valuable technological advancements that were made.

Greatly improved survival rates made the prospect of providing transplantation services more appealing. Excessive media coverage helped to heighten the awareness that transplantation had come of age. The perception of these procedures as experimental heroics, to be used only after all conventional interventions had failed, began to dissipate. The acceptance of transplantation as a viable treatment option significantly escalated patient inquiries and physician referrals. This is evidenced by the increasing number of transplants being performed annually (Table 18–1).

TABLE 18–1. NUMBER OF ORGAN TRANSPLANTS PERFORMED

ORGAN	1981	1982	1984	1985	1986
Kidney	7885	5358	6968	7695	8973
Liver	26	62	308	605	924
Heart	62	103	346	731	1368
Heart and lung	5	7	22	30	45
Pancreas	—	135	87	133	140

From American Council on Transplantation. 1987. Washington, D.C.

Initially, transplantation was available at a limited number of centers. Consumers demanded easier geographical access to this lifesaving technology. The result was a rampant proliferation of transplant centers (Table 18–2). Taking into account the less altruistic incentive of economics, Monaco (1987) identified two additional catalysts behind this proliferation: (1) "the desire frequently to get what is euphemistically called the market share of new patients" and (2) "the need for many surgeons . . . to expand into clinical transplantation as their own particular field of interest diminishes in scope and importance" (p. 3).

FUNDING AND DESIGNATION OF CENTERS

A discussion of limited resources would not be complete without recognizing issues related to funding. Transplantation is expensive. The ESRD program alone cost over $2.4 billion to serve 120,060 patients in 1986 (K. Sagel, personal communication, February 1, 1988).

The United States now faces tough decisions in allocation of economic resources for health care. The technology exists, but where are the resources necessary to sustain the enormous financial burden associated with this endeavor? Health care has been assumed to be available to all, cost being secondary, especially in lifesaving innovations. The two primary issues are (1) can the nation afford it? and (2) will other factions of health care that service a larger portion of society be sacrificed in order to service a comparatively few?

If financial restriction becomes a factor in the process of recipient selection, transplantation becomes a lifesaving commodity available only

TABLE 18–2. NUMBER OF CENTERS PERFORMING ORGAN TRANSPLANTS

ORGAN	1984	1985	1986
Kidney	170	178	184
Liver	25	36	45
Heart	37	74	94
Heart and lung	5	9	14
Pancreas	8	23	34

From American Council on Transplantation. 1987. Washington, D.C.

to those who can pay. Recourse has been to seek coverage through health insurance and federal programs. However, in the absence of knowledge regarding long-term costs and projected reimbursement risks, few states or third-party payers have been willing to adopt a formal payment policy. They are currently making these financial coverage decisions based on a case-by-case assessment of potential outcome. This assessment is an effort to determine if the procedure is "reasonable and necessary" and if it is experimental or an accepted therapeutic intervention. This approach has made third-party coverage quite inconsistent thus far. Of some help is the improvement of one- and five-year graft survival rates to greater than 50 per cent. As a result, the therapeutic value of these procedures is slowly being recognized as justification for reimbursement.

Kidney transplants are currently funded through the ESRD program and private insurers. Medicare also pays for corneal and bone marrow transplants. As of October 1986 Medicare expanded its coverage to include immunosuppressive therapy for the first 12 months post transplant for patients who qualify. Beyond this program, there is no formal method of payment uniformly available. After major assessment of heart transplantation a limited number of heart transplants are now funded through the Health Care Financing Administration. Medicaid currently pays for liver transplants in 33 states, heart transplants in 24 states, heart and lung transplants in 13 states, and pancreas transplants in 3 states (Health Resource Services Administration, 1986). Civilian Health and Medical Program of the Uniformed Services (CHAMPUS) pays for liver, kidney, and bone marrow transplants to their beneficiaries, and military medical programs provide for kidney, heart, and bone marrow transplants.

State Medicaid programs have pursued this independently. For example, Pennsylvania has incorporated a diagnostic-related group system for payment of liver and bone marrow transplants. Illinois will pay up to 60 per cent of transplantation charges for heart, heart and lung, and liver transplants. Ohio has developed a statewide consortium for reimbursement of heart, heart and lung, liver, and pancreas transplants (Davis, 1987). After participation in the task force, the Association of Blue Cross and Blue Shield developed a national organ transplant insurance pool that has been incorporated by more than 10 million health maintenance organization enrollees (Mayers, 1987). The Association is maintaining a data base of cost and outcome rates per center, establishing a plan to extend coverage only for services provided by transplant centers that meet explicit criteria (Mayers, 1987). This concept was initially recommended by the task force. After reviewing data on the diffusion of technology, coupled with economic possibility, it was decided that designation of transplant centers was the best method of ensuring quality of care. The Health Care Financing Administration is currently implementing a formal process of center designation. Those centers that meet well-defined criteria will qualify for reimbursement.

RECIPIENT CANDIDACY

Acceptance of transplantation as a therapeutic option by the lay and medical communities significantly increased the number of patient referrals. The previously restrictive criteria for candidate selection were expanded. The number of candidates awaiting transplantation grew much more rapidly than the supply of donor organs.

Because there are not enough transplantable organs for all who medically qualify, a reassessment of who will receive them is necessary. The task of deciding who will and who will not benefit from this technology is fraught with controversy. Who should decide? Should the candidate, or a candidate advocate, have the opportunity to plead her case? Should age be a criterion? Are retransplants in one patient justified when many are waiting for their first chance? Should a candidate's character, accomplishments, and "estimated worth to the community" (Munson, 1979, p. 398) be factors? The questions are endless. Individual transplant centers have addressed these and many other issues as they arose on a case-by-case basis. Ultimately health care providers must juggle professional responsibility for the welfare of their patients with the social responsibility of not wasting the limited national resource with which they have been entrusted.

As the severity of this allocation problem grows, an increasing demand for standardization of recipient selection is likely. Equity is the issue. Donated organs are a gift to the community. Thus they must be distributed fairly, without bias or discrimination, and in a manner that yields the greatest good.

Patient selection is a three-phase process. The first phase deals with objective medical data. Investigations are geared toward confirming diagnosis, surgical candidacy, and anatomical feasibility of the procedure. Although seldom used as grounds for exclusion, a financial assessment is also conducted. After transplantation, recipients are faced with expensive medications, frequent laboratory work, follow-up visits, and a heightened potential morbidity. Patients and their families must know the financial ramifications of pursuing transplantation.

The phase-two criteria are predominantly subjective and attempt to determine the potential for long-term benefit. Do the patients understand how consuming follow-up can be? Will they keep doctors' appointments and continue daily medication once they are well? Will they resume behaviors that originally contributed to their illness? Are they capable of being well, or have they become dependent on the role of being ill?

These determinations, although critical, are not easily made. Many centers use psychiatric evaluations of both the candidates and their families in hopes of gaining an educated, unbiased third-party opinion.

The first and second phases of evaluation are intended to yield a competent candidate pool through a process of exclusion. Were donor supplies adequate, all patients in this pool would receive transplants and the third phase of selection would not be necessary. However, they are not. As each donor organ becomes available, transplant teams must often apply what have been called "rules of final selection" (Evans, 1983, p. 2211). First, all who match the donor are identified. If there are several candidates, the team assesses who is the worst or whose condition would least tolerate waiting for another donor. Should this fail to narrow the field to one candidate, most advocate introducing some form of chance or randomization (Evans, 1983). The OPTN has significantly standardized this process. The efforts have been to develop criteria that are fair, definable, nondiscriminatory, of public knowledge, and uniformly applicable (Caplan, 1987).

Transplantation is not without risk. For most end-stage organ failure patients, however, the options are limited. Patients with kidney disease may choose dialysis, but it too has significant long term risks; including significant life-style restrictions. Those in end-stage liver and heart failure do not have such an alternative. Without transplantation, death is certain. In short, do these patients really believe that there is a choice to be made? Are sick, often frightened patients capable of making unencumbered decisions about their care? Are they able to focus on and weigh the long lists of risks, expenses, side effects, and experimental protocols they may encounter, or are they only able to focus on not dying? Dickman (1980) questions whether health care providers are honestly able to provide patients with information that does not reflect their own biases and values. Despite their best intentions, it is unlikely that patients and families assimilate the information in the same way it is given (Pennock, McCormick, Thomasma, & Haddoow, 1986). This dilemma is not new to medicine and is not likely to be remedied in the complex arena of transplantation. However, all who have contact with these patients have a responsibility to provide thorough, honest information regarding the long- and short-term implications of transplantation to the candidates and their families.

The potential benefits of transplantation far outweigh the risks for most candidates. An important aspect of making this determination is an assessment of the quality of life the patient and family can expect post transplant. Evans (1985) points out that offering extended life without reasonable quality does not qualify transplantation as a successful intervention. Quality of life, however, is an intangible asset that is elusive and difficult to define (Woolley, 1984). Evans (1985) also suggests that there are objective and subjective dimensions to be considered. Objective indicators include functional status, ability to work, and general health. Subjective indicators include psychosocial effect, sense of wellness, and life satisfaction. More important, however, is that this issue should not be assessed without patient and family input. Their personal value systems and framework are critical elements. For this reason, timely and thorough explanations of the long-term commitments and potential outcomes are vitally important. Ultimately it is they who must find the quality of life acceptable.

According to Peters and Strong (1987), bioethics emerge as an attempt to resolve conflicts between treasured human values. The goal is to facilitate the social process of developing and implementing an agreeable, rational, and defensible resolution to a societal dilemma. Key is that these are issues society must decide—not physicians, attorneys, or politicians. The process of achieving widespread acceptance of bioethical conflict resolutions is long and challenging. Although education and awareness are the foundation, there are five principles that McCullough and associates (1982) believe must be applied when deciding these issues: (1) respect for life—reverence for death, (2) promotion of good, (3) justice and fairness, (4) honesty, and (5) individual freedom.

CONCLUSION

Technology has forced us to deal with these issues. Maintaining a moral, ethical balance as we approach resolve is paramount. As we search for guidance in the formation of policy, the responsibility of the medical professionals and society is to provide the necessary checks and balances. The goal we continue to strive for during the evolution of ethical issues in organ and tissue transplantation is to maintain the highest dignity in human values while furthering society's accomplishments in science and research.

References

Bart, K.J., Macon, E.J., Whittier, F.C., Baldwin, R.J., & Blount, J.H. (1981). Cadaveric kidneys for transplant. *Transplantation, 31*(5), 279–287.

Brant, J. (1984). Legal issues involving bone marrow transplants in minors. *American Journal of Pediatric Hematology/Oncology, 6*(1), 89–91.

Caplan, A.L. (1983, December). Organ transplants: The costs of success. *Hastings Center Report, 75*(1), 23–32.

Caplan, A.L. (1987, January). Equity in the selection of recipients for cardiac transplants. *Hastings Center Report, 75*(1), 10–19.

Capron, A.M. (1987, February). Anencephalic donors: Separate the dead from the dying. *Hastings Center Report, 75*(1), 5–9.

Capron, A.M. & Kass, L.R. (1972, 1973). Statutory definition of the standards in determining human death: An appraisal and a proposal. *University of Pennsylvania Law Review, 121,* 87–118.

Davis, C.K. (1987). Paying for organ transplants under Medicare. In D.H. Cowan, J.A. Kantorowitz, J.A. Moskowitz, & P.H. Rheinstein (Eds.). *Human Organ Transplantation: Societal, Medical-Legal, Regulatory and Reimbursement Issues.* Ann Arbor: Health Administration Press.

Dickman, R.L. (1980, May-June). The ethics of informed consent. *Nurse Practitioner, 5*(3), 25–26.

Evans, R.W. (1983, April). Health care technology and the inevitability of resource allocation and rationing decisions: Part II. *Journal of American Medical Association, 249*(16), 2208–2217.

Evans, R.W. (1985, December). The socioeconomics of organ transplantation. *Transplantation Proceedings, 17*(6), 129–136.

Gore, A. (1986, November). National Transplantation Network: UNOS or NBC? Symposium conducted at Loma Linda University, Loma Linda, Calif.

Harrison, M.R. (1986, April). The anencephalic newborn as organ donor. *Hastings Center Report, 74,* 21–22.

Health Resource Services Administration (1986). *Organ Transplantation.* Report of the Task Force on Organ Transplantation (DHHS Publication No. 181–350–814153554). Washington, D.C.: Government Printing Office.

Irwin, B.C. (1986, December). Ethical problems in organ procurement and transplantation. *ANNA Journal, 13*(6), 305–310.

Levey, A.S., Hou, S., & Bush, H.L. (1986, April). Kidney transplantation from unrelated living donors: Time to reclaim a discarded opportunity. *New England Journal of Medicine, 314*(14), 914.

Lombardo, P.A. (1981, December). Consent and donations from the dead. *Hastings Center Report, 50,* 9–11.

McCullough, J., Bach, F.M., Coccia, P., Crisham, P., Dardis, M., Diehl, J., Goeken, J., Gocken, N., Graves, R., Hansen, J., Kersey, J., McElligott, M., Menitove, J., Meryman, M.T., Rodney, G., Sandler, S.G., & Warkentin, P. (1982). Bone marrow transplantation from unrelated volunteer donors. *Transfusion, 22*(1), 78–81.

Mahowald, M.B., Silver, J., & Ratcheson, R.A. (1987, February). The ethical options in transplanting fetal tissue. *Hastings Center Report, 75,* 9–15.

Manninen, D.L. & Evans, R.W. (1985). Public attitudes and behavior regarding organ donation. *Journal of the American Medical Association, 253*(21), 3111–3116.

Martin, A. (1983). *Legal and Ethical Issues in Organ Procurement.* Unpublished manuscript.

Mayers, B.W. (1987). Blue Cross and Blue Shield coverage for major organ transplants. In D.H. Cowan, J.A. Kantorowitz, J.A. Moskowitz, & P.H. Rheinstein (Eds.). *Human Organ Transplantation: Societal, Medical-Legal, Regulatory, and Reimbursement Issues.* Ann Arbor: Health Administration Press.

Monaco, A.P. (1987). Problems in transplantation—ethics, education and expansion. *Transplantation, 43*(1), 1–4.

Morris, P.J. (1987, February). Problems facing the society today. Presidential address, The Transplantation Society, 1986. *Transplantation Proceedings, 19*(1), 16–19.

Moskop, J.C. (1987, February). Organ transplantation in children: Ethical issues (special article). *Journal of Pediatrics, 110*(2), 175–180.

Munson, R. (1979). Competition and allocation. In K. King (Ed.). *Intervention and Reflection: Basic Issues in Medical Ethics,* (pp. 397–437). Belmont, CA: Wadsworth.

National Conference of Commissioners on Uniform State Laws (1987). Uniform Anatomical Gift Act. Annual conference meeting in its Ninety-Sixth Year in Newport Beach, California, July 31-August 7, 1987.

Office of Inspector General (1986). *The Access of Foreign Nationals to U.S. Cadaver Organs.* (DHHS Control No. P–01–86–00074). Washington, D.C.: U.S. Government Printing Office.

Overcast, T.D., Evans, R.W., Bowen, L.E., Moe, M.M., & Livak, C.L. (1984). Problems in the identification of potential organ donors: Misconceptions and fallacies associated with donor cards. *Journal of the American Medical Association, 251*(12), 1559–1562.

Overcast, T.D., Merriken, K.J., & Evans, R.W. (1985). Malpractice issues in heart transplantation. *American Journal of Law & Medicine, 10*(4), 363–395.

Pennock, J.L., McCormick, R., Thomasma, D., & Haddoow, C.M. (1986, December). Bioethical issues in organ transplantation. In Chancellaro, L.A. (mod.). *Proceedings of the 79th Annual Scientific Assembly of the Southern Medical Association, 17*(12), 1471–1484.

Peters, T.G. & Strong, C. (1987, July). Bioethics and transplantation. *Southern Medical Journal, 80*(7), 805–807.

Schneider, A. & Flaherty, M.P. (1985). Loan shark organ broker. In *The Challenge of a Miracle: Selling the Gift*, (pp. 22–23). Pittsburgh, Pa.: The Pittsburgh Press Co.

Slemenda, M.B. (1983). Brain death determination and management in children. *Critical Care Nurse*, May/June, 63–66.

Starzl, T.E. (1985, April). Will live organ donations no longer be justified? *Hastings Center Report, 15*(2), 5.

Stuart, F.P., Veith, F.J., & Cranford, R.E. (1981). Brain death laws and patterns of consent to remove organs for transplantation from cadavers in the United States and 28 other countries. *Transplantation, 31*, 238–244.

Stuart, F.P. (1984, February). Need, Supply, & Legal Issues Related to Organ Transplantation in the United States. *Transplantation Proceedings, 16*(1), 87–94.

Woolley, F.R. (1984, February). Ethical issues in the implantation of the total artificial heart. *New England Journal of Medicine, 310*(5), 292–296.

19

Transcultural Nursing and Transplantation

Joanne Bartosh and Patricia Chalupsky

Nursing is a special science, not only because of its scientific associations, but also because of its unique position in dealing with the humanities. Nursing educators teach students to consider the whole person when planning care for clients. The primary focus has been on the biological, psychological, and social aspects of the client.

Today the field of transcultural nursing, pioneered by Madeleine M. Leininger, encourages nurses to examine cultural differences and to alter nursing care to accommodate these differences. The once "difficult" patient can now be understood from a different vantage point as nurses begin to develop cultural sensitivity.

Depending on the area of employment, type of institution, and geographical location, nurses are more likely to deal with clients from cultures different than their own. For example, in New York the Puerto Rican culture is prominent, whereas in Florida there may be more Cubans, or in Texas and California, more Mexican clients.

Wherever nurses practice or interact with others they must be attuned to the differences between themselves and the people with whom they are interacting. In our communications we often assume that certain aspects of perception, understanding, judging, and thinking occur. At times we think that the other person will automatically have the same perceptions as we do. We especially think this if the person is from the same cultural background. However, there can be enormous differences between individuals who have had completely different backgrounds (e.g., childhood experiences, education, and age). In such instances interactions can be uneasy. Common examples of these types of interactions are adolescents communicating with their parents, or the uneducated person from a lower socioeconomic status communicating with an educated person from a higher socioeconomic status. This type of difficulty in communication is compounded in interactions with a person from a different culture.

A multicultural approach to health care is seen as essential in providing quality care to the foreign client who is a transplant recipient. To identify the unique needs, ideas, and beliefs of this client, assessment of cultural characteristics is discussed. Communication patterns, dress and appearance, dietary preferences, time awareness, relationships, and religious beliefs are reviewed in the Arabic and Latin cultures. Specific cultural issues of the Arabic kidney transplant patient are addressed.

CULTURE

Culture is learned socialization passed down from generation to generation, whereby a person learns behavior by incorporating societal values, beliefs, and meaning. Behavioral patterns of problem solving and coping also develop in this socialization process (Varricchio, 1987).

When people become clients in a hospital or health care setting they are immediately placed in an environment that has cultural expectations that are quite different from those of their own home environment. For example, the patient must adapt to the hospital's routine for meals and must sacrifice a large measure of privacy. In this setting a sensitivity to cultural backgrounds becomes essential at the very onset of the relationship between the health care provider and client. Even the way the nurse greets the client can influence future interactions. This initial interaction can also influence the health care provider's perception of the patient in all other interactions. For example, a new patient who has just arrived from a foreign country after a long and delayed trip may be hungry, tired, and frightened. The nurse who is admitting this patient needs to be aware that the patient may be grumpy and short-tempered, and to be sensitive to what the patient has been through and must be experiencing, especially if the patient and the nurse cannot communicate in the same language. One must also exercise caution, in terms of attitudes, compliance, or demands, before making assumptions about the patient and significant others. The health care provider must consciously think about the situation before responding to or judging the patient. The nurse's sensitivity and knowledge of cultural values, beliefs, and practices will make a difference in the patient's satisfaction, promotion of health, and ultimate recovery from illness or disability (Leininger, 1979, 1984).

Cultural Characteristics

We identify with our own culture, and our cultural characteristics identify us. Insight into a person's cultural background will help the health care provider to establish a therapeutic relationship, reduce misunderstandings, and increase the success of the client's progress (Collins, Mathure, & Risher, 1984). Assessment of the following characteristics will be helpful in providing the basis for mutual understanding.

Communication Patterns. Communication can be verbal or nonverbal. There are many foreign languages, yet even within the same language there can be different dialects, slang words, and accents. There can also be subcultural languages. An example of this is the language that health care providers use in their everyday work. The type of communication style is also related to the social customs of the patient. Certain nonverbal gestures are used to accent verbal communications, and these also vary from culture to culture.

Dress and Appearance. This includes not only the major outward dress, but also the type of makeup. Decorations or other distinguishing aspects of appearance are also included.

Nutrition and Eating Habits. The type of food and customs associated with its consumption reveal a great deal about a culture. Some foods may be accepted in some countries that are totally rejected in others. Pork, for example, is popular with Americans and Chinese, but may be totally unacceptable to people of Jewish and Muslim faith. Every culture has its preferences and taboos.

Time Awareness. Concern about time varies from culture to culture. Some cultures are strict about adhering to appointments, whereas others cannot understand such time constraints. Typically, Americans and Germans are known to be precise about the clock, whereas Latins and Arabs are much more flexible.

Relationships. The family is the most revealing example of this cultural characteristic. Included in this characteristic would be family dynamics, decision making, life-style, and living arrangements. The dynamics of family relations vary from culture to culture. Some cultures incorporate the extended family into their familial nucleus. The authoritarian head of the family may be a male or an elder. Some cultures allow polygamy or polyandry, although polyandry is uncommon. Many cultures place women in an inferior position.

Religion. Every culture has its religious preferences. Many cultures have a variety of religions. In dealing with clients, health care providers must realize that there are religious beliefs with associated rituals and taboos that must be recognized and respected.

Health care providers frequently think that their own culture is superior, and on this basis they may believe that they know what is best for their clients. This attitude is called "ethnocentrism." Ethnocentrism creates misunderstanding and friction between cultures because of the implication that one culture and understanding of life is somehow superior compared with another (Dawes, 1986). Becoming aware of this attitude is the beginning of understanding cultural differences and the importance of dealing with them. This understanding will help to alleviate health care providers' tendency to impose their values on the client without being aware of the client's values, feelings, and beliefs (Leininger, 1973). Without awareness of one's ethnocentrism, it is possible for the client who is silent or unexpressive to be labeled as lazy, apathetic, hostile, or stupid (White, 1977). As health care providers become more experienced with different cultures, they develop a greater understanding and sensitivity, resulting in less of a cultural shock for both the client and the health care provider.

Cultural Assessment

Many cultural assessment tools have been developed. Tripp-Reimer and co-workers (1984) have proposed that cultural information should be obtained only as it relates to a specific health problem.

The nurse may find the following questions helpful in eliciting problem-specific information:

- What do you think has caused your problem?
- Why do you think it started when it did?
- What does your sickness do to you? How does it work?
- How severe is your sickness? Will it have a long or short duration?
- What kind of treatment do you think you should receive?
- What are the most important results you hope to receive from this treatment?
- What are the chief problems your sickness has caused you?
- What do you fear about your sickness? (Tripp-Reimer, Brink, & Saunders, 1984).

Two additional questions used at Long Island Jewish–Hillside Medical Center are:

- How has your illness changed your family life?
- Is there anyone or anything else other than the hospital and the doctors that could help you get better? (Redlin, Roy, & Atcherson, 1985)

The data collected from these questions can give health care providers an idea of the client's perceptions and expectations, and this information should be used in planning the client's health care. Cultural assessment functions to identify deviations in cultural parameters, to modify the client's system, or to modify the health care professional's system in order to increase similarity between them. If there are inconsistencies between these two systems, the health care provider should determine if the client's system is adaptive, neutral, or maladaptive.

Examples of behavior that may be different from the health care provider's culture are food preferences and pain expression. These areas should be considered during treatment planning with the client's background in mind. However, if there are areas that are detrimental to achieving the desired health outcome, the health care provider must determine methods of persuasion that will aid in adapting the client's system, if the client is agreeable to these adaptations, or ways of understanding the client who will not change (Tripp-Reimer et al., 1984).

Assessing cultural characteristics is a complex process that encompasses many aspects of life. Although the characteristics described above are not all-inclusive, they are helpful in identifying areas of potential conflict between the foreign client and health care provider.

THE ARABIC CULTURE

The Arabic culture is found in countries of the Middle East, such as Saudi Arabia, United Arab Emirate, Lebanon, Syria, and Jordan.

Communication Patterns

The common language is Arabic. This language has many dialects and accents. The language is read and written from right to left. It is considered to be a divine language by Arabs, since it is the language of the Koran. The Koran is a holy text that is considered to be the word of God as presented by the great prophet Muhammad.

During verbal communications, Arabs of the same sex usually maintain a proximity of about 15 inches. They also tend to speak at length without immediately getting to the point. They repeat their message several times for emphasis, and tend to overassert themselves (Shouby, 1951). One should show patience during this phase of communication, for impatience is interpreted as rudeness. A yes or no answer cannot be taken at face value from an Arab. Offers or questions must be repeated and emphasized numerous times. Maintaining eye contact is usual for Arabs. They shake hands frequently. Serving food, eating, or gesturing with the left hand is considered by some Arabs to be impolite, as is crossing one's legs so that the sole points toward someone.

When an Arab greets another Arab of the same sex they embrace and kiss cheeks; however, this type of greeting is not acceptable between members of the opposite sex. Men and women will greet with only a nod of recognition.

Time Awareness

Arab culture does not emphasize strict adherence to time considerations. It is therefore recommended that appointments for these clients have a certain amount of flexibility to take this cultural aspect into account.

Nutrition and Eating Habits

The Arab diet consists of lamb, chicken, rice, cracked wheat, pita bread, fresh fruit, and vegetables. Chicken is prepared with oil, allspice, lemon juice, and garlic. Lamb is prepared with oil, onion, beef stock, black pepper, thyme, basil, and cornstarch. Pork and alcohol are prohibited in the Muslim religion. Fresh fruits and vegetables are preferred over canned or frozen items. One should note that Arab clients often prefer a vegetarian diet unless they are assured that their meat has been specially prepared by allowing the animal to die peacefully. Hot tea and warm milk are the preferred beverages. Arabs do not typically drink iced drinks or eat salads.

Relationships

There is strong loyalty to the family because it is the most important and prominent social unit. The father is considered the leader of the family, and affiliation follows the male line. There is masculine authority and subordination of women. Owing to these factors there is a strong emphasis on having male children. Marriages are usually arranged, and marriage to cousins is common as an attempt to strengthen family ties (Reizian & Meleis, 1986). Polygamy is often accepted in the Muslim culture.

When an Arabic client is in the hospital there are usually many visits from family and friends. Their involvement in health care is usually limited, not only because of a lack of communication and understanding of treatment, but also because they believe that this is the responsibility of the health care provider. If the participation of family and friends is necessary, one should explain the importance of their role in the client's ultimate recovery.

Dress and Appearance

Female attire consists of long dresses in any color covered with a black coat. A veil covers the face, and a head covering is also worn. They are usually black, although if an Arab woman is in the United States, different colored headdresses may be worn. In the Arabic culture only the woman's eyes, face, hands, and feet should be exposed to the public. Women use henna for decorative purposes to color their soles, faces, nails, and palms. They do not use nail polish because this does not allow water to wash the outside of their nails. Before they pray they must be "cleansed," so they wash their hands and their body.

Males wear floor-length gowns that are usually white, brown, or gray. They wear a headdress, usually white, with a band to hold it in place. They also wear a coat over their gown that can be decorated with silk or gold threads. Men may change into western-style clothing when traveling through Europe or the United States.

Religion

Most Arabs are of the Muslim faith. The Muslims revere two holy places: Mecca, which is the birthplace of Muhammad, the Great Prophet, and Medina, which is the city where the prophet is buried. Muhammed is considered to be the last and greatest of God's prophets, and the one who introduced the Muslims to their holy book, the *Koran*. The main pillars of the Muslim faith are (a) the recitation of the profession of faith; (b) canonical prayer repeated five times a day; (c) fasting during Ramadan, a religious period lasting approximately one month; (d) payment of a tax of purification on certain kinds of property; and (e) the pilgrimage to Mecca, or haj, some time during one's lifetime.

Friday is considered a holy day, and prayer is of particular importance. Prayer is always preceded by cleansing. While praying, Muslims must always face Mecca, which is toward the southeast in the United States. If a patient cannot adhere to these religious responsibilities, distress can occur (Walker, 1982). The prayers are short. Even bedridden clients may be expected to pray, if only with their hearts and fingers; however, they are forgiven if they cannot fast or pray.

Health Care Expectations

Arab clients believe in Western medicine. They believe that there will be immediate postoperative pain relief, and that pain can be taken care of by modern technology. If Arabs must tolerate pain, they do better if they know the consequences will be positive. In planning care more compliance will be seen when short-term goals are set.

Arab clients also believe that modern technology can cure most illnesses, and they do not anticipate complications. If complications do arise, they may be blamed on negligence or lack of expertise (Reizian & Meleis, 1986). Therefore, informing the client of potential risks needs to be addressed from the beginning. Many Arabs are not familiar with detailed informed consent forms (Meleis & Jansen, 1983). In the United States detailed informed consent is mandatory, and all risks, if not stated in the consent, are discussed in detail. When dealing with an Arab client it may be best to discuss the informed consent in general terms, and to emphasize the potential positive results of a procedure instead of focusing solely on the risks involved.

Pain may be described by the Arab patient in constellations that include more than the immediate, direct pain (Reizian, 1984). For example, chest pain may be described as "I have pain in my chest and feel dizzy." Pain can also be expressed as a generalized experience even though it may be localized (Reizian & Meleis, 1986).

LATIN CULTURE

The Latin culture is found in countries located in Central and South America and in Spain. There are many similarities in their cultural characteristics. In this section only the Latin culture as seen in Mexico is addressed.

Communication

The national language of Mexico is Spanish. However, other languages are also spoken: English, Arabic, Chinese, Yiddish, and more than 200 Indian languages.

When communicating, Mexicans stand close to each other. Women often greet with a kiss on the cheek and an embrace. Men greet each other with a handshake when they first meet, but if there has been a long absence between long-time male friends, a handshake occurs and flows smoothly into a full embrace, ending with another handshake. Usually there is a lively and joyful verbal exchange. A male may shake a female's hand, give her a kiss on the cheek (if they know each other quite well), and even embrace if she is a close friend or relative. Otherwise, females and males only offer a handshake to each other.

Time Awareness

Mexicans have a fluid concept of time. They generally feel that if a friend or a business associate passes by to chat, they will give that person time. This in turn may cause them to be late for a scheduled appointment. Because Americans are viewed as prompt and expecting promptness, most Mexicans who interact with Americans attempt to respect the American concept of time. In the health care environment, if Mexican patients are scheduled for tests at a particular time, they expect to receive those tests at the designated time. If they do not, they may become frustrated or worried or even feel neglected because of their idea that Americans are organized and prompt. Therefore, if tests are being delayed or canceled, explanations should be given to the client without delay.

Nutrition and Eating Habits

The Mexican diet consists largely of carbohydrates. Foods include corn or flour tortillas (a flat type of bread), rolls, rice, beans, fresh vegetables, and fruit. All types of meats are eaten. The food is usually hot and spicy. Appetizers (antojitos) are especially appreciated in this culture.

Meals usually consist of light breakfasts, heavy lunches around 2 P.M., and a moderate dinner at 9 or 10 P.M. When eating, both hands may be used simultaneously. After lunch and dinner a long chat over coffee often occurs (sobremesa). Iced tea and milk are not served with lunch or dinner. Wine, beer, carbonated soda, and mineral drinks are commonly served with main meals. For dessert, a sweet custard or fresh fruit is served with strong coffee. Siestas are common after lunch.

Relationships

The Mexican family is usually large. Close ties exist with the immediate and extended family. The father is considered the family leader who makes most decisions. The mother is in charge of the household. There is a strong sense of belonging among family members. Family comes first, for it is seen as the greatest resource to fulfill one's needs. Divorce is relatively infrequent because of the influence of the

Catholic Church. There are several restrictions regarding dating. A single girl should usually not be out alone after dark, for this symbolizes poor character. Mexican children usually continue to live in their parents' home until they marry. These characteristics of the Mexican family have been slowly changing as American customs and values have been incorporated into the Mexican culture.

Dress and Appearance

Dress is much the same as in the United States. There are, however, more restrictions on the type of clothing considered appropriate for the Mexican woman. For example, shorts would be acceptable apparel only on the beach or at sporting events.

Religion

Most Mexicans are Roman Catholic, although some follow other Christian religions. Even though most are Christians, the Jewish faith is quite active in Mexico.

A Mexican is usually religious and asks for God's help and guidance during illness. Catholics often pray the rosary, offer novenas (petitions to the Virgin Mary or a particular saint), or want to attend Mass.

Health Care Expectations

Mexicans are usually open and emotional. When a family member is ill other members of the family need a great deal of support. The family may be quite protective of the client despite the health care provider's emphasis on independence in health care activities. Explanations of treatment to the family will enable the health care provider to elicit family support and participation in the client's recovery.

When a Mexican client has a fatal disease invariably family members do not want the client to be made aware of the prognosis. They may request that the physician withhold this information. In dealing with a Mexican client it is helpful to establish a close relationship not only with the client, but with the client's family as well.

NURSING IMPLICATIONS AND TRANSPLANTATION

Cultural characteristics are important tools in the assessment of the foreign client; however, this assessment is not complete unless standard care plans are altered to fit the client's special needs. Areas of particular concern during kidney transplantation are the client's expectations, communication patterns, dietary preferences, perceptions of medication, body issues, and feelings of depression and loneliness. A discussion of these areas with potential solutions for the Arab client are discussed below.

Expectations

Arab clients who come to this country seeking transplantation expect nothing less than a cure. They also expect the transplant team to make all of the decisions involving their care and to assume the responsibility for these decisions. They acquiesce and appear passive in encounters with physicians because they view the physician as the authority. The transplant team, however, expects clients to understand all of their treatment options and to make informed decisions regarding transplantation. The nursing staff is trained to educate clients about the process of transplantation, including frank discussion of the benefits and risks. Arab clients experience feelings of mistrust when presented with this detailed information. They perceive the health care provider as knowledgeable and educated, and themselves as incapable of making health care decisions. They may also believe that because their fate is predetermined by God, a discussion of what might happen is irrelevant.

Arabs question the necessity of consent forms for invasive procedures or surgery because their verbal agreement is, to them, sufficient and just as binding as a written agreement. Again, they may believe that their consent is irrelevant because this is the health care provider's domain.

The pretransplant psychosocial evaluation is interpreted as intrusive because it is unclear to them how detailed personal information could have any bearing on their health status. The social worker finds that their answers are brief and often designed to please. In the Arab culture privacy is vehemently guarded until a relationship has been developed.

These expectations are problematic because they conflict with our emphasis on individual self-determination, independence, and informed consent. The first step in alleviating the potential conflicts surrounding the Arab client's expectations is to have the transplant team meet with the client and interpreter to explain each member's roles and responsibilities. This helps to clarify the hospital's and the team's philosophy of health care for the client.

Many of these issues are best addressed by a patient representative who is familiar with the expectations of both cultures. Some institutions provide this service through an International Patient Services Department. A trained worker is assigned to every foreign client and is on call

24 hours a day for any needs or concerns expressed by the client, family, or staff. The patient representative can also provide interpretation as needed. A special telephone device can be placed at the bedside to provide this service by telephone around the clock.

The positive benefits of procedures and medications should be emphasized in patient teaching. It must be understood that Arab clients may not attain the same level of understanding as American clients. Their knowledge develops over time and is supplemented by their own experience postoperatively. The positive relationship that often develops between the Arab client and the health care team member goes a long way in establishing trust and increasing the client's knowledge base.

Communication Patterns

Arab clients come from a highly contextual culture. This means that they are very aware of nonverbal messages and examine all of the circumstances around an event in order to understand it. They need to know a great deal about a person before a relationship develops. Expression tends toward overemphasis, hyperbole, and exaggeration (Racy, 1970). Arabs tend to repeat themselves for emphasis. When passing by their hospital rooms you may hear what sounds like agitated conversation as they visit with friends and family.

More time is needed for effective communication with these clients because their emphasis is more on personal contact and much less on procedures. A warm-up period is helpful before addressing the business at hand. Offering personal information helps the Arab begin to know the health care provider and will go a long way in establishing trust. They watch others carefully for nonverbal cues in order to develop feelings about those people. They are sensitive to thermal, olfactory, and kinesthetic cues as they form their impressions (Hall, 1979). An interpreter is essential in caring for Arab clients. Family members, when asked to interpret, edit and reinterpret the communication into messages they deem appropriate for the client to hear. Illness is a family affair, and family members manifest their caring by guarding the client from any responsibility or bad news.

Communication will be more successful with this client if a primary caretaker is assigned. Continuity of care is important in establishing trust.

Dietary Preferences

Food is important to Arab clients for both religious and social reasons. They believe that a disruption or imbalance in the preparation or eating of food causes illness. A poor appetite, *mafish nefs*, may be considered a manifestation of the illness or an indication that one's life is not as it should be (Meleis, 1981).

American food is considered bland, which presents quite a problem in attempting to find acceptable menus for the calorie-deficient and malnourished client. The restrictive pretransplant diet for patients with kidney disease is an added challenge. Preparing appealing dishes that meet caloric, protein, and potassium content guidelines in a hospital setting requires commitment from the dietitian to work closely with this client. Even with the aid of an interpreter menu selection is confusing for the Arab client because of the fancy names given to food choices.

In order to design a rational dietary plan a dietary history and the client's usual daily food intake must be elicited. Family members, if present, can be encouraged to bring ethnic dishes from home when posttransplant restrictions are relaxed. When decreased food intake is noted the nurse or dietitian should ask why clients are not eating well and establish their perception of the consequences of their eating habits. The answer often lies in the food that is being offered and, sometimes, in the absence of mealtime socialization.

Medications

Medications are an essential part of the posttransplant period. Commonly for the rural, less educated Arab, medications given intravenously are preferred over intramuscular injections. The more intrusive procedure is seen as having the greatest potential to aid in recovery. Colored pills may be preferred over uncolored ones, and larger pills over smaller ones (Racy, 1969). If the physician fails to prescribe medication, it is thought that he did not do anything to remedy the client's complaint. Medication is heavily used in the Arab culture, and both pharmacists and nurses prescribe drugs. The Arab client is often resentful of the limited number of available over-the-counter drugs and the need for professional, written prescriptions (Meleis, 1981).

Establishing trust is an essential component of ensuring medication compliance in the Arab client. Recent data suggest that the health care provider who demonstrates an orientation toward the patient and a desire to influence compliance, and one who is able to communicate nonverbal sensitivity and warmth, improves the odds in favor of compliance (Becker, 1985). The care plan must address ways to foster mutual respect between the health care provider and client. Because the Arab already believes in the authority and expertise of the physician, the main ingredient for the development of trust is already there. As long as the medical team remains sensitive to the client's cultural needs, noncompliance usually does not become an issue.

Body Issues

An important part of communication in the Arab world is touching. Not only do Arabs position themselves closer to each other when conversing, than do Americans, but members of the same sex tend to touch each other. However, they are reluctant to be touched by members of the opposite sex. This poses obvious difficulties for the female nurse working with the male patient. On one hand, the Arab client may expect the nursing staff to perform all of his activities of daily living, but on the other hand he is likely to refuse to be bathed unless the nurse fits the older female, "mother" role.

Cold and dampness are seen as causes of illness; therefore, the Arab client will refuse cold drinks and refuse to bathe when ill. The nurse will discover the patient wrapped up in her covers without even her head showing. The nurse who disturbs her to assess respiratory status, intravenous lines, and surgical wounds is resented for exposing her to drafts and cold. If a cooling blanket is used for a febrile client, this is very upsetting because the families prefer to keep the feverish person warm. These issues are important to Arab clients and should be sensitively considered by the health care staff. Patient but firm explanations are required to ease the client's distress.

Female Arab clients often fear examination by male physicians. A gynecologic examination can be problematic as part of the pretransplant medical evaluation for the young Arab female, especially if she is a virgin. Same-sex staffing is encouraged whenever possible.

It is expected that extraordinary measures should always be taken to save a terminally ill patient. To give up hope is diametrically opposed to Middle Eastern values. This event is in God's hands, and to prepare for death by terminating life support or asking for organ donation is tantamount to forfeiting God's help. This view is currently changing. Religious and social leaders are beginning to encourage cadaveric organ donation. The Arab family will also refuse autopsy because in Islam a person is not considered to be the owner of his body (Walker, 1982).

Depression and Loneliness

Middle Eastern clients come from a culture in which the extended family is the most important social institution. Their need for affiliation is strong, and they cope with the stresses of everyday life by turning to others for counsel and support. As previously mentioned, Arab clients rely exclusively on family members to make health care decisions. Often family members are seen by the health care team to be excessively demanding; however, to the Arab family this demanding attitude is merely an indication of the intensity of their caring.

Arab clients who must go through the process of transplantation alone are vulnerable to intense feelings of loneliness and depression. Western behavior and symbols have little meaning to them. They suffer anxiety and feelings of loss without their intimate circle of family and friends to turn to in coping with their illness and treatment. Because they guard their privacy with people who are not part of their intimate circle, Arab clients do not reach out to establish a relationship. This effort is up to members of the transplant team. Although this process can be exhausting, it usually alleviates a great deal of frustration for both the health care provider and client.

The care plan must provide for a primary caretaker whenever possible. A business-like, hurried attitude is discouraged because the Arab client sees the emotional and subjective approach as evidence of caring. Sharing personal information fosters trust, as does the sharing of food.

Health care professionals have the capacity to make a substantial impact in lessening the Arab client's anxiety, loneliness, and feelings of loss when a few simple measures are used in keeping with Arabic cultural values. In many ways, establishing a truly therapeutic alliance with an Arab is not that much different than establishing a similar alliance with an American.

CONCLUSION

Nursing teaching and practice will achieve the desired outcomes more often when they are congruent with the client's culture. Assessing the client's cultural characteristics is the first step in identifying potential areas of differences. Although the client's values may at first appear absurd or irrational to the health care provider, understanding and empathy can only grow when the client's and the health care provider's cultural values and beliefs are respected and understood. A multicultural approach in the complex field of organ transplantation is essential if these clients are expected to return home capable of independence and self-care.

References

Becker, M.H. (1985). Patient adherence to prescribed therapies. *Medical Care, 23*(5), 539–563.

Collins, J.L., Mathure, C.B., & Risher, D.L. (1984). Training psychiatric staff to treat a multicultural patient population. *Hospital and Community Psychiatry, 35*(4), 372–375.

Dawes, T. (1986). Multicultural nursing. *International Nursing Review, 33*(5), 148–150.

Hall, E.T. (1979, August). Interview with Kenneth Friedman. *Psychology Today,* 45–54.

Leininger, M. (1973). Becoming aware of types of health practitioners and cultural imposition (summary). *Proceedings of the 48th Convention of the American Nurses Association,* 9–15. Kansas City, Mo.

Leininger, M. (1979). Transcultural nursing. *Proceedings from Four Transcultural Nursing Conferences* (p. 742). New York: Masson.

Leininger, M. (1984). *Care II: The Essence of Nursing and Health.* Thorofare, N.J.: Charles B. Slack.

Meleis, A.I. (1981). The Arab-American in the health care system. *American Journal of Nursing, 81*(2), 1180–1183.

Meleis, A.I. & Jansen, A.R. (1983). Ethical crises and cultural differences. *Western Journal of Medicine, 138*(6), 889–893.

Racy, J. (1969). Death in an Arab culture. *Academic Sciences, 164,* 871–880.

Racy, J. (1970). Psychiatry in the Arab east. *Acta Psychiatrica Scandinavia [Suppl], 221*:1.

Redlin, J., Roy, C., & Atcherson, E. (1985). Dialysis of foreign nationals: A new challenge. *Journal of Nephrology Nursing, 2*(3), 135–138.

Reizian, A. (1984). *Illness Behavior and Help-Seeking Behavior Among Arab-Americans.* Ph.D. diss., University of California, San Francisco.

Reizian, A. & Meleis, A.F. (1986). Arab-Americans' perceptions to pain. *Critical Care Nurse, 6*(6), 30–37.

Shouby, E. (1951). The influence of the Arabic language on the psychology of the Arab. *Middle East Journal, 5,* 284.

Tripp-Reimer, T., Brink, P.J., & Saunders, J.M. (1984). Cultural assessment helps nurses meet their patients' needs. *Nursing Outlook, 32*(2), 78–82.

Varricchio, C. (1987). Cultural and ethnic dimensions of cancer nursing care. *Oncology Nursing Forum, 14*(3), 57–58.

Walker, C. (1982). Attitudes to death and bereavement among cultural minority groups. *Nursing Times, 78*(12), 2106–2109.

White, E. (1977). Giving health care to minority patients. *Nursing Clinics of North America, 12*(1), 27–39.

INDEX